Antiemetic Therapy

Antiemetic Therapy

Editor

Josef Donnerer *Graz*

39 figures, 1 in color, and 28 tables, 2003

KARGER

Basel · Freiburg · Paris · London · New York ·
Bangalore · Bangkok · Singapore · Tokyo · Sydney

Prof. Dr. Josef Donnerer
Institut für Experimentelle und
Klinische Pharmakologie
Karl-Franzens-Universität Graz (Austria)

Library of Congress Cataloging-in-Publication Data

Antiemetic therapy / editor, Josef Donnerer.
p. ; cm.
Includes bibliographical references and indexes.
ISBN 3–8055–7547–5 (hard cover : alk. paper)
1. Antiemetics. 2. Vomiting–Treatment. 3. Nausea–Treatment. I. Donnerer, Josef.
[DNLM: 1. Antiemetics–therapeutic use. 2. Vomiting–drug therapy. 3. Nausea–drug therapy. 4. Nausea–physiopathology. 5. Vomiting–physiopathology. WI 146 A629 2003]
RB150.N38A58 2003
616′.047–dc21

2003040097

Bibliographic Indices. This publication is listed in bibliographic services, including Current Contents® and Index Medicus.

Drug Dosage. The authors and the publisher have exerted every effort to ensure that drug selection and dosage set forth in this text are in accord with current recommendations and practice at the time of publication. However, in view of ongoing research, changes in government regulations, and the constant flow of information relating to drug therapy and drug reactions, the reader is urged to check the package insert for each drug for any change in indications and dosage and for added warnings and precautions. This is particularly important when the recommended agent is a new and/or infrequently employed drug.

www.karger.com
Printed in Switzerland on acid-free paper by Reinhardt Druck, Basel
ISBN 3–8055–7547–5

Contents

Preface

Prevention and treatment of nausea and emesis are very important issues for the patient's well-being under different clinical as well as outpatient situations. This multidisciplinary book on this topic should bridge the gap between basic research and clinical practice, and we hope that many scientists will be able to benefit from it. In this context I am very grateful to everybody who was involved in the preparation and completion of this book.

Various and partly still unresolved pathomechanisms play roles in nausea and emesis in humans, and appropriate animal models are not always available for preclinical research on antiemetic drugs. Therefore, only the results from studies in the clinical setting can decide a new compound's utility. Basically, we have a rather small number of drugs in the established treatment regimens, however some new interesting compounds are being studied in clinical trials.

The aim of this book on the one hand is to lead to a better understanding of the pathophysiology of nausea and emesis under different conditions, and on the other to provide an update of the treatment regimens. Specifically, the increasing use of emetogenic anti-cancer chemotherapy needs the best prevention and treatment strategies to control its nausea- and emesis-provoking side effects. Vomiting might also be a complicating factor in radiation therapy and surgery. On the other hand, in women affected by nausea and vomiting in early pregnancy, the question of drug treatment versus non-treatment has to be answered.

Essentially, this book should serve the clinician. In collecting the articles we aimed at providing a 'state-of-the-art' overview of the selection of antiemetic drugs available and their dosages and routes of administration under specific clinical conditions. After a few decades of intense research, we are in the fortunate situation that in almost every relevant clinical condition of nausea and emesis, a collection of investigations has put forward clear conclusions for the best treatment modalities.

Whereas the main task of collecting these papers was to serve the clinician when making the right choice for every patient's needs, the book also pays significant attention to the interests of scientists in basic research as well as academic teachers.

Josef Donnerer
September 2002

Donnerer J (ed): Antiemetic Therapy.
Basel, Karger, 2003, pp 1–10

The Emetic Reflex Arc

Josef Donnerer

Institute of Experimental and Clinical Pharmacology, University of Graz, Austria

The emetic reflex is an autonomous defense reaction of the gastrointestinal tract, aimed at eliminating noxious agents, in a similar way as the cough reflex or sneezing is aimed at eliminating irritating particles from the respiratory tract. Therefore, in many instances, nausea and emesis are evoked by ingestion of spoiled food, too much alcohol, or simply by eating too much. Under these circumstances the ability to detect and to eject potential toxic substances from the gastrointestinal tract can be regarded as a useful reaction. However, nausea and emesis can also represent general symptoms of a disease or they are side effects of certain drug actions. Under these latter circumstances, the emetic reflex has to be regarded as a more general defense reaction against potential toxic substances; the toxic substances are, however, in the bloodstream and cannot be eliminated anymore by vomiting. These conditions are very stressful for the patient and need efficient therapy. Examples represent chemotherapeutic agents inducing nausea and emesis for hours and days without eliminating any toxins from the body, postoperative nausea and vomiting, hyperemesis gravidarum and nausea in the course of opioid therapy.

Neuronal Structures Involved in the Emetic Reflex Arc

The receptive pathway of the emetic reflex is a build-up of different sensors and receptors in the periphery as well as within the CNS [1]. Sensory impulses are conveyed by afferent neurons towards a medullary control center. In the so-called ‘vomiting center’, impulses are integrated and transmitted onto motor and autonomic output limbs to elicit either the feeling of nausea, retching or emesis. Although the receptive pathways may be different, all sensory pathways converge on a common preprogrammed motor and autonomic output to the digestive tract.

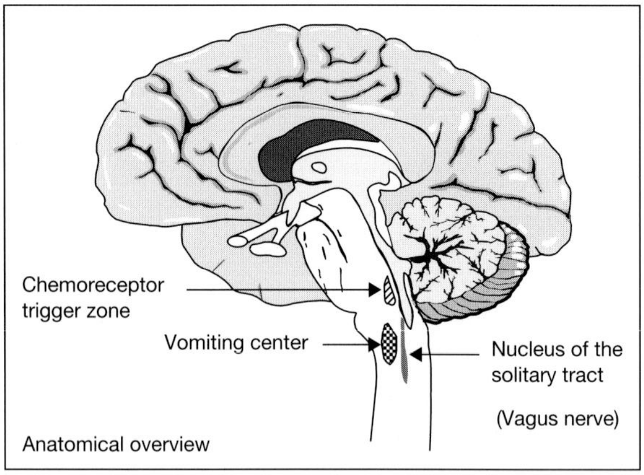

Fig. 1. Structures within the CNS that can be regarded as central coordination areas of the emetic reflex.

Many neurotransmitter receptors are present on this reflex arc, which can be selectively influenced by antiemetic drugs. Depending on the noxious agents and the anatomical location of the pathways, different receptors may be involved and different therapeutic drugs are effective.

Within the CNS there are three structures that can be regarded as central coordination areas of the emetic reflex (fig. 1). They are located in the medulla/brainstem region. Vomiting is coordinated by a distributed medullary control system rather than a unique, well-defined vomiting center. Neurons involved are embedded in an arc of neurons radiating from the area postrema and nucleus of the solitary tract (NTS) through the intermediate reticular zone of the lateral tegmental field to the ventrolateral medulla. These functional areas are located close to or are integrated into nuclei of the vagus nerve, the most important input for the emetic reflex. The vomiting center represents the central connection between sensory afferents and motor and autonomic efferents [2–4].

The 'chemoreceptor trigger zone' (CTZ) of the area postrema is situated nearby, which serves the central detection of noxious agents that circulate in the bloodstream and in the cerebrospinal fluid. This area on the floor of the fourth ventricle is on the one hand directly exposed to the cerebrospinal fluid, and can detect noxious agents that are present in it, and on the other hand it contains a dense vascular network of fenestrated capillaries. In this way, substances circulating in the blood can be detected that would not penetrate the blood-brain barrier. Chemoreceptors in the area postrema, which are outside the blood-brain barrier, are sensitive to circulating emetic agents such as apomorphine, cytotoxic drugs and dopamine.

Furthermore, the CTZ is integrated into the afferent pathway of emetic signals from the periphery and from the vestibular labyrinth. Apomorphine, a dopamine agonist, is a very specific stimulus for the CTZ, and can be used as an emetic agent. The area postrema is a chemoreceptive area for triggering vomiting. The area postrema projects to the vomiting center and to the NTS.

The NTS is the sensory nucleus of the vagus nerve and of the glossopharyngeus nerve, and transmits the afferent signals from the pharynx and from the gastrointestinal tract to the CNS. In the NTS, there is a close correspondence between neurons activated by emetic drugs and sites of afferent input from the area postrema and abdominal vagus nerve. Some NTS neurons receive convergent input from the vestibular labyrinth and abdominal vagus nerve. Thus the NTS may represent the beginning of a final common pathway by which different emetic inputs produce vomiting. The region of the retrofacial nucleus contains pre-motor and motor neuronal circuitry critical for generating the pattern of the respiratory-related components of vomiting. Emetic stimuli activate neurons in the dorsal vagal complex; these neurons also control swallowing, baroreceptor reflexes, respiration, tone and motility of the stomach and lower esophageal sphincter.

In short, the emetic reflex arc connects sites of primary sensory input (nodose ganglia, NTS, area postrema) to pre-motor (nucleus retroambiguus) and motor (dorsal vagus, phrenic nuclei) output limbs (fig. 2).

Serotonin 5-HT_3, dopamine D_2, histamine H_1 and muscarinic (M) acetylcholine receptors are located within the described three brain nuclei receptors important for the initiation of nausea and emesis [5, 6]. Corresponding antagonists can therefore have an inhibitory effect within these areas to prevent or inhibit emesis.

The efferent part of the vomiting reflex includes coordinated control of the diaphragm, inspiration, blood pressure, heart rate, larynx, pharynx, tongue, lower esophageal sphincter and gastric fundus (fig. 3). A rapid and distinctive firing pattern from vagal motor nerve fibers is essential for emesis.

Brain regions essential for vomiting or thought to be involved in the emetic motor response are known from animal experiments during fictive vomiting [3]. These include the retrofacial nucleus of the brainstem and the dorsolateral medullary reticular formation of the obex. Cells are activated in the ventral medulla – they control larynx and pharynx, respiration, sympathetic outflow to maintain blood pressure and parasympathetic neurons that innervate the heart. The respiratory components of the vomiting arc are also controlled from the ventrolateral medulla. Extensive activation also occurs in the dorsal motor nucleus of the vagus. In the reticular formation, activation occurs of neurons in distinct columns corresponding to the locations both of swallowing reflex interneurons and of the inferior salivatory nucleus. Activity is also seen in the

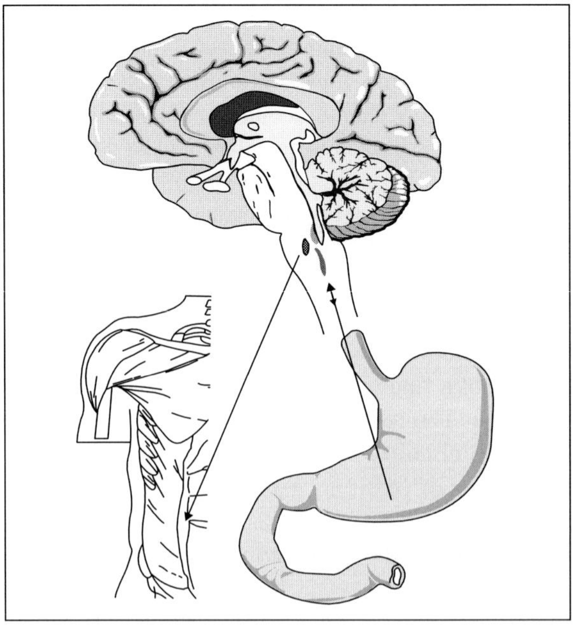

Fig. 2. The emetic reflex arc connects sites of sensory input to motor output limbs.

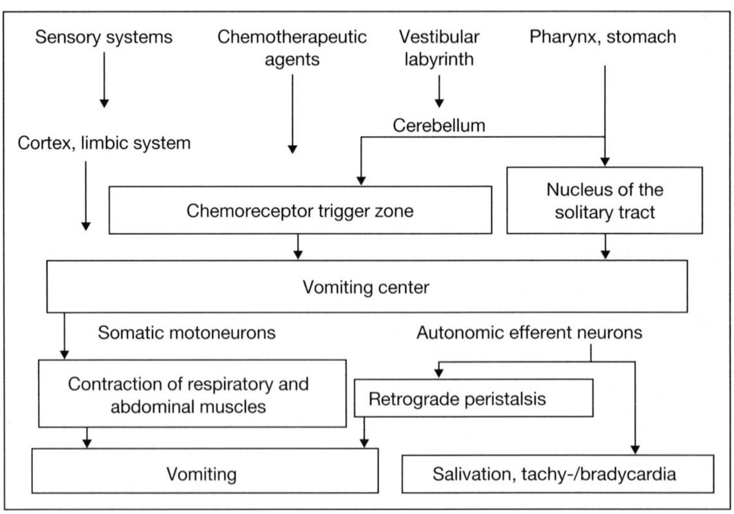

Fig. 3. Schematic diagram of the vomiting reflex.

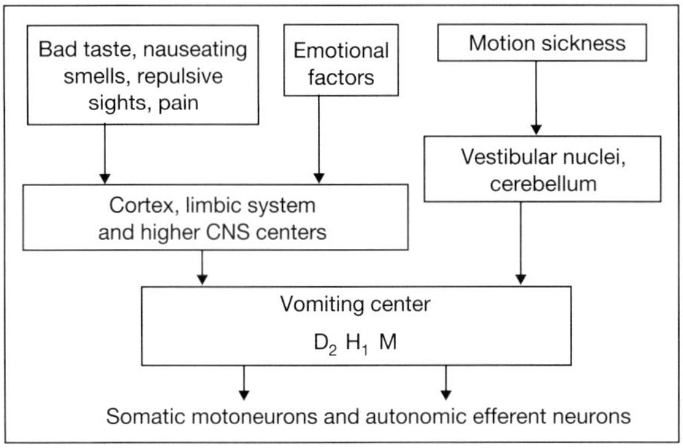

Fig. 4. Emetic reflexes evoked by the first line of defense. D_2 = Dopamine D_2 receptor, H_1 = histamine H_1 receptor, M = muscarinic cholinergic receptor.

subretrofacial nucleus, which conveys sympathoexcitatory signals to spinal preganglionic neurons.

The efferent motor output is mediated by the motor nerves to the respiratory and abdominal muscles [7]. Efferent autonomic impulses are conveyed to the smooth muscles of the gastrointestinal tract, to the salivary glands and to the heart. The neural reflexes in emesis evoke a contraction of the respiratory and abdominal muscles and a reversal of the normal function programs of esophagus and stomach: relaxation of the lower esophagus sphincter and of the proximal stomach, and retroperistalsis. The heart rate can be influenced towards bradycardia or towards tachycardia.

The Emetic Reflex as a Defense Reaction

With regard to the receptors and afferent pathways, that convey information to the emetic reflex center, three different lines of defense can be distinguished [1]: (1) a first line of defense before enteral intake of toxins; (2) a second line of defense before absorption of toxins, and (3) a third line of defense after the absorption of noxious substances.

The relevant sensors of the first line of defense include taste, smell, hearing, eyesight and the vestibular labyrinth (fig. 4). Bad taste (taste aversion), nauseating smells and repulsive sights, even thinking of it can evoke emesis. The afferent signals are transmitted via higher CNS centers. An important sensor for several types of nausea and emesis is the vestibular labyrinth. The receptors there are stimulated by increment of speed (motion-induced vomiting) or

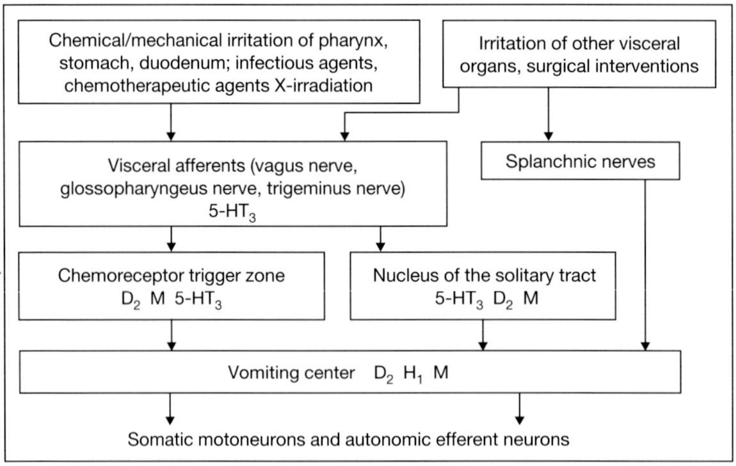

Fig. 5. Emetic reflexes evoked by the second line of defense in the digestive tract. D_2 = Dopamine D_2 receptor, H_1 = histamine H_1 receptor, M = muscarinic cholinergic receptor, 5-HT_3 = serotonin 5-HT_3 receptor.

by the position of the body (vestibular-induced vomiting). A disharmony between the messages from the eye and the vestibular apparatus can evoke oculovestibular system-induced motion sickness [7]. The afferent signals to the vomiting center travel via the vestibular nuclei and the cerebellum. In motion sickness, histamine H_1 and muscarinic receptors are thought to be involved.

The second line of defense is carried by sensory systems in the digestive tract that sense swallowed noxious substances and represent the preabsorptive response (fig. 5). The sensory neural pathways include the vagus nerve which mediates responses from the stomach, and the splanchnic nerves which mediate responses from the entire small intestine. The vagus nerve innervates almost all parts of the upper digestive organs and conveys its afferent signals to the NTS, which is located close to the vomiting center. The receptors on the vagal nerve can detect chemical or mechanical stimuli within the visceral organs [8].

Mechanical stimulation of the digestive tract from pharynx to small intestine can activate nausea and emesis. Similarly, chemoreceptors in the mucosa and possibly also in the serosa respond to a variety of stimuli. The distal stomach and duodenum are the most sensitive regions. Visceral mechanoreceptors react very sensitively to a distension of the distal parts of the stomach and of the small intestine as it occurs in motility disorders. Mechanical stimuli on the mesenterium, the peritoneum and on many visceral organs can evoke nausea and emesis [9]. Other sensory nerves in the trigeminus nerve or in the

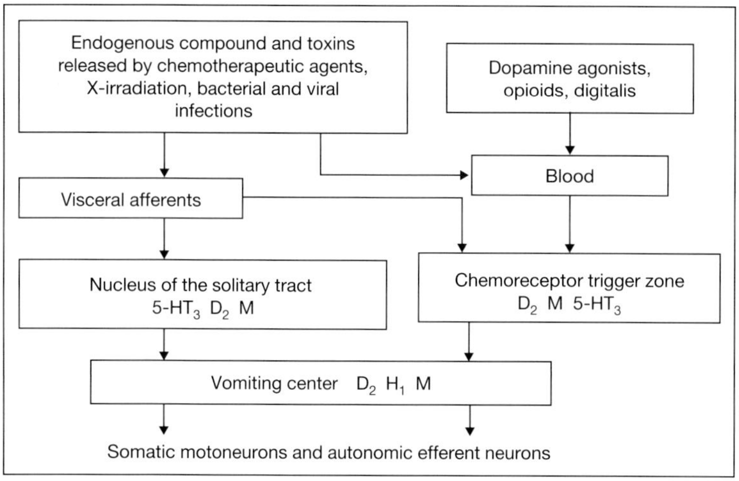

Fig. 6. Emetic reflexes from the third line of defense. D_2 = Dopamine D_2 receptor, H_1 = histamine H_1 receptor, M = muscarinic cholinergic receptor, $5\text{-}HT_3$ = serotonin $5\text{-}HT_3$ receptor.

glossopharyngeus nerve can also transmit emetogenic signals, e.g. mechanical stimuli from the eye or stimuli from the pharynx.

Polymodal receptors in the stomach can be stimulated by a variety of chemical agents, like hypertonic saline or ipecacuanha. When chromaffin-like cells of the upper gastrointestinal tract are damaged by X-irradiation or by chemotherapeutic agents, they release serotonin (5-hydroxytryptamine, 5-HT), which can stimulate $5\text{-}HT_3$ receptors on the vagus nerve. Released 5-HT can also reach the CTZ directly via the bloodstream and stimulate $5\text{-}HT_3$ receptors. Additionally, a direct stimulation of vagal afferents by the antineoplastic agents or by the X-irradiation could be responsible for the induction of emesis. Strong emetogenic agents include cisplatin, dacarbazine, cyclophosphamide, melphalan and actinomycin [10]. Toxins produced by infectious agents can also activate the emetic reflex.

$5\text{-}HT_3$ receptors are widespread receptors activated primarily by toxic stimuli. 5-HT depolarizes the vagus nerve through $5\text{-}HT_3$ receptors and is a noxious stimulant for vagal afferents. Other receptors in the intestine that might be activated by chemical stimulation include the $5\text{-}HT_4$ receptor and the dopamine D_2 receptor.

The third line of defense representing the postabsorptive response includes the CTZ of the area postrema, which senses noxious substances in the circulation (fig. 6). The CTZ can be stimulated by a variety of compounds, that also stimulate the vagal afferents like 5-HT, by toxins released from damaged cells or by antineoplastic agents themselves. Within the CTZ, agents like nicotine, digitalis and opioids can also produce emetogenic signals. Dopamine agonists like apomorphine can evoke nausea and emesis by stimulation of central D_2 dopamine receptors, and opioids by stimulation of centrally located opioid receptors. Cisplatin produces vomiting by a cascade of mechanisms that probably involve parallel activation of abdominal visceral (vagal and splanchnic) afferents and the emetic CTZ in the area postrema.

Nausea and Emesis Response

Immediate and Indirect Consequences

Nausea is a subjective sensation (the feeling of nausea), often combined with autonomic reactions: hypersecretion in the upper digestive system, cold sweat, pallor, epigastric awareness, tachycardia or bradycardia with a relaxation of the proximal parts of the stomach. A discussion is still going on whether there is a distinct nausea center close to the emetic reflex center, or alternatively if nausea corresponds only to a subthreshold activation of the emetic reflex center. Emesis can follow, but this does not have to be the case; vomiting can occur without any preceding phase of nausea.

Nausea symptoms are often followed by a retching phase. This is characterized by convulsive, rhythmic inspiratory movements and contractions of the abdominal muscles, however during the inspiration the pressure evoked by the abdominal muscles is neutralized by the negative pressure within the thorax, so that the content of the stomach is only moved forward and backward. When the stomach is filled with food after a meal, vomiting will follow rapidly. However, when the stomach is empty, the retching episodes are unproductive and a relief by emesis cannot follow; these situations are specifically stressful, e.g. in antineoplastic therapy.

During the emetic phase a coordinated activation of various groups of muscles occurs: respiratory, abdominal, oral, trunk and head muscles are activated and lead to the typical posture during vomiting. A wave of high intra-abdominal pressure is combined with a phase of high intrathoracic pressure. Expulsion is a response to changes in intra-abdominal and intrathoracic pressure generated by the respiratory muscles. Vomitus expulsion consists of the simultaneous contraction of the diaphragm, abdominal muscles, and expiratory intercostalis muscles. Retrograde giant contractions of the small intestine and gastric antrum are accompanied by relaxation of the gastric fundus and corpus and thoracic esophagus, and a retrograde contraction of the cervical esophagus to expel gastrointestinal content orally. The smooth muscles of the stomach itself do not contract, the pressure onto the stomach is solely produced by the abdominal wall and the diaphragma. During emesis the gum and the glottis close the respiratory tract to protect it from aspiration. The coordinated activation of oropharyngeal and laryngeal motoneurons is an integral component of the vomiting response.

Dopamine receptors in the stomach mediate the inhibition of gastric motility during nausea and emesis – this is one of the targets of the dopamine D_2 receptor antagonists. Newly developed tachykinin NK_1 receptor antagonists act at a site in the dorsal vagal complex. Part of their effectiveness may be the result of inhibition of the NK_1 receptors on vagal motor neurons to prevent fundic relaxation, which is a prodromal event essential for emesis.

The immediate consequences of vomiting are a loss of water and electrolytes with fluid depletion and electrolyte changes likely to occur following prolonged vomiting. This can be particularly dangerous for young children. There is always a danger of aspiration, specifically when CNS-depressing drugs are taken concomitantly by the patient. The psychological stress can lead to lifelong aversions or conditioning, e.g. to the refusal of curative antineoplastic therapy.

Among the indirect consequences of vomiting there are effects on the heart rate and on the circulatory system, as well as a high pressure in certain organs. It can lead to mechanical injury of the esophagus or the stomach, such as ruptures of the mucosal or inner muscular layers of these organs. The increase in the cranial blood pressure could lead to the rupture of an aneurysm. Postoperative vomiting can endanger the results of the preceding surgical interventions, in the case of aspiration there is a danger of pneumonia.

As already stated above, several well-defined receptor sites can serve as targets for effective antiemetic drug therapy. In view of the considerable stress exerted on a person by nausea and vomiting, antiemetic therapy should, whenever possible, already be a preventive measure. A selection of drugs for specific clinical situations are given in the following chapters.

References

1 Waldvogel HH, Aapro MS, Beubler E, Schneck H, Widmer W, Wilder-Smith C, Wilder-Smith OHG: Antiemetische Therapie – Nausea und Emesis. Stuttgart, Thieme, 1995.

2 Miller AD, Ruggiero DA: Emetic reflex arc revealed by expression of the immediate-early gene c-fos in the cat. J Neurosci 1994;14:871–888.

3 Miller AD, Nonaka S, Jakus J: Brain areas essential or non-essential for emesis. Brain Res 1994; 647:255–264.

4 Fukuda H, Nakamura E, Koga T, Furukawa N, Shiroshita Y: The site of the anti-emetic action of tachykinin NK_1 receptor antagonists may exist in the medullary area adjacent to the semicompact part of the nucleus ambiguous. Brain Res 1999;818:439–449.

5 Hornby PJ: Central neurocircuitry associated with emesis. Am J Med 2001;111:106S–112S.
6 Hasler WL: Serotonin receptor physiology: Relation to emesis. Dig Dis Sci 1999;44:108S–113S.
7 Lang IM, Sarna SK, Shaker R: Gastrointestinal motor and myoelectric correlates of motion sickness. Am J Physiol 1999;277:G642–G652.
8 Lang IM: Noxious stimulation of emesis. Dig Dis Sci 1999;44:58S–63S.
9 Gan TJ: Postoperative nausea and vomiting – Can it be eliminated? JAMA 2002;287:1233–1236.
10 Veyrat-Follet C, Farinotti R, Palmer JL: Physiology of chemotherapy-induced emesis and antiemetic therapy. Predictive models for evaluation of new compounds. Drugs 1997;53:206–234.

Prof. Dr. Josef Donnerer
Institut für Experimentelle und Klinische Pharmakologie
Karl-Franzens-Universität Graz
Universitätsplatz 4, A–8010 Graz (Austria)
Tel. +43 316 3804509, Fax +43 316 3809645, E-Mail Josef.Donnerer@uni-graz.at

Donnerer J (ed): Antiemetic Therapy.
Basel, Karger, 2003, pp 11–21

Receptive Mechanisms of Noxious Stimulation of Emesis

Ivan M. Lang

Department of Medicine, Medical College of Wisconsin, Milwaukee, Wisc., USA

This chapter will address the receptive mechanisms of vomiting initiated by noxious substances or forces acting through the digestive tract and the chemoreceptor trigger zone (CTZ). Some may consider motion sickness a noxious form of emesis, but this subject will not be addressed here.

Emesis caused by noxious substances serves a protective function and involves receptors located at different levels within the neuraxis. Pre-absorptive noxious receptors are located in the mucosa of the digestive tract [1] and the post-absorptive noxious receptors are located in the CTZ of the brain [2]. Clinically relevant agents or forces, e.g. radiation [3] or cytotoxic drugs [4], may cause emesis by activating receptive mechanisms for noxious stimulation-induced vomiting. Before describing the receptive mechanisms of noxious stimulation-induced emesis, a brief description of the motor events of emesis will be provided in order to better understand functions of the emetic response.

Characterization and Function of Emetic Responses

The emetic process involves coordinated changes in respiratory, gastrointestinal and cardiovascular systems [5, 6], but vomitus expulsion is comprised of two separately controlled but related sets of motor events of the respiratory and digestive tracts [7, 8]. The first set of events involves most of the digestive tract, and the first digestive tract response is increased salivation and swallowing [9]. The swallowing of salivary secretions has been found to buffer acid refluxed into the esophagus [10], similarly, the increased swallowing before vomiting may act to buffer acidic gastric contents before passage through the esophagus during vomiting. This buffering of gastric contents may be an important function because the esophagus is not well protected against acid exposure [11].

After this period of increased swallowing, separate sets of intestinal contractions expel the contents of the small intestine into the stomach and colon [12, 13]. The primary function of these contractions is to remove the offending noxious substance from the absorbing areas of the digestive tract and to allow elimination of the substance orally and anally. The upper half of the small intestine is emptied by a single large amplitude contraction that propagates retrogradely [12, 14]. However, the retrograde contraction also occurs during types of vomiting, e.g. motion sickness [15], when there is no offending noxious substance to expel. Perhaps the retrograde contraction serves an additional function. In all vomiting acidic gastric juice must be expelled through a weakly protected esophagus [11]. The retrograde contraction probably causes intraluminal release and gastric deposition of mucous and bicarbonate from the Brunner's glands as it passes from duodenum to stomach, because strong duodenal contractions have been shown to cause Brunner's gland secretion [16]. Therefore, the retrograde contraction may function not only to protect the organism from offending noxious substances, but also to assist in protection of the esophagus from damage by acidic gastric contents.

The contents of the lower half of the small intestine are emptied into the colon by a series of anally propagating contractions [12, 13]. While the size of these contractions is not larger than those that occur during the fed or fasted states, the propagation distance of these phasic contractions is longer [6, 12]. The longer propagation distance and repetitive nature of these distal intestinal contractions act to quickly milk distal intestinal contents into the colon. Defecation often follows emesis [15], and if significant amounts of the offending substance reach the colon defecation may be as important as vomitus expulsion in eliminating the offending noxious substance from the organism.

After the intestinal contents are refluxed back to the stomach, the respiratory phase of vomiting begins. The lower esophageal sphincter relaxes and the esophagus contracts longitudinally pulling the gastroesophageal junction into the thoracic cavity [9, 17]. This action removes the primary physical barrier, i.e. the esophagofundic angle which forms the fundic pouch [17], to gastroesophageal reflux. Retching begins as the entire diaphragm contracts pulling the stomach caudad [18, 19]. At this time the esophagus and upper esophageal sphincter (UES) relax and the glottis closes [7]. While some gastric contents may be expelled into the esophagus during retching [18, 19], this reflux is limited by contraction of the diaphragmatic hiatus [8, 9]. Between retches the diaphragm relaxes as the esophagus contracts pulling the stomach orad [9]. Both the UES and glottis close [7–9] preventing esophagopharyngeal reflux and aspiration. These events are repeated once per second which causes the gastric contents to mix together while being thrown cranially and caudally during retching [7, 9]. Finally, during the contractile phase of the last retch, vomiting occurs [7, 9]. The vomit is similar to the contractile phase of retching except that the diaphragmatic hiatus and the UES relax allowing gastro-oral reflux. In addition, the UES and pharynx are maximally pulled rostrally and anteriorly by contraction of the suprahyoid and suprapharyngeal muscles [7, 9]. At this time the gastric contents enter the esophagus [18, 19] and a retrograde contraction of the striated muscle portion of the esophagus assists the orad progression of the bolus through the maximally opened and relaxed UES to the pharynx [9]. It is unknown whether this retrograde contraction of the esophagus is a centrally controlled patterned motor event or a series of myostatic reflexes. If it is a patterned event then it actively pushes the bolus orad, and if it is a series of reflexes then it probably acts to prevent the bolus from moving caudad.

Receptive Mechanisms

Digestive Tract

Physiological Receptors. The digestive tract is the source of the pre-absorptive receptors for the activation of vomiting by noxious substances or forces. These receptors may be mechano- or chemoreceptors. Mechanical stimulation of the digestive tract from the pharynx to the small intestine by stroking the mucosa, distention, compression or obstruction activates nausea and vomiting [20–22].

Gastrointestinal mechanoreceptors have been found in all three layers of the digestive tract [23]. The mucosal mechanoreceptors are primarily rapidly adapting and many are also chemosensitive [23]. These receptors may be free nerve endings as no specific receptor organ has been identified [24]. The mechanoreceptors of the muscularis are primarily slowly adapting in-series tension receptors which are located within the muscular plexus and have been termed intraganglionic laminar endings [23, 25, 26]. The mechanoreceptors of the serosa are also slowly adapting tension receptors which may be free nerve endings, however, the threshold for activation of these receptors is greater than that for receptors of the muscularis [23]. Considering that the physiological mechanical stimulus most likely to activate vomiting is a slow but strong distention due to obstruction [22, 23, 27], it is possible that one of the mechanoreceptors mediating vomiting may be the high threshold slowly adapting mechanoreceptors of the serosa. These serosal receptors may also be responsible for peritonitis-induced emesis [28, 29].

The chemoreceptors mediating emesis have been found mostly [22, 30] in the distal stomach and proximal small intestine and are probably located in the mucosa. These receptors respond to a variety of noxious substances including

HCl [14, 21], alkaline solutions [21], $CuSO_4$ [1, 31–33], acetic acid [34], hypertonic saline [21, 34], potassium myltartrate [34], syrup of ipecac [35], mustard [34] and mercuric chloride [34]. Two types of chemoreceptive mechanisms have been identified in the digestive tract wall: chemoreceptors of the mucosa [23, 36] and enterochromaffin (EC) cells [37, 38]. The mucosal chemoreceptors may be free nerve endings [24], are found in all areas of the digestive tract [23], and may be either polymodal or chemospecific [23]. The EC cells span the mucosa, secrete neuroactive substances, are richly innervated, and are found in the stomach, duodenum and colon [39]. Both the chemoreceptors and the EC cells are found in greatest abundance in areas of the digestive tract [39], i.e. upper digestive tract, that are most sensitive to chemical stimulation of emesis [22, 30].

The specific physiological receptor responsible for emesis caused by noxious chemical stimulation of the digestive tract is unclear. Peripherally stimulated emesis caused by intraluminal administration of noxious chemicals, e.g. $CuSO_4$, is blocked by vagotomy [1]. The most sensitive areas of the digestive tract to luminal stimulation are the stomach and duodenum, and the ileum is insensitive to $CuSO_4$ [22, 30]. However, intraluminal administration of $CuSO_4$ releases 5-HT from EC cells of the ileum, but not the stomach [40, 41]. Therefore, evidence suggests that $CuSO_4$-induced emesis and perhaps all noxious chemical (intraluminally administered) induced emesis is mediated by vagal chemoreceptors of the digestive tract mucosa rather than release of 5-HT from EC cells. The specific receptive mechanisms mediating cytotoxin- or radiation-induced emesis are unknown. While cytotoxin, radiation or $CuSO_4$ can release 5-HT from EC cells of the lower small intestine [40, 41, 42], cytoxin- but not $CuSO_4$-induced emesis is blocked by 5-HT_3 antagonists [31, 32, 40, 41, 43, 44]. These findings suggest that radiation- or cytotoxin-induced emesis causes vomiting by the release of 5-HT from EC cells rather than activation of chemoreceptors.

Neural Pathways. The afferent pathways for digestive tract noxious stimulation-induced emesis comprise the vagus and splanchnic nerves, and possibly a co-sympathetic nerve mediated spinal cord pathway. These pathways can be through direct innervation of the chemoreceptors [23] or through synaptic contact with EC cells as the EC cells are innervated by the vagus nerves [37, 38]. The afferent pathway is more related to the location of the stimulus in the digestive tract than to the specific type of stimulus. The vagus nerves mediate emetic responses from the stomach [21], and the splanchnic nerves and spinal cord mediate emetic responses from the small intestine [27]. Correspondingly, $CuSO_4$-induced (intraluminally administered) emesis is blocked by vagotomy [1], but stimuli, i.e., radiation and cytotoxins (i.v. or i.p.), that affect both stomach and small intestine can be blocked only by transection of the vagus, and splanchnic nerves or spinal cord [43–46]. Regardless of the noxious stimulus, the vagus nerves are the primary afferents for activation of emesis as vagotomy, but not splanchnectomy, block emesis due to low doses [47, 48] or significantly inhibits emesis due to higher doses of these stimuli [43, 44]. However, non-vagal afferents, i.e. sympathetic or co-sympathetic afferents, have a significant role in these forms of emesis as transection of these pathways enhances the effects of vagotomy [43–46]. Although the splanchnic nerves mediate some of the noxious-induced sensory information from the digestive tract, only electrical stimulation of the vagus nerves [49, 50] activate retching and vomiting. Emesis may be mediated by noxious stimulation of receptors in the abdomen not projecting through the vagus or splanchnic nerves, as radiation-induced emesis is blocked only after vagotomy and high dorsal column cordotomy [45]. Perhaps the physiological receptors involved in this non-splanchnic nerve but spinal cord-mediated emetic response are those involved in emesis due to peritonitis, because peritonitis-induced emesis is not blocked by vagus and splanchnic nerve section, but is blocked by spinal cord transection [28].

Neuropharmacology. Many studies have concluded that receptors for noxious substance-induced emesis are located peripherally or centrally, but identifying specific sites of drug action is difficult. Techniques to distinguish between central and peripheral sites of action of agents include observing the effects of agonists before and after afferent denervation, comparison of responses to central versus peripheral administration of agonists or antagonist, and comparison of the effects of peripherally versus centrally acting agonists or antagonists. None of these techniques is without drawbacks.

Many pharmacological agents cross the blood-brain barrier slowly, therefore, at lower doses their effects are peripherally mediated, however, at higher doses the response may be centrally mediated. Some emetic agonists, e.g. $CuSO_4$, act at the peripheral level when administered orally or intraluminally at or below about 5 mg/kg, but at or above 15 mg/kg $CuSO_4$ also activates emesis by stimulation of the CTZ [1, 2]. Many recent studies of $CuSO_4$-induced emesis have used oral doses ranging from 10 to 25 mg/kg. Peripheral denervation is only effective when used with doses of agonists that act exclusively at the peripheral level, but demonstration of this exclusiveness is rarely performed. In addition, complete peripheral deafferentation is very difficult and rarely performed as it requires spinal cord section [45]. The comparison of the effects of peripherally versus centrally administered agonists or antagonists is often difficult to interpret. One may inject an agent into the ventricular system of the brain to bypass the blood-brain barrier or to preferentially stimulate circumventricular organs, but the agent may not readily diffuse to all parts of the brain and the investigated receptors of the circumventricular organs may not be readily accessible from the cerebral ventricles. All of the above problems have made the localization of the receptors mediating noxious stimulation-induced emesis difficult.

The serotonergic receptors are perhaps the most studied of those mediating the noxious stimulation of the digestive tract. Serotonergic receptors have been found at many levels of the digestive tract including the enteric nervous system, interstitial cells of Cajal and the enteroendocrine cells [51]. The role of each of these sources of serotonergic receptors in noxious stimulation of emesis is unknown, but cyotoxin or $CuSO_4$ can induce the release of 5-HT from EC cells of the digestive tract [40, 41].

The specific subtypes of serotonergic receptors involved in the emesis-induced noxious stimulation of the digestive tract have been studied. Multiple subtypes of serotonergic receptors have been found to mediate different forms of noxious stimulation of emesis suggesting that different noxious agents or forces may activate emesis through different mechanisms. The emesis activated by oral administration of copper sulfate was inhibited [32] or blocked [31] by 5-HT_4 receptor antagonists, but not 5-HT_3 receptor antagonists [31, 32]. However, the dose of $CuSO_4$ (100 mg/kg) used in the study in which only inhibition of emesis was observed was well above the threshold dose capable of activating the CTZ [1]. Vagotomy blocked the effects of low dose $CuSO_4$ [1], and vagal stimulation-induced emesis was not blocked by 5-HT_3 antagonist [52]. These results suggested that low dose of $CuSO_4$ activated emesis through a peripheral 5-HT_4 receptor on vagal afferents. $CuSO_4$ may also act at the CTZ to activate emesis but the receptor mediating this action is unknown.

Cytotoxin- or radiation-induced emesis, which is mediated by visceral afferents, is blocked by 5-HT_3 antagonists [40, 41, 43, 44], and emesis induced by intravenous administration of 5-HT_3 agonist is significantly inhibited by vagotomy and splanchnectomy [53, 54]. Therefore, evidence suggests that peripheral 5-HT_3 receptors mediate radiation or cytotoxin-induced emesis. On the other hand, digestive tract mechanical stimulation-induced emesis is not blocked by 5-HT_3 receptor antagonists [20], but the role of other digestive tract serotonergic receptors in this response has not been investigated.

Conclusion. The stimulation of emesis by noxious stimuli may be mediated by different types of physiological receptors located at different levels and different regions of the digestive tract. Chemical stimulation of emesis may be mediated by mucosal receptors of the upper digestive tract, mechanical stimulation of emesis may be mediated by receptors of the mucosa and/or serosa of the upper and lower digestive tract, and radiation- or cytotoxin-induced emesis may be mediated by the release of 5-HT from EC cells of the distal small intestine. The afferent pathways mediating different noxious emetic stimuli may be similar and observed differences may be more related to the location of the stimulus in the digestive tract rather than the type of noxious substance.

Regardless, the vagus nerves are probably the major afferent pathway, but spinal cord pathways may be facilitatory.

Chemoreceptor Trigger Zone

Borison and Brizzee [2] observed about 50 years ago that ablation of the area postrema (AP) blocked the emetic effects of some agents administered intravenously, but did not block the ability of the animal to vomit. They concluded that the AP, which has no blood-brain barrier, contains the CTZ for vomiting and that the CTZ acted as a second line of defense, i.e. post-absorptive defense, against the ingestion of a toxic or noxious substance.

The investigation of the role of the CTZ and AP in various forms of emesis has resulted in numerous contradictory findings primarily because of technical differences. The AP lies adjacent to the primary vagal afferent nuclei (nucleus tractus solitarius (NTS)), therefore ablation or stimulation of the AP is difficult without affecting the NTS. In addition, anatomical studies have revealed that some vagal afferents project through the AP en route to the NTS [55, 56]. In addition, there may be species differences [55, 56] regarding the separation of chemosensitive cells from brainstem-integrative neurons within the AP such that separation of functions by ablative techniques is difficult or impossible. Considering that the CTZ is a physiologically defined entity, the only way to accurately determine the role of the CTZ is to confirm through physiological techniques that the area destroyed or stimulated affected only the CTZ and not the emetic control areas of the dorsal brainstem. Many studies of the role of the CTZ have failed to confirm this distinction, and therefore, the results of these studies are difficult to interpret. Therefore, while the AP may contain the CTZ, it may also contain other pathways and neurons mediating other forms of emesis.

Chemosensitivity. The AP is one of the circumventricular organs and it contains many elements of neural tissue like neurons, nerve fibers and neuroglia, but the unique features of the AP are the lack of a blood-brain barrier and the vascular sinusoids similar to chemoreceptive organs of the cardiovascular system [55]. Numerous AP structures could act as chemosensors including the microvilli and microvillous tufts of ependymal cells, tanocyte-like cells of the ependyma which extend to the sinusoids, or the nerve endings in the perivascular space of the sinusoids [55], but the specific role of each structure is unknown.

Numerous neurotransmitters and neuroactive substances have been found in the AP [56], but the role of most of these agents in mediating emesis is unknown. Ablation of the CTZ (ablation of the AP which preserves the emetic response to veratrum alkaloids, $CuSO_4$, naloxone, phenylbiguanide, vagal stimulation, or motion sickness) blocked the emetic effects of angiotensin II, apomorphine, cisplatin, digitalis, epinephrine, histamine, levodopa, lobeline, neurotensin, nicotine, xylazine, etc. [55, 56]. Considering that specific antagonists to these agents block emesis activated by these agents only, this effect may be on the chemosensitive cells of the CTZ rather than on the neural elements of the AP [55, 56]. Similarly, neurons of the AP [57, 58] respond to cholinergic, adrenergic, GABA-ergic, opioid, serotonergic, histaminergic and numerous peptidergic agents as well as hormones, but it is unknown which of these agents are neurotransmitters of the AP and which are stimulants of the chemoreceptors. However, serotonin-binding sites have been found in the AP [59] and injection of 5-HT_3 antagonist into the AP blocks cisplatin-induced emesis [60]. The serotonin-binding sites are dependent upon the vagal afferent input, suggesting that these were on presynaptic vagal afferent terminals [59]. Although the AP injection of antagonist may not have been limited to the AP, these results suggest an important role for 5-HT_3 receptors of the AP mediating cytotoxin-induced emesis.

The role of the CTZ or AP in radiation-induced emesis is controversial. Almost all of the studies in cats have found that ablation of the CTZ does not affect radiation-induced emesis [3, 61]. In these studies, it was confirmed that the lesions of the AP affected only the CTZ-activated emesis. On the other hand, all of the studies using dogs [46, 55, 56, 63] or monkeys [55, 56, 62] have found that AP ablation blocked radiation-induced emesis. However, while in all of these experiments the ablation of the CTZ was confirmed, the sparing of the non-CTZ brainstem pathways was not confirmed. The only explanation consistent with all studies is that the CTZ does not mediate radiation-induced emesis, but that in the dog and monkey studies non-CTZ areas of the AP or adjacent dorsal brainstem nuclei or fibers mediating radiation-induced emesis were damaged by these AP lesions.

The mechanisms of cytotoxin- and radiation-induced emesis seem contradictory. Both stimuli are mediated by the same receptive mechanisms (EC cells), neurotransmitter (5-HT_3) and afferent pathways (vagal and spinal), but only cytotoxin-induced emesis is mediated by the CTZ. This difference may be due to the ability of cytotoxins to stimulate the CTZ directly as does $CuSO_4$ or technical differences. No studies of the role of the AP or CTZ in emesis investigated both cytotoxins and radiation in the same animals. Considering the significant technical problems and differences associated with this type of research, differences in techniques may explain the observed differences in results.

Conclusion. The CTZ is a physiologically defined entity which provides the second line of defense against noxious substances and is responsive to numerous endogenous and exogenous agents. The CTZ mediates cytotoxin- but not radiation-induced emesis. The CTZ resides within the AP of the brain and is structurally similar to the cardiovascular chemoreceptors. The AP may also contain neural pathways independent of the CTZ, therefore, ablation studies of the AP are difficult to interpret. Distinguishing between chemosensitive and neurotransmitter receptors of the CTZ is difficult, but 5-HT_3 vagal presynaptic receptors may comprise one of the neurotransmitter receptors of the CTZ mediating vomiting.

References

1 Wang SC, Borison HL: Copper sulphate emesis: A study of afferent pathways from the gastrointestinal tract. Am J Physiol 1951;164:520–526.
2 Borison HL, Brizzee KR: Morphology of emetic chemoreceptor trigger zone in cat medulla. Proc Soc Exp Biol Med 1951;77:38–42.
3 Borison HL: Site of emetic action of X-radiation in the cat. J Comp Neurol 1957;107:439–453.
4 McCarthy LE, Borison HL: Cisplatin-induced vomiting eliminated by ablation of the area postrema in cats. Cancer Treat Rep 1984;68:401–404.
5 McCarthy LE, Borison HL: Respiratory mechanics of vomiting in decerebrate cats. Am J Physiol 1974;26:738–743.
6 Lang IM: Digestive tract motor correlates of vomiting and nausea. Can J Physiol Pharmacol 1990; 68:242–253.
7 Lang IM, Dana N, Medda BK, Shaker R: Mechanisms of airway protection during retching, vomiting and swallowing. Am J Physiol 2002;283:G529–G536.
8 Monges H, Salducci J, Nandy B: Dissociation between the electrical activity of the diaphragmatic dome and crural muscular fibers during esophageal distension, vomiting and eructation. An electromyographic study in the dog. J Physiol 1978;74:541–554.
9 Lang IM, Dodds WJ, Sarna SK: The pharyngeal, esophageal and gastric responses associated with vomiting. Am J Physiol 1993;265:G963–G972.
10 Helm JF, Dodds WJ, Hogan WJ: Salivary response to esophageal acid in normal subjects and patients with reflux esophagitis. Gastroenterology 1987;93:1393–1397.
11 Pope CE: Pathophysiology and diagnosis of reflux esophagitis. Gastroenterology 1976;70:445–454.
12 Lang IM, Sarna SK, Condon RE: Gastrointestinal motor correlates of vomiting in the dog: Quantification and identification as an independent phenomenon. Gastroenterology 1986;90: 40–47.
13 Code CF, Steinbach JH, Schlegel JF, Amberg JR, Hollenbeck GA: Pyloric and duodenal motor contribution to duodenogastric reflux. Scand J Gastroenterol Suppl 1984;92:13–16.
14 Ehrlein HJ: Retroperistaltism and duodenogastric reflux in dogs. Scand J Gastroenterol Suppl 1981;67:29–32.
15 Lang IM, Sarna SK, Shaker R. Gastrointestinal motor and myoelectrical correlates of motion sickness. Am J Physiol 1999;277:G642–G652.
16 Lang IM, Tansy MF: Mechanisms of the secretory and motor responses of the Brunner's gland region of the intestine to duodenal acidification. Pflügers Arch 1983;396:15–120.
17 Lunsden K, Holden WS: The act of vomiting in man. Gut 1969;10:173–179.
18 Hesse O: Zur Kenntnis des Brechaktes. Nach Röntgenversuchen an Hunden. Pflügers Arch Ges Physiol 1913;152:1–22.
19 Smith CC, Brizzee KR: Cineradiographic analysis of vomiting in the cat. I. Lower esophagus, stomach and small intestine. Gastroenterology 1961;40:654–664.
20 Andrews PLR, Torii Y, Saito H, Matsuki N: The pharmacology of the emetic response to upper gastrointestinal tract stimulation in *Suncus murinus*. Eur J Pharmacol 1996;307:305–313.

21 Andrews PLR, Wood KL: Vagally mediated gastric motor and emetic reflexes evoked by stimulation of the antral mucosa in anesthetized ferrets. J Physiol 1988;395:1–16.
22 Lang IM: Noxious stimulation of emesis. Dig Dis Sci 1999;44:58S–63S.
23 Grundy D, Scratcherd T: Sensory afferents form the gastrointestinal ract; in Wood JD (ed): The Gastrointestinal System. Section 6: Alimentary Canal. Bethesda, American Physiological Society, 1989, vol 1, pp 593–620.
24 Rodrigo J, Hernandez CJ, Vidal MA, Pedrosa JA: Vegetative innervation of the esophagus. III. Intraepithelial endings. Acta Anat Basel 1975;92:242–258.
25 Rodrigo J, Hernandez CJ, Vidal MA, Pedrosa JA: Vegetative innervation of the esophagus. II. Intraganglionic laminar endings. Acta Anat Basel 1975;92:79–100.
26 Zagorodnyuk VP, Chen BN, Brookes SJ: Intraganglionic laminar endings are mechano-transduction sites of vagal tension receptors in the guinea pig stomach. J Physiol 2001;534:255–268.
27 Sharma RN, Dubey PC, Dixit KS, Bhargava KP: Neural pathways of emesis associated with experimental intestinal obstruction in digs. Indian J Med Res 1972;60:291–295.
28 Walton FE, Moore RM, Graham EA: The nerve pathways in vomiting of peritonitis. Arch Surg 1931;22:829–837.
29 Sugiyama H, Hayama T, Yagasaki O: Emetic action of bacterial endotoxin in the cat. Proc Soc Exp Biol Med 1966;121:278–281.
30 Kayashima N, Tarraka M, Iwasaki M, Hayama T: Site of emetic action of oral copper sulfate in dogs. I. Threshold of various portions of gastrointestinal tract to locally applied copper sulfate. Jpn J Pharmacol 1978;98:775–781.
31 Bhandari P, Andrews PLR: Preliminary evidence for the involvement of the putative 5-HT_4 receptors in zacopride- and copper sulphate-induced vomiting in the ferret. Eur J Pharmacol 1991;204: 273–280.
32 Fukui H, Yamamoto M, Sasaki S, Sato S: Possible involvement of peripheral 5-HT_4 receptors in copper sulfate-induced vomiting in dogs. Eur J Pharmacol 1994;257:47–52.
33 Lang IM, Marvig J: Functional localization of specific receptors mediating the GI motor correlates of vomiting. Am J Physiol 1989;256:G92–G99.
34 Hatcher RA: The mechanisms of vomiting. Physiol Rev 1924;4:479–504.
35 Wolf S: Studies on nausea. Effect of ipecac and other emetics on the human stomach and duodenum. Gastroenterology 1949;12:212–218.
36 Andrews PLR: Vagal afferent innervation of the gastrointestinal tract; in Morison JFB (ed): Progress in Brain Research. Amsterdam, Elsevier, 1986, vol 67, pp 65–86.
37 Lundberg J, Dahlstrom A, Bylock A, Ahlman H, Peterson G, Larsson I, Hansson HA, Kewenter J: Ultrastructural evidence for an innervation of epithelial enteroendocrine cells in the guinea pig duodenum. Acta Physiol Scand 1978;104:3–12.
38 Ahlman H, Bhargava HN, Donahue PE, Newson B, Das Gupta TH, Nyhus LM: The vagal release of 5-hydroxytryptamine from enterochromaffin cells in the cat. Acta Physiol Scand 1978;104:262–270.
39 Solcia E, Capella C, Buffa R, Uselini L, Fiocca R, Sessa F: Endocrine cells of the digestive system; in Johnson LR (ed): Physiology of the Gastrointestinal Tract. New York, Raven Press, 1981, vol 1, pp 39–58.
40 Endo T, Minami M, Hirafuji M, Ogawa T, Akita K, Nemoto M, Saito H, Yoshioka M, Parvez SH: Neurochemistry and neuropharmacology of emesis – Role of serotonin. Toxicology 2000;153: 189–201.
41 Gale JD: Serotonergic mediation of vomiting. J Pediatr Gastroenterol Nutr 1995;21(suppl 1): 22–28.
42 Fukui H, Yamamoto M, Ando T, Sasaki S, Sato S: Increase in serotonin levels in the dog ileum and blood by cisplatin as measured by microdialysis. Neuropharmacology 1993;32:959–968.
43 Hawthorn J, Ostler KJ, Andrews PLR: The role of the abdominal visceral innervation and 5-hydroxytryptamine M-receptors in vomiting induced by the cytotoxic drugs cyclophosphamide and cisplatin in the ferret. J Exp Physiol 1988;73:7–21.
44 Fukui H, Yamamoto M, Sato S: Vagal afferent fibers and peripheral 5-HT_3 receptors mediate cisplatin-induced emesis in dogs. Jpn J Pharmacol 1992;59:221–226.
45 Borison HL, McCarthy LE, Johnson JR: High dorsal column cordotomy plus subdiaphragmatic vagotomy prevents acute ionizing radiation sickness in cats. Exp Neurol 1987;98:645–658.

46 Wang SC, Renzi AA, Chinn HI: Mechanisms of emesis following X-irradiation. Am J Physiol 1958;193:335–339.
47 Fukui H, Yamamoto M, Sasaki S, Sato S: Involvement of 5-HT_3 receptors and vagal afferents in copper sulfate- and cisplatin-induced emesis in monkeys. Eur J Physiol 1993;249:13–18.
48 Ito J, Okada M, Abo T, Okamoto Y, Yamashito T, Takahashi K: Experimental study on the control of cisplatin-induced emesis in dogs. Jap J Cancer Chemother 1987;14:706–710.
49 Chapman WP, Wilkins EW, Von Heuber F: Electrical stimulation of the central end of the vagus nerve in the anesthetized dog. Surg Gynecol Obstet 1954;98:579–595.
50 Zabara J, Chaffee RB, Tansy MF: Neuroinhibition in the regulation of emesis. Space Life Sci 1972;3:282–292.
51 Glatzle J, Sternini C, Robin C, Zittel TT, Wong H, Reeve JR, Raybould HE: Expression of 5-HT_3 receptors in the rat gastrointestinal tract. Gastroenterology 2002;123:217–226.
52 Milano S, Grelot L, Chen Z, Bianchi AL: Vagal-induced vomiting in decerebrate cat is not suppressed by specific 5-HT_3 receptor antagonists. J Autonom Nerv Syst 1990;31:109–118.
53 Miller AD, Nonaka S: Mechanisms of vomiting induced by serotonin-3 receptor agonists in the cat: Effect of vagotomy, splanchnectomy or area postrema lesion. J Pharmacol Exp Ther 1992; 260:509–517.
54 Torii Y, Saito H, Matsuki N: 5-Hydroxytryptamine is emetogenic in the mouse shrew, *Suncus murinus*. Naunyn Schmiedebergs Arch Pharmacol 1991;344:564–567.
55 Miller AD, Leslie RA: The area postrema and vomiting. Front Neuroendocrinol 1994;15:301–320.
56 Borison HL: Area postrema: Chemoreceptor circumventricular organ of the medulla oblongata. Prog Neurbiol 1989;32:351–390.
57 Borison HL, Hawken MJ, Hubbard JI, Sirett NE: Unit activity from area postrema influenced by drugs. Brain Res 1975;92:153–156.
58 Carpenter DO, Briggs DB, Knox AP, Strominger N: Excitation of area postrema neurons by transmitters, peptides and cyclic nucleotides. J Neurophysiol 1988;59:358–369.
59 Leslie RA, Reynolds DJM, Andrews PLR, Graham-Smith DG, Davis CJ, Harvey JM: Evidence for presynaptic 5-hydroxytryptamine-3 recognition sites in vagal afferent terminals in the brainstem of the ferret. Neuroscience 1990;38:667–673.
60 Higgins GA, Kilpatrick GJ, Bunce KT, Jones BJ, Tyers MB: 5-HT_3 receptor antagonists injected into the area postrema inhibit cispaltin-induced emesis in the ferret. Br J Pharmacol 1989;97: 247–255.
61 Borison HL, McCarthy LE, Douple EB, Johnson J, Borison R: Acute radiation-induced vomiting in area postrema-ablated cats. Radiat Res 1987;109:430–439.
62 Brizzee KR: The effect of localized brain lesions and supradiaphragmatic vagotomy on X-irradiation emesis in the monkey. Am J Physiol 1956;187:567–570.
63 Harding RK, Hugenholtz H, Keany M, Kucharczyk J: Discrete lesions of the area postrema abolish radiation-induced emesis in the dog. Neurosci Lett 1985;53:95–100.

Dr. Ivan M. Lang
Dysphagia Research Laboratory, Medical College of Wisconsin
Milwaukee, WI 53226 (USA)
Tel. +1 414 4568138, Fax +1 414 4566215, E-Mail imlang@mcw.edu

Donnerer J (ed): Antiemetic Therapy.
Basel, Karger, 2003, pp 22–32

5-HT$_3$ Receptor Antagonists in Antiemetic Therapy

J. Donnerer, E. Beubler

Institute of Experimental and Clinical Pharmacology, University of Graz, Austria

Serotonin (5-hydroxytryptamine, 5-HT) exerts its physiological effects on a wide variety of receptor subtypes in the central and peripheral nervous system, gastrointestinal tract, and other sites. The 5-HT$_3$ receptor as one subtype belongs to the family of receptors directly coupled to membrane cation channels, whereas all the other 5-HT receptor subtypes are G-protein-coupled receptors. The 5-HT$_3$ receptor is located primarily pre- and postsynaptically on neurons and its prime function is modulation of neuron excitability and neurotransmitter release.

5-HT$_3$ receptor activation on central and peripheral autonomic sensory and enteric neurons has shown that it mediates a rapid depolarizing response, associated with an increase in membrane conductance consequent on the opening of cation-selective channels [1]. Single cell studies employing intracellular recording of 5-HT$_3$ receptor-mediated depolarization in several preparations have indicated that an inflow of sodium and potassium ions contributes to the response [2]. The channels are also permeable to divalent cations such as Ca^{2+} and Mg^{2+}. Whereas the endogenous compound 5-HT itself excites all different subtypes of 5-HT receptors, 2-methyl-5-HT and the amidine derivatives 1-phenylbiguanide and metachlorophenylbiguanide have relatively selective affinity for the 5-HT$_3$ receptor [3].

5-HT$_3$ Receptor Localization

5-HT$_3$ receptors are present especially in high density in the lower brainstem, i.e. the dorsal vagal complex, nucleus of the solitary tract, spinal trigeminal nucleus and around the area postrema, extending to the dorsal horn of the spinal cord [4]. Several other brain areas like the cerebral cortex and limbic regions have a lower density of 5-HT_3 receptors. In the peripheral nervous system 5-HT_3 receptors occur on nociceptive sensory neurons, on autonomic and enteric neurons, on which 5-HT exerts a strong excitatory effect [3, 5]. It remains an interesting observation that no 5-HT_3 receptor mRNA was detected in the area postrema/nucleus tractus solitarius, the area of highest 5-HT_3 receptor density. This suggests a presynaptic location of 5-HT_3 receptors on peripheral, i.e. vagal afferent modulating transmitter release from these neurons [5, 6]. With regard to the emetic reflex, 5-HT receptors are located pre- and postsynaptically at peripheral and central terminals of vagal and other visceral afferents, in the emetic reflex center, the chemoreceptor trigger zone in the area postrema as well as on efferent pathways [7]. They are mainly involved in inducing nausea and emesis by chemotherapeutic agents, X-irradiation, chemical or mechanical gastrointestinal irritation.

In addition to the vagal afferent 5-HT_3 receptors, the presence of 5-HT autoreceptors on chromaffin cells has been demonstrated. The enterochromaffin cell 5-HT_3 receptor is a low affinity site that responds to high levels of 5-HT, such as those which occur following highly emetogenic antineoplastic therapy. This then results in increasing surges of 5-HT, in what amounts to a positive feedback loop that further contributes to the pathophysiology of emesis [8, 9].

Specific 5-HT_3 Receptor Antagonists

From a historical view the use of 5-HT_3 receptor antagonists as antiemetics is due largely to the use of metoclopramide. There was evidence that the efficacy of high-dose metoclopramide might be due to an additional action beside the well-known D_2 receptor blocking action, and it was revealed that the compound has also antagonistic properties at the 5-HT_3 receptor. The new developed selective 5-HT_3 antagonists displayed a much higher affinity for 5-HT_3 receptors (pA_2 values between 9.8 and 10.7) and a great selectivity [2]. The affinity for other 5-HT receptors, as well as for other transmitter receptors, is at least several hundred times less or even lacking. Within the 5-HT system, granisetron and ondansetron display weak agonistic activity at the 5-HT_4 receptor, whereas tropisetron is a weak antagonist; these effects most probably play no significant role in their antiemetic activity.

Whereas the depolarizing effect of 5-HT_3 receptor stimulation induces neuronal firing and enhances neurotransmitter release, the 5-HT_3 antagonists can attenuate neuronal excitation and moderate transmitter release. These activities may relate to their attenuation of emetic responses [5]. The clinically used

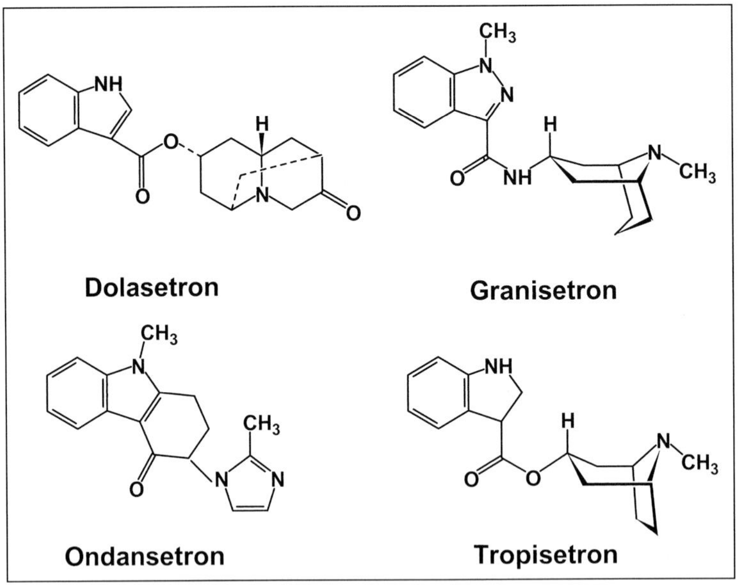

Fig. 1. Clinically used 5-HT_3 antagonists. Structures derived from indole (tropisetron, dolasetron), carbazole (ondansetron) and indazole (granisetron).

specific 5-HT_3 antagonists include ondansetron, granisetron, tropisetron, and dolasetron.

The structures are derived from indole (tropisetron, dolasetron), carbazole (ondansetron), and indazole (granisetron) rings (fig. 1). From the use of several in vitro models it became clear that, with the possible exception of ondansetron, 5-HT_3 antagonists may attenuate the effects of 5-HT through competitive and non-competitive mechanisms. Whereas the receptor blockade induced by tropisetron, granisetron and dolasetron cannot be reversed even at high 5-HT concentrations, the effect of ondansetron can be abolished by high 5-HT concentrations [9]. Due to the fact of a partly insurmountable non-competitive antagonism and possibly due to high receptor affinity by these compounds their activity in vivo lasts much longer than their plasma concentration would indicate (see also table 5).

Site of the Antiemetic Action of 5-HT_3 Receptor Antagonists

5-HT hypothesis in chemotherapy- and radiotherapy-induced emesis: Whereas there is an agreement that 5-HT plays an important role in nausea and vomiting induced by chemotherapeutic agents, the site of involvement is still unresolved. Most of the 5-HT in humans (and mammals in general) is present in the gastrointestinal tract within the enterochromaffin cells. 5-HT secretion from enterochromaffin cells is controlled by a complex pattern of receptor-mediated mechanisms [10]. Upon administration of highly emetogenic agents like cisplatin there is possibly a release of gastrointestinal 5-HT from the enterochromaffin cells by exocytosis. This has been documented by biochemical and histological changes in the intestine and by increases in the mucosa levels of 5-HT and its metabolite 5-hydroxyindolacetic acid (5-HIAA). The 5-HT metabolite can also be found elevated in plasma and there is an increased urinary excretion of 5-HIAA detected after high dose cisplatin [11].

The increased turnover of gastrointestinal 5-HT would then activate 5-HT_3 receptors on visceral afferent fibers, increasing the afferent input to the brain and stimulating the CTZ and the vomiting center. It was discussed as unlikely that the 5-HT released from the gut mucosa into the systemic circulation being involved in the direct activation of the area postrema, because most of the 5-HT is taken up in platelets or is metabolized during the passage through the liver. In addition, intravenous 5-HT fails to induce emesis. Possibly the release of 5-HT by chemotherapeutic agents has certain specific dynamics, because a 'regular' release during the carcinoid syndrome does not induce emesis. It is also likely that the peripheral 5-HT release evoked by chemotherapeutic agents is accompanied by a local neuronal release of 5-HT in the region of the area postrema. This synergistic action triggers the emetic reflex [12, 13].

Irrespective of the exact mode of action, clearly chemotherapeutic drugs and/or irradiation activate central and vagal afferent nerve fibers, increasing the input to the CTZ and the vomiting center, and 5-HT_3 receptors stimulation is responsible for this. Blockade of central and peripheral 5-HT_3 receptors suppresses nausea and emesis [14]. It has also become clear that the selective 5-HT_3 antagonists are much more effective against certain types of emesis than against others. They are far superior against vomiting associated with chemotherapy and radiation therapy, whereas they are not effective against motion sickness, or against delayed emesis [15, 16].

In general, there is still conflicting evidence whether peripheral or central sites of action, or both, are implicated in the 5-HT_3 antagonists antiemetic action. Animal studies employing direct injection of 5-HT_3 antagonists into the area postrema or fourth ventricle showed inhibition of cisplatin-induced emesis. Based on the above presented 5-HT hypothesis, an activation or sensitization of abdominal vagal afferents known to terminate in close proximity to enterochromaffin cells plays an important role in chemotherapy-induced emesis. In addition to the 5-HT_3 receptor, other 5-HT receptors could also be involved. The 5-HT_3 antagonists would block the peripheral activation of vagal afferents.

There is a consensus that the 5-HT_3 antagonists block the emetic reflex arc on different specific locations [14, 17]: (1) by blocking the 5-HT autoreceptors on the enterochromaffin cells they prevent excessive release of 5-HT; (2) by presynaptic vagal 5-HT_3 receptor blockade they prevent the initiation of an afferent emetic signal; (3) they prevent the transmission and integration of emetic signals within the central relay nuclei of the vagus nerve and the vomiting reflex center, and (4) they block the 5-HT_3 receptors in the chemoreceptor trigger zone.

These various sites of antiemetic actions of 5-HT_3 antagonists have been elucidated by selective local central application of the drugs, by vagotomy, and by the use of compounds with an inability to cross the blood-brain barrier. The concept from the available data would include a peripheral and a central site of antiemetic action of these compounds. The multifactorial nature of the chemotherapy-induced emesis necessitates in severe cases a combination antiemetic therapy (see also following chapters).

Clinical Utility of 5-HT_3 Antagonists

Ondansetron and the other related compounds are used as antiemetic drugs particularly for controlling the severe nausea and vomiting that occurs with many forms of cancer chemotherapy within the first 24 h following treatment [18–21]. A line of clinical investigations has demonstrated that 5-HT_3 antagonists are superior to metoclopramide in the treatment of acute emesis in response to severely emetogenic cancer chemotherapy [5, 14, 22]. They represent the most efficacious drugs for the prevention of acute emesis induced by highly emetogenic chemotherapy and by moderately emetogenic chemotherapy (tables 1–4). In a series of open trials and double-blind clinical studies, response rates in highly emetogenic chemotherapy have been determined to be in the range of 45–60%, in moderately emetogenic chemotherapy in the range of 65–80% [23, 24]. Response rates vary with the number of risk factors for developing chemotherapy-induced nausea and vomiting, and with the emetogenic potential of the chemotherapeutic agents. Usually, response rates can be improved by the addition of dexamethasone to the antiemetic treatment [25]. In the same way, acute nausea and retches are responsive to prophylaxis with 5-HT_3 antagonists. Their use is already standard preventive care in cancer chemotherapy, in many instances in combination with highly potent glucocorticoids such as dexamethasone. Anticipatory and delayed emesis occurring 1 or more days after cancer chemotherapy is less effectively relieved by this class of drugs.

5-HT_3 antagonists have not only a documented utility in preventing cancer chemotherapy-induced emesis, they also display efficacy in radiation

Table 1. Ondansetron

Indications	Recommended dosage (adults)	Recommended dosage (children)
Highly emetogenic chemotherapy[1]	3 × 8 mg i.v. or 3 × 0.15 mg/kg i.v.; first dose of 8 mg given before chemotherapy; max. daily dose 32 mg; treatment for 2–5 days	4–18 years: 5 mg/m² or 0.15 mg/kg i.v., repeated after 4 and 8 h, or 2 × 4 mg p.o. for up to 5 days
Moderately emetogenic chemotherapy[1]	2–3 × 8 mg i.v. first day; or 8 mg i.v. followed by 8 mg p.o. every 8 h; treatment for up to 2–5 days	4–11 years: 3 × 4 mg/day p.o. 12 years up: 2 × 8 mg/day p.o.
Radiation-induced nausea and emesis	2 × 8 mg p.o./day; first dose 1–2 h before radiation; treatment for up to 3–5 days	4–11 years: 3 × 4 mg/day p.o. 12 years up: 2 × 8 mg/day p.o.
Prevention of PONV	4–8 mg i.v. before anesthesia or 16 mg p.o. before anesthesia	2–12 years: 0.1 mg/kg i.v./i.m., max. dose 4 mg 12 years up: 4 mg i.v.
Existing PONV	4 mg i.v./i.m.	0.1 mg/kg i.v./i.m., max. dose 4 mg

Patients with significant disturbance of liver function: maximum daily dose of 8 mg; impaired renal function: no dose adjustment necessary.

Note: All intravenous applications are given as short infusions (15 min) or as injections lasting more than 30 s; alternatively, continuous infusions with the indicated doses can be given.

[1]Response rate can be improved by the combination with dexamethasone, 10–20 mg i.v. prior to chemotherapy.

therapy-induced nausea and postoperative nausea. Specifically, ondansetron has shown good efficacy in the prevention of acute nausea and vomiting in children receiving moderately or highly emetogenic chemotherapy and/or irradiation, particularly when combined with dexamethasone. It is also an effective first-line antiemetic in children undergoing surgery [18].

Pharmacokinetic Data and Possible Side Effects

The basic pharmacokinetic data of the available compounds are given in table 5. The properties of all four compounds are very similar, clinically

Table 2. Granisetron

Indications	Recommended dosage (adults)	Recommended dosage (children)
Highly emetogenic chemotherapy[1]	1–3 × 3 mg i.v. first dose given before chemotherapy; max. 9 mg/day (1 × 10 μg/kg i.v.: USA)	1 × 40 μg/kg i.v.; max. 3 mg; one additional oral dose of 40 μg/kg within 24 h
Moderately emetogenic chemotherapy[1]	1–3 × 3 mg i.v. or 1 × 2 or 2 × 1 mg/day p.o. treatment up to 5 days (1 × 10 μg/kg i.v.: USA)	1 × 40 μg/kg i.v.; max. 3 mg; one additional oral dose of 40 μg/kg within 24 h
Radiation-induced nausea and emesis	1 × 2 or 2 × 1 mg/day p.o. treatment up to 5 days	–
Prevention of PONV	1 × 1–3 mg i.v.	–
Existing PONV	1–3 mg i.v.	–

Impaired liver or renal function: no dose adjustment necessary.

Note: All intravenous applications are given as short infusions (15 min) or as injections lasting more than 30 s; alternatively, continuous infusions with the indicated doses can be given.

[1]Response rate can be improved by the combination with dexamethasone, 10–20 mg i.v. prior to chemotherapy.

Table 3. Tropisetron

Indications	Recommended dosage (adults)	Recommended dosage (children)
Highly emetogenic chemotherapy[1]	Day 1: 1 × 5 mg i.v. Days 2–5: 1 × 5 mg p.o.	Day 1: 0.2 mg/kg i.v., max. 5 mg Days 2–5: 0.2 mg/kg p.o.
Moderately emetogenic chemotherapy[1]	Day 1: 1 × 5 mg i.v. Days 2–5: 1 × 5 mg p.o.	Day 1: 0.2 mg/kg i.v., max. 5 mg Days 2–5: 0.2 mg/kg p.o.
Radiation-induced nausea and emesis	Day 1: 1 × 5 mg i.v. Days 2–5: 1 × 5 mg p.o.	–
Prevention of PONV	2 mg i.v.	–
Existing PONV	2 mg i.v.	–

Impaired liver or renal function: no dose adjustment necessary.

Note: All intravenous applications are given as short infusions (15 min) or as injections lasting more than 30 s; alternatively, continuous infusions with the indicated doses can be given.

[1]Response rate can be improved by the combination with dexamethasone, 10–20 mg i.v. prior to chemotherapy.

Table 4. Dolasetron

Indications	Recommended dosage (adults)	Recommended dosage (children)
Highly emetogenic chemotherapy[1]	1 × 1.8–2.4 mg/kg i.v. or 1 × 100 mg i.v.; treatment for up to 4 days	2–16 years: 1 × 1.8 mg/kg i.v. or p.o., max. 100 mg
Moderately emetogenic chemotherapy[1]	1 × 1.8–2.4 mg/kg i.v. or 1 × 100 mg i.v. or 1 × 200 mg p.o.; treatment for up to 4 days	2–16 years: 1 × 1.8 mg/kg i.v. or p.o., max. 100 mg
Radiation-induced nausea and emesis	–	–
Prevention of PONV	12.5 mg i.v. or 50 mg p.o.	–
Existing PONV	12.5 mg i.v.	–

Impaired liver or renal function: no dose adjustment necessary.

Note: All intravenous applications are given as short infusions (15 min) or as injections lasting more than 30 s; alternatively, continuous infusions with the indicated doses can be given.

[1]Response rate can be improved by the combination with dexamethasone, 10–20 mg i.v. prior to chemotherapy.

Table 5. Pharmacokinetic data of clinically used $5\text{-}HT_3$ receptor antagonists

Compound	Oral bioavailability %	Plasma half-life, h	Duration of action, h
Ondansetron	60	3–5	12 (24)
Granisetron	60	5–9	24
Tropisetron	60–100	7–9	24
Dolasetron	70–90	5–9 (active metabolite hydrodolasetron)	24

relevant differences exist mainly between the half-lives [9]. Dolasetron also has a particular characteristic insofar as it is a prodrug that has to be converted in vivo to its active metabolite hydrodolasetron before exerting its effects.

Early clinical studies of dosage regimens took into consideration these differences in half-life; thus, ondansetron was initially administered 3 times daily compared with once daily for the other $5\text{-}HT_3$ antagonists. It has now been demonstrated that ondansetron, as well as the other compounds, can be effectively administered once daily and that antiemetic efficacy persists long after one or two plasma half-lives. This indicates that interactions at the receptor level, not plasma pharmacokinetics, are the most important criteria for defining efficacy.

The compounds are readily absorbed after oral administration; the blood-brain barrier is easily crossed. After intravenous injection the antiemetic effect is observed within a few minutes. The drugs are almost completely metabolized in the liver by different subtypes of the cytochrome P_{450} (CYP) enzyme system and the metabolites are excreted by the renal or biliary route. Ondansetron and granisetron are metabolized by CYP3A, tropisetron and dolasetron by CYP2D6. Although due to genetic variability in a low percentage of the population the elimination rates of tropisetron and dolasetron are slowed, a dose adjustment is not necessary in these patients. Usually at standard doses there is no need for dosage adjustment in impaired renal function. For ondansetron, in patients with significant disturbances of liver functions, a maximum daily dose of 8 mg is recommended.

Since the compounds exhibit only moderately plasma protein binding, no interactions due to displacement from the binding site are to be expected. There are also no relevant interactions to be expected by cytochrome P_{450} enzyme inducers or inhibitors.

Their great advantage is the lack of unwanted sedative, extrapyramidal or cardiovascular side effects as seen with other antiemetics, notably with dopamine D_2 receptor antagonists or histamine H_1 receptor antagonists [8, 14]. 5-HT_3 receptor antagonists fail to cause any overt changes in the behavior of animals and humans. The administration of millions of doses of ondansetron and the other antagonists has been without behavioral effect in the cancer patient or postoperatively. Recently it has however been proposed that they might have an anxiolytic profile of action which is a matter of investigation per se.

Headache is a rather frequent confirmed side effect, and lightheadedness or dizziness may occur. Since 5-HT_3 receptor activity might control intestinal propulsive peristalsis and fluid secretion [26–28], ondansetron and the other antagonists in high dosage can slow down intestinal transit and lead to constipation; rarely abdominal pain or cramping is observed. Discrete, clinically insignificant changes in cardiac conduction have been reported. Elevations of hepatic transaminases are mostly due to the chemotherapy and not due to the 5-HT_3 antagonists.

Conclusion

5-HT_3 receptor antagonists are highly effective and well-tolerated agents. All drugs can be administered as a single dose or in a short-term dosage regimen. The review of publications, which have compared the efficacy of the available compounds, has yielded no important differences in clinical outcomes [29].

References

1 Derkach V, Surprenant A, North RA: 5-HT_3 receptors are membrane ion channels. Nature 1989; 339:706–709.
2 Jackson MB, Yakel JL: The 5-HT_3 receptor channel. Annu Rev Physiol 1995;57:447–468.
3 Hoyer D, Clarke DE, Fozard JR, Hartig PR, Martin GR, Mylecharane EJ, Saxena PR, Humphrey PPA: VIIth International Union of Pharmacology classification of receptors for 5-hydroxytryptamine (serotonin). Pharmacol Rev 1994;46:157–203.
4 Costall B, Naylor RJ: Neuropharmacology of 5-HT_3 receptor ligands; in Baumgarten HG, Göthert M (eds): Handb Exp Pharm. Berlin, Springer, 1997, vol 129, pp 409–438.
5 Kilpatrick GJ, Bunce KT, Tyers MB: 5-HT_3 receptors. Med Res Rev 1990;10:441–475.
6 Boess FG, Martin IL: Molecular biology of 5-HT receptors. Neuropharmacology 1994;33: 275–317.
7 Hasler WL: Serotonin receptor physiology. Relation to emesis. Dig Dis Sci 1999;44(suppl): 108–113.
8 Perez EA: A risk-benefit assessment of serotonin 5-HT_3 receptor antagonists in antineoplastic therapy-induced emesis. Drug Saf 1998;18:43–56.
9 Wolf H: Preclinical and clinical pharmacology of the 5-HT_3 receptor antagonists. Scand J Rheumatol 2000;29(suppl 113):37–45.
10 Racké K, Reimann A, Schwörer H, Kilbinger H: Regulation of 5-HT release from enterochromaffin cells. Behav Brain Res 1996;73:83–87.
11 Barnes NM, Ge J, Jones WG, Naylor RJ, Rudd JA: Cisplatin-induced emesis: Preliminary results indicative of changes in plasma levels of 5-hydroxytryptamine. Br J Cancer 1990;62:862–864.
12 Waldvogel HH, Aapro MS, Beubler E, Schneck H, Widmer W, Wilder-Smith C, Wilder-Smith OHG: Antiemetische Therapie – Nausea und Emesis. Stuttgart, Thieme, 1995.
13 Veyrat-Follet C, Farinotti R, Palmer JL: Physiology of chemotherapy-induced emesis and antiemetic therapy. Predictive models for evaluation of new compounds. Drugs 1997;53:206–234.
14 Hesketh PJ, Gandara DR: Serotonin antagonists: A new class of antiemetic agents. J Natl Cancer Inst 1991;83:613–620.
15 Gregory RE, Ettinger DS: 5-HT_3 receptor antagonists for the prevention of chemotherapy-induced nausea and vomiting. Drugs 1998;55:173–189.
16 Kovac AL: Prevention and treatment of postoperative nausea and vomiting. Drugs 2000;59: 213–243.
17 Freeman AJ, Cunningham KT, Tyers MB: Selectivity of 5-HT_3 receptor antagonists and anti-emetic mechanisms of action. Anticancer Drugs 1992;3:79–85.
18 Culy CR, Bhana N, Plosker GL: Ondansetron: A review of its use as an antiemetic in children. Paediatr Drugs 2001;3:441–478.
19 Balfour JA, Goa KL: Dolasetron. A review of its pharmacology and therapeutic potential in the management of nausea and vomiting induced by chemotherapy, radiotherapy or surgery. Drugs 1997;54:273–298.
20 Hesketh PJ: Comparative review of 5-HT_3 receptor antagonists in the treatment of acute chemotherapy-induced nausea and vomiting. Cancer Invest 2000;18:163–173.
21 Simpson K, Spencer CM, McClellan KJ: Tropisetron. An update of its use in the prevention of chemotherapy-induced nausea and vomiting. Drugs 2000;59:1297–1315.
22 Marty M, Pouillart P, Scholl S, Droz JP, Azab M, Brion N, Pujade-Lauraine E, Paule B, Paes D, Bons J: Comparison of the 5-hydroxytryptamine-3 (serotonin) antagonist ondansetron (GR 38032F) with high-dose metoclopramide in the control of cisplatin-induced emesis. N Engl J Med 1990;322:816–821.

23 Roila F, Ballatori E, Tonato M, Del Favero A: 5-HT_3 receptor antagonists: Differences and similarities. Eur J Cancer 1997;33:1364–1370.
24 Walton SM: Advances in use of the 5-HT_3 receptor antagonists. Exp Opin Pharmacother 2000;1:207–223.
25 Roila F and The Italian Group for Antiemetic Research: Dexamethasone alone or in combination with ondansetron for the prevention of delayed nausea and vomiting induced by chemotherapy. N Engl J Med 2000;342:1554–1559.
26 Beubler E, Horina G: 5-HT_2 and 5-HT_3 receptor subtypes mediate cholera toxin-induced intestinal fluid secretion in the rat. Gastroenterology 1990;99:83–89.
27 Beubler E, Schirgi-Degen A, Gamse R: Inhibition of 5-hydroxytryptamine- and enterotoxin-induced fluid secretion by 5-HT receptor antagonists in the rat jejunum. Eur J Pharmacol 1993; 248:157–162.
28 Haga K, Asano K, Fukuda T, Kobayakawa T: The function of 5-HT_3 receptors on colonic transit in rats. Obes Res 1995;3(suppl 5):801–810.
29 Morrow GR, Hickok JT, Rosenthal SN: Progress in reducing nausea and emesis. Comparisons of ondansetron (Zofran), granisetron (Kytril) and tropisetron (Navoban). Cancer 1995;76:343–357.

Prof. Dr. Josef Donnerer
Institut für Experimentelle und Klinische Pharmakologie
Karl-Franzens-Universität Graz, Universitätsplatz 4, A–8010 Graz (Austria)
Tel. +43 316 3804509, Fax +43 316 3809645, E-Mail josef.donnerer@uni-graz.at

Donnerer J (ed): Antiemetic Therapy.
Basel, Karger, 2003, pp 33–77

The Site of the Antiemetic Action of NK_1 Receptor Antagonists

Hiroyuki Fukuda[a,b], *Tomoshige Koga*[c], *Naohiro Furukawa*[a], *Emi Nakamura*[a], *Mizue Hatano*[a], *Mamoru Yanagihara*[d]

[a]Department of Physiology, Kawasaki Medical School; [b]Department of Clinical Nutrition, Kawasaki University of Medical Welfare; [c]Department of Restorative Science, Kawasaki University of Medical Welfare; [d]Junior College, Okayama Prefectural University, Kurashiki, Japan

Introduction

Tachykinin NK_1 receptor antagonists have been shown to suppress vomiting caused by various emetic stimuli, i.e., cisplatin [1–7], radiation [1–3, 5], copper sulfate [1–3, 7], ipecacuanha [1–3, 7], morphine [1–3], apomorphine [7, 8], loperamide [7] and motion [9, 10]. Tattersall et al. [6] compared the antiemetic effects of an NK_1 receptor antagonist, L-741,671, which can permeate into the brain, and its quaternary compound, L-743,310, which cannot, and demonstrated that the intravenous administration of L-741,671 produces dose-dependent inhibition of retching and vomiting induced by cisplatin, while L-743,310 is inactive, and that both drugs have equivalent activity when injected centrally. These results clearly indicate that NK_1 receptor antagonists act centrally and produce antiemetic activity. However, the precise site of the antiemetic effects had not been identified when we studied this subject in 1999. We found the site on the neuronal pathway (fig. 1) that was presumed to be involved in the induction of vomiting based on our electrophysiological results. Therefore, we first explain the neuronal pathway for convenience of explanation of the site of antiemetic action of NK_1 receptor antagonists.

The Neuronal Circuit for the Induction of Vomiting

Borison and Wang [11] first demonstrated that stimulation of the solitary tract and nucleus and the dorsolateral border of the lateral reticular formation

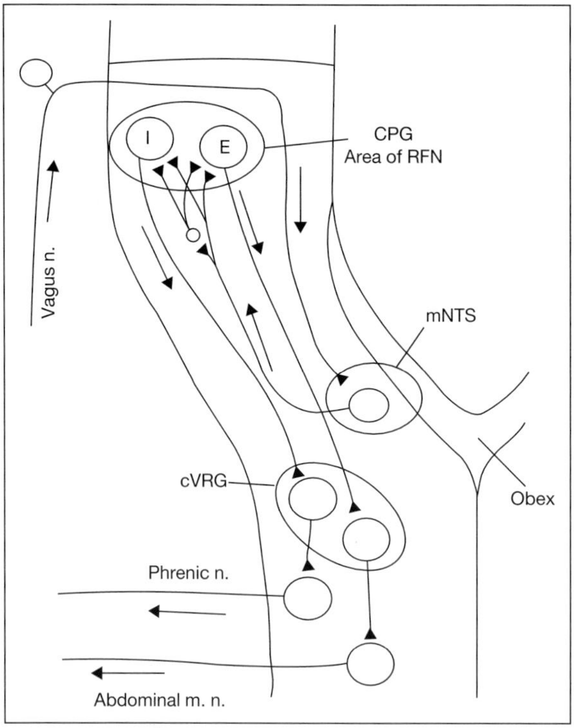

Fig. 1. The reflex arc for vomiting caused by the activity of abdominal vagal afferents. Schematic representation of the dorsal view of the canine medulla oblongata. CPG = The central pattern generator for vomiting motion; cVRG = inspiratory and expiratory premotoneurons in the caudal part of the ventral respiratory group area; E = CPG neurons that exhibit a firing pattern similar to the vomiting activity of the abdominal muscle nerve; I = CPG neurons that produce a firing pattern that resembles the vomiting activity of the phrenic nerve; mNTS = the medial solitary nucleus; m = muscle; n = nerve. These explanations and abbreviations also apply to the following figures.

(the area ventrolaterally adjacent to the solitary complex) induced vomiting in decerebrate cats. Subsequently, they attempted to make chronic lesions in the corresponding reticular area by implantation of glass and/or gold beads containing radioactive radon in 11 dogs, and demonstrated that retching and vomiting responses to apomorphine and copper sulfate were attenuated in 5 dogs and disappeared in 2 dogs [12, 13]. Based on these results, they postulated that the 'vomiting center' that coordinates other neural tissues to produce complicated emetic activities exists in the medullar area. Their concept of the vomiting center is still referred to in many recent textbooks. Miller and Wilson [14] elicited vomiting responses by stimulating the solitary tract and reticular formation in decerebrate cats. However, they could not identify the limited area in which stimulation produces reproducible vomiting responses, and concluded that neurons involved in the control of vomiting are diffusely distributed in the effective region described by Borison and Wang [11].

We were enticed by such confusion and started experiments to define the central neuronal circuit that produced vomiting. Before we determined the site of the antiemetic action of NK_1 receptor antagonists, we assumed that vomiting caused by afferent activities of abdominal vagal fibers is induced through the pathway shown schematically in figure 1. While each part of the scheme will be precisely explained below, a brief explanation may be useful for understanding the complicated experiments. Abdominal vagal afferents activate the second-order neurons in the medial solitary nucleus (mNTS). Outputs of mNTS neurons are mediated through their direct and/or indirect projections to the reticular area dorsomedial to the retrofacial nucleus (RFN) and activate non-respiratory reticular neurons comprising the central pattern generator (CPG) for vomiting motions. The CPG neurons generate temporal neuronal activity patterns of rhythmic retching and expulsive motions of the inspiratory and expiratory muscles. The vomiting activity patterns of the CPG neurons activate phrenic and abdominal muscle motoneurons via respiratory premotoneurons in the caudal medulla, and finally produce vomiting motions.

Stimulation Experiments to Elucidate Bulbar Areas Involved in the Induction of Vomiting

At first, we systematically stimulated the medulla oblongata in decerebrate paralyzed dogs [15]. Efferent discharges from the phrenic branch of the fifth cervical nerve and an abdominal muscle branch of the first lumbar nerve were simultaneously recorded in all dogs. Discharge patterns of both nerves in response to bulbar stimulation were compared with the characteristic patterns in fictive vomiting induced by stimulation of abdominal vagal afferents, and fictive retching and expulsion were recognized in accordance with the definitions proposed by Miller et al. [16] (see schematic representation in figure 2). To confirm this recognition, firing patterns were also observed in efferent discharges recorded from the phrenic branches to the hiatal and dorm parts of the diaphragm, the recurrent nerve branches to the adductors and abductor of the glottis, the vagal esophageal branch and the trigeminal branch to the digastrics in some dogs, as shown in figure 3.

Electrical stimulation at 175 of 2,092 points in the medulla oblongata of 23 dogs produced fictive retching responses, and fictive expulsion occurred as the final episode of retching at 42 of the 175 points. Retching responses were reproducibly produced by stimulation at an effective point in a dog, and by stimulation of the corresponding medullar area in other dogs (fig. 4). The effective points in figure 4 showed that vomiting could be produced by stimulation

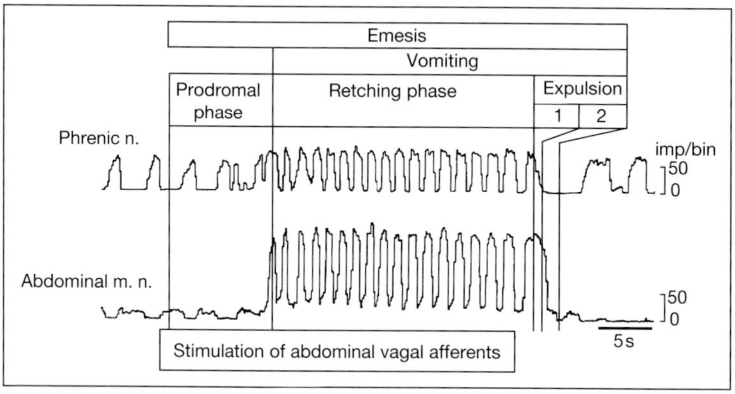

Fig. 2. Vomiting activity patterns of the phrenic and abdominal muscle nerves. The centrifugal activities recorded from both nerves are represented as frequency histograms with 100-ms bins. The terms emesis, vomiting, prodromal phase, retching (phase) and expulsion are used in this chapter to express the phases of emesis as shown. Expulsion consists of the first and second phases. Both phrenic and abdominal muscle nerves discharge during the first phase, but only abdominal muscle nerves discharge during the second phase. 1 and 2 represent the first and second phase of expulsion respectively.

of the intrabulbar bundle of vagal afferent fibers, solitary tract, medial and commissural parts of the solitary nucleus, the area postrema and the reticular areas between the caudal parts of the solitary complex and nucleus ambiguus. Except for the intrabulbar bundle, all of these effective regions may be consistent with the effective areas reported by Borison and Wang [11], Ikeda and Yamanaka [17], Iwase et al. [18] and Miller and Wilson [14]. However, the horizontal columnar area of the ventrolateral reticular formation adjacent medially to the semicompact part of the nucleus ambiguus and dorsomedially to the RFN had not been reported. Thus, we performed partial knife-cutting of the medulla oblongata to clarify the role of the reticular area in 10 dogs.

Lesions Made to Elucidate the Participation of the Reticular Area Adjacent to the RFN in the Induction of Vomiting

In these dogs, a fictive retching response was produced by stimulation of the solitary complex at the point indicated by S1 or S2 in figure 5 [15]. The responses persisted after a hemisection of the right half of the bulb was manually made first at the level indicated by a thick horizontal line in figure 5 in all dogs. Several transverse cuts of the left half of the rostral medulla were then performed in each dog, and the most caudal cut after which retching response still persisted is represented by a thin horizontal line. The most rostral section

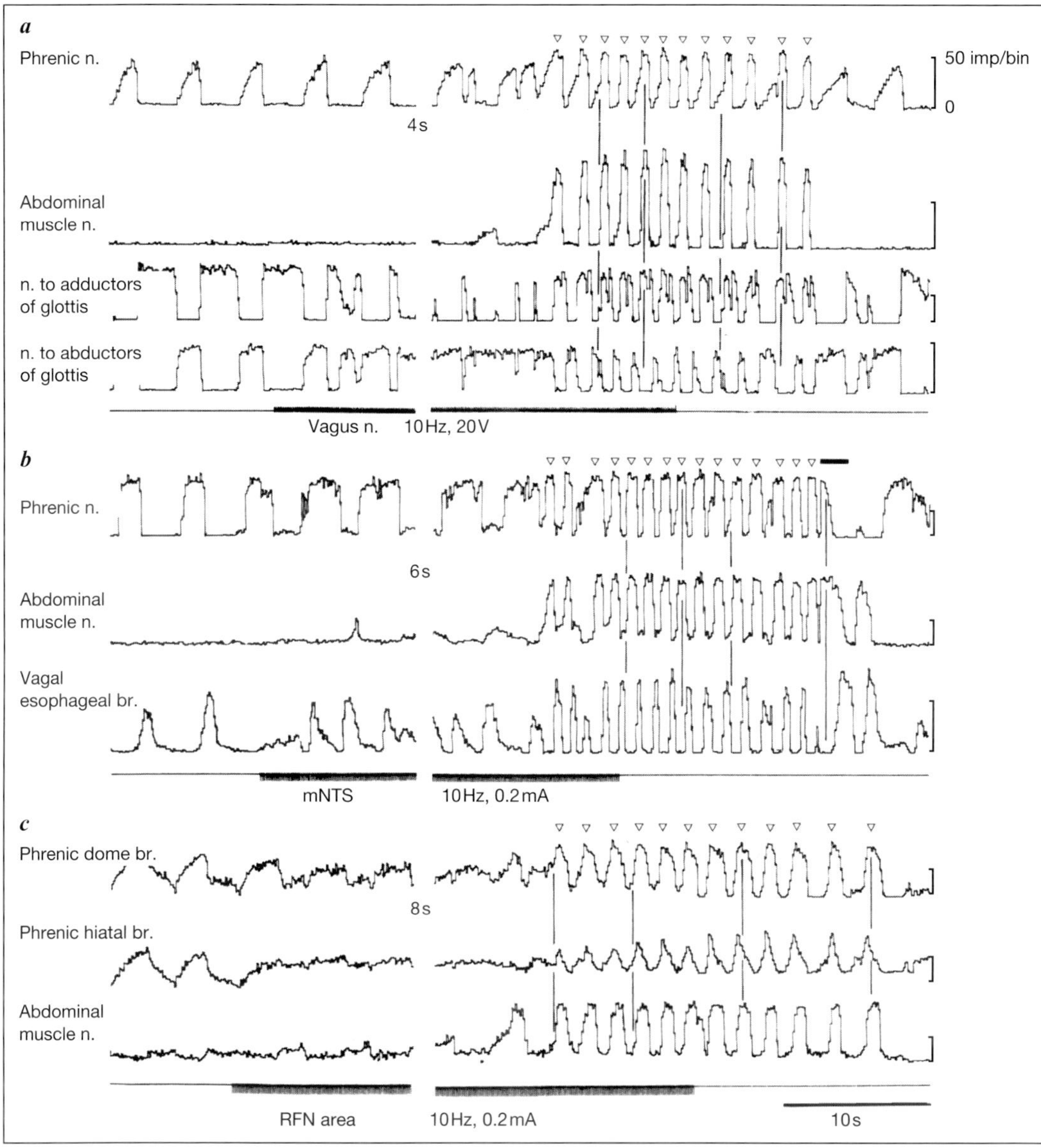

Fig. 3. Discharge patterns exhibited during retching by the muscle nerves indicated. ***a*** Retching induced by stimulation of abdominal vagal afferents. ***b*** Retching and expulsion induced by stimulation of the medial solitary nucleus. ***c*** Retching induced by stimulation of the reticular area adjacent to the retrofacial nucleus (RFN). Traces of the indicated lengths of time were omitted at the interrupted regions. br = Branch.

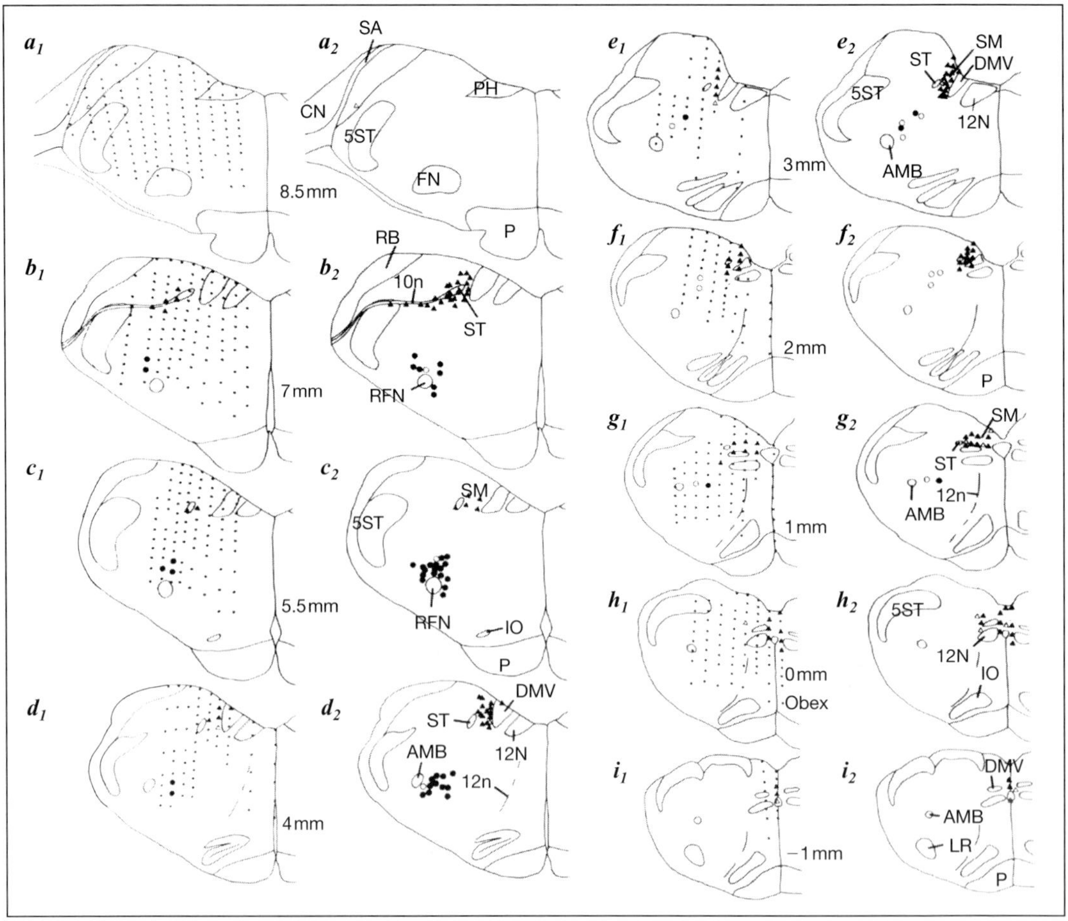

Fig. 4. Bulbar structures in which stimulation elicited retching and vomiting. $\boldsymbol{a_1}$–$\boldsymbol{i_1}$ Each sketch shows the results of systematic stimulation performed at 9 different levels in the bulb with pulses of 10 Hz, 0.2 mA, and 0.5 ms duration. The levels are indicated by the distance from the obex. Filled circles and triangles: points at which retching was induced during stimulation. Open circles and triangles: points at which retching was induced just after stimulation was stopped. Dots: points at which stimulation did not elicit retching. $\boldsymbol{a_2}$–$\boldsymbol{i_2}$ The sum of the results in 17 dogs. 5ST = Spinal trigeminal tract; 10n = vagus nerve; 12N = hypoglossal nucleus; 12n = hypoglossal nerve; AP = area postrema; CN = cochlear nucleus; DMV = dorsal motor nucleus of the vagus; FN = facial nucleus; IO = inferior olive; LR = lateral reticular nucleus; P = pyramidal tract; PH = nucleus prepositus hypoglossi; RG = restiform body; SA = stria medullaris; RFN = retrofacial nucleus; SM = medial solitary nucleus; ST = solitary tract.

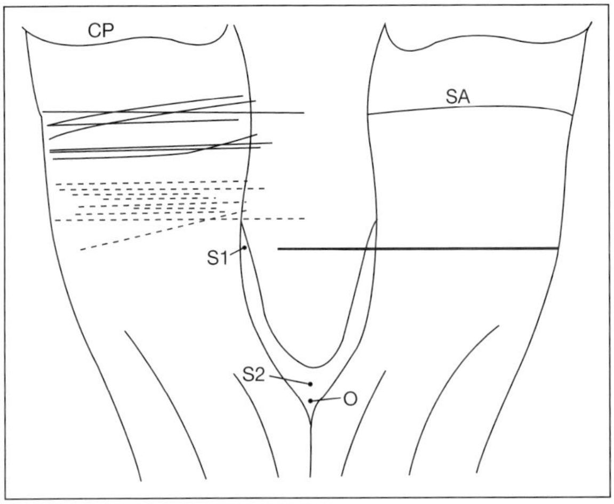

Fig. 5. Locations of transverse cuts performed in 10 dogs. The horizontal line on the right side represents the average position of the hemisection first performed in each dog. The continuous lines on the left side indicate the position of the most caudal cut in each dog after which retching and vomiting responses to stimulation of the caudal part of the solitary complex (S1, S2) still appeared. The broken lines on the left side show the position of the most rostral cut in each dog after which the retching and vomiting responses disappeared. CP = cerebella peduncle; O = obex; SA = stria medullaris.

after which the response disappeared is shown by a broken line. Histological observation of these bulbar preparations revealed that the bulbar levels indicated by the thin and broken lines correspond, respectively, to the caudal end of the facial nucleus and the caudal portion of the RFN. Miller et al. [19] made similar transections in the bulb of 4 cats and reported consistent results.

The results of these cutting and stimulation experiments suggest that the reticular area dorsomedially adjacent to the RFN plays some essential role(s) in the induction of vomiting. To confirm this supposition, we made electrical lesions in the neural tissue on the left side in 6 dogs in which we had first sectioned the right bulb and then chemically destroyed neuronal cell bodies in the area by a microinjection of kainic acid (4.7 mmol/l, 0.5 or 1.0 μl) in 5 dogs [20]. These lesions eliminated the fictive retching in response to vagal stimulation in all of the dogs. Similarly, Miller et al. [19] reported that the fictive vomiting in response to emetics was abolished by large bilateral injections of kainic acid in bulbar areas including the RFN in 2 cats. However, precise delimitation of the extent of these lesions was difficult. Therefore, we used pontamine sky blue, which stains neurons and acts as an excitatory neurotoxin [pers. unpubl. results], to produce lesions in the bulbar area.

Pontamine sky blue (20–30 mg/ml, 0.5 or 1.0 μl) was injected into the area on the left side in 9 dogs in which the right bulb was first severed. The retching response to stimulation of abdominal vagal afferents disappeared in all but 1 dog [pers. unpubl. results]. In 8 dogs, the areas stained by the injections commonly covered a medullar area including the RFN and the reticular area dorsally adjacent to the nucleus, as shown by the shaded area in figure 6. In the other dog, a retching response appeared throughout the observation period for 65 min after the injection. The stained area in this case (indicated by the No. 608 in figure 6) did not fully cover the common reticular area, but almost completely covered the RFN included in the common area. The results in one dog (No. 602) are shown in figure 7. The retching in response to vagal stimulation disappeared within 5 min after injection of the dye (0.5 μl) (fig. 7b), and the frequency of inspiratory discharges of the phrenic nerve and a facilitating response in salivation from the submandibular gland was attenuated at 12 min after injection (fig. 7c). These results suggest that an essential neuronal element for the induction of vomiting exists in the reticular part dorsomedial to the RNF, and that this essential element is adjacent to the neuronal tissue involved in salivation in the prodromal phase of vomiting. We next observed neuronal activity in this essential area to elucidate the role of neurons in this area in the induction of vomiting.

Recording of Neuronal Firings to Define Emetic Roles of Neurons in the Reticular Area Adjacent to the RFN

We explored neurons that responded to pulse-train vagal stimulation in the RFN area using a glass microelectrode filled with 3% pontamine sky blue, and detected unitary firings as shown in figure 8b [21]. The mean latency (387.4 ms) of the responses of 78 non-respiratory neurons to pulse-train vagal stimulation was longer than that (306.5 ms, n = 40) of neurons in the mNTS [22]. When 10-Hz vagal stimulation was applied to induce retching, 30 of the 78 non-respiratory neurons exhibited firing patterns similar to that in the example shown in figure 8a. The firing of these neurons gradually increased during the prodromal phase of vomiting. When the firing frequency reached a threshold, rhythmic bursts occurred synchronously with retching bursts of the phrenic and abdominal muscle nerves (synchronous high-frequency firing type, SH type). Nineteen of the 78 neurons similarly produced bursts of high-frequency discharges during retching. However, in contrast to the SH-type, the bursts occurred between retching bursts of the phrenic and abdominal muscle nerves (BH-type). The recording sites of these non-respiratory neurons were marked by an electrophoretic injection of pontamine sky blue. These sites were located near the RFN, as shown in figure 9.

Based on these locations and firing patterns, we proposed that these non-respiratory neurons in the RFN area comprise the CPG for retching.

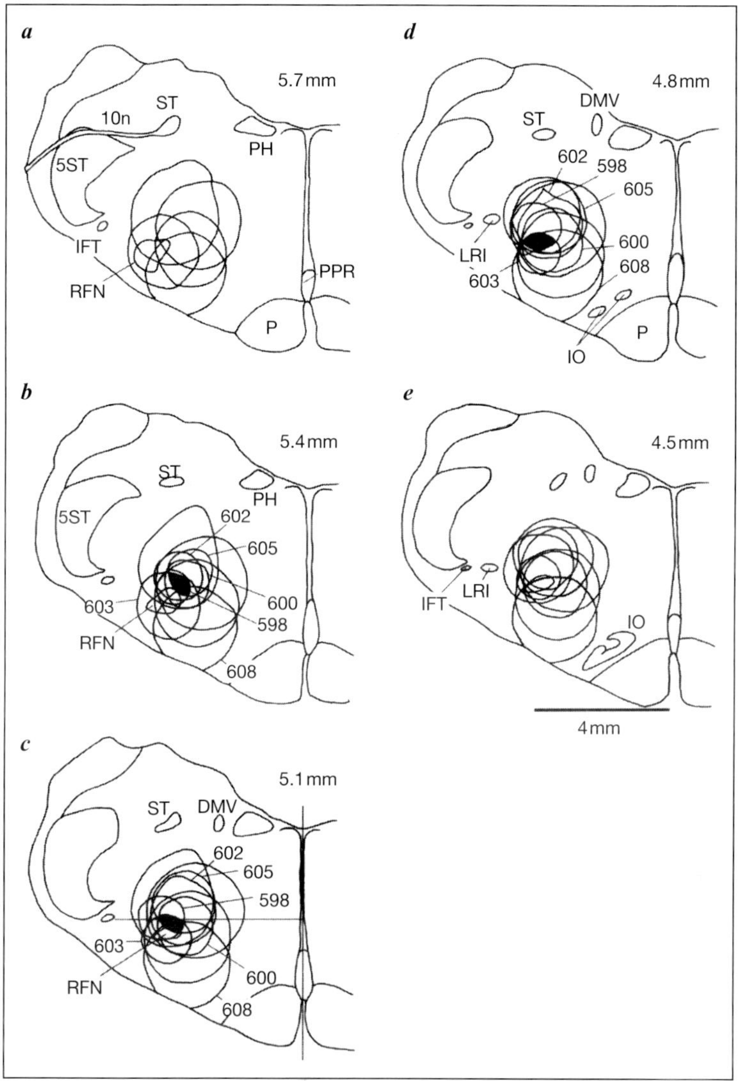

Fig. 6. a–e The areas stained by pontamine sky blue (20–30 mg/ml, 0.5 or 1.0 μl) injected in the left bulb for dysfunction of the CPG for vomiting in 9 dogs in which the right bulb was preliminary severed. Retching in response to stimulation of abdominal vagal afferents disappeared in 8 dogs, but not in the other. The area commonly covered by the stained areas in the 8 dogs is shaded. IFT = Infratrigeminal nucleus; LRI = lateral reticular nucleus; PPR = post-pyramidal nucleus of the raphe.

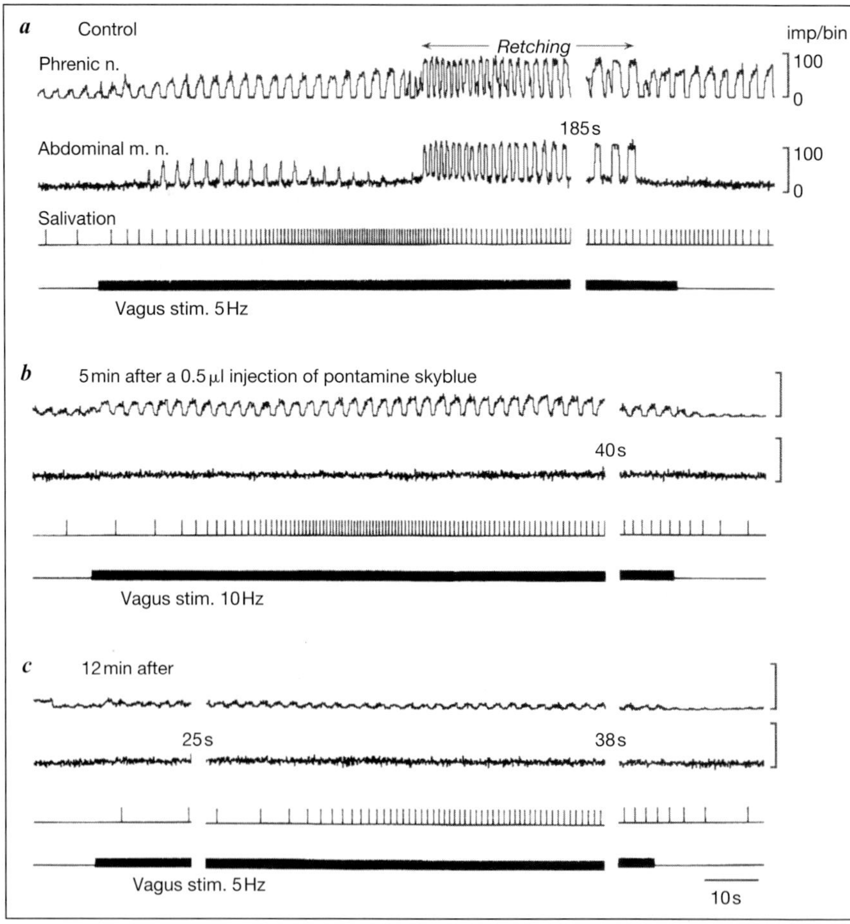

Fig. 7. a–c Effects of a microinjection of pontamine sky blue on retching and salivation in response to stimulation of abdominal vagal afferents. Salivation from the submandibular gland is represented by pulses from a drop counter. The retching response disappeared 5 min after injection (***b***) and salivation was markedly attenuated 12 min after injection (***c***).

Projection from the Solitary Nucleus to the Central Pattern Generator

Stimulation of the mNTS produced a retching response as shown in figure 4, and mNTS neurons fired during the application of vagal stimulation to induce vomiting, as shown in figure 8. Both results suggest that mNTS neurons relay emetic vagal afferent activities to the CPG for vomiting. To examine this possibility, the effects of focal cooling of the mNTS were observed in 11 CPG SH-type neurons recorded in 7 dogs [21]. The typical result shown in figure 10 was obtained from a neuron located in the right CPG area. The response to

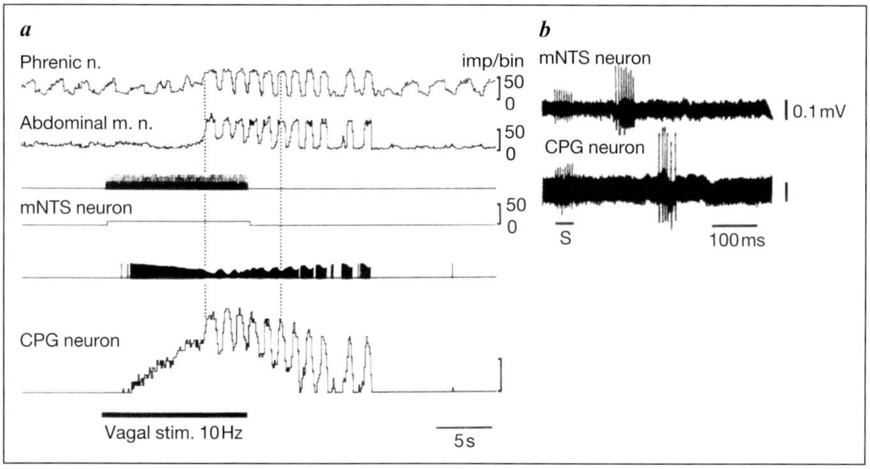

Fig. 8. Temporal relationships between firings of a neuron of the medial solitary nucleus (mNTS) and a CPG SH-type neuron in response to vagal stimulation. ***a*** Firings of both neurons during the emetic response to continuous vagal stimulation. The 3rd and 4th traces show pulses representing firings of the mNTS neuron and a frequency histogram. The 5th and 6th traces show pulses representing firings of the CPG neuron and a frequency histogram. ***b*** A raw photograph of the responses of both neurons to pulse-train vagal stimulation.

pulse-train stimulation of the thoracic vagal trunk as well as SH-type neuronal activities and concomitant retching activities of the phrenic and abdominal muscle nerves were completely and reversibly abolished by the application of focal cooling to the vagal triangle ipsilateral to the stimulated vagal trunk. Bentina and Conde [23] reported that it is impossible to block conduction along fibers by cooling to a temperature above 0°C, and that trans-synaptic excitation is reversibly blocked at 10°C or above. Therefore, these results suggest that emetic vagal afferent fibers make synapses on mNTS neurons, which directly and/or indirectly project to the CPG on either side.

To examine direct projection, antidromic responses to stimulation of the CPG area was examined in 289 neurons in the mNTS area [22]. Antidromic action potentials were elicited in only 13 mNTS neurons. These directly-projecting neurons may mediate emetic afferent activities to the CPG. This assumption, however, does not exclude the possibility that polysynaptic pathways mediate the activities, since polysynaptic pathways seem to favor the small number of directly-projecting neurons and the large difference (80 ms; see fig. 8) between the latencies in the responses of mNTS neurons and CPG SH-type neurons to pulse-train vagal stimulation.

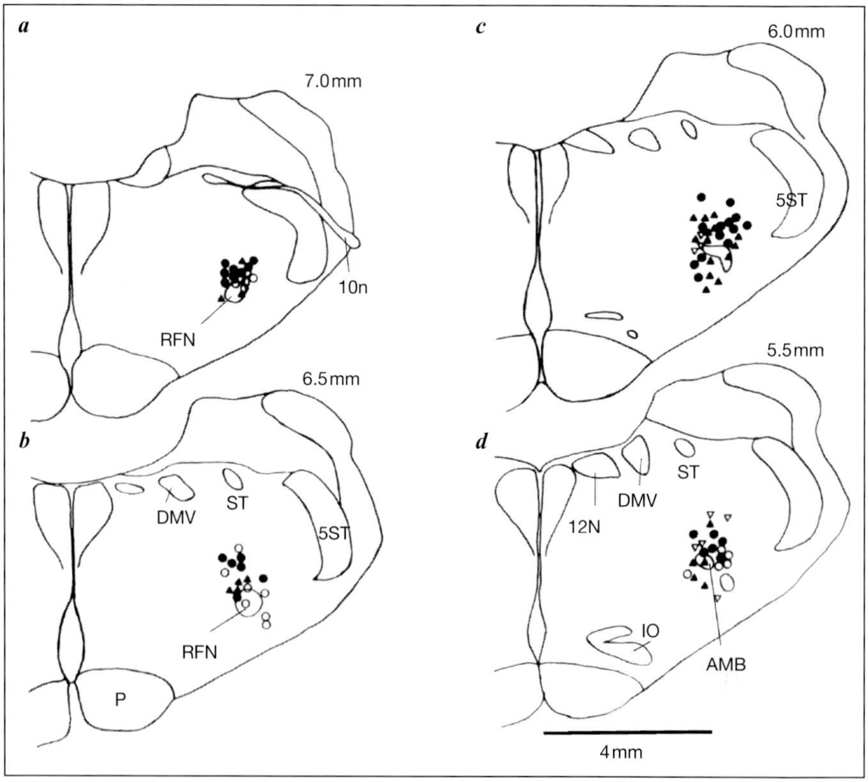

Fig. 9. ***a–d*** Recording sites of CPG SH-type (filled circles) and BH-type (filled triangles) neurons. Recording sites of other neurons, which responded to vagal stimulation, are shown by open symbols.

Convergence of Emetic Afferent Activities on mNTS Neurons

Neurons in the mNTS have been shown to express c-fos immunoreactivity after animals were subjected to various emetic stimuli, e.g., cisplatin in ferrets [24], cisplatin, lobeline, protoveratrine, naloxone, apomorphine in cats [25], stimulation of abdominal vagal afferents in ferrets [26] and dogs [pers. unpubl. results], loperamide in ferrets [27], X-ray irradiation in rats [28] and veratrine in musk shrews [29]. Since the area postrema is known to lack a blood-brain barrier, so that it can act as the chemoreceptor trigger-zone for vomiting, these results suggest that afferent activities from the abdominal viscera and area postrema elicited by these various emetic stimuli converge on mNTS neurons.

To examine this supposition, unitary firings in response to pulse-train vagal stimulation were recorded from 14 neurons in the mNTS, as well as the

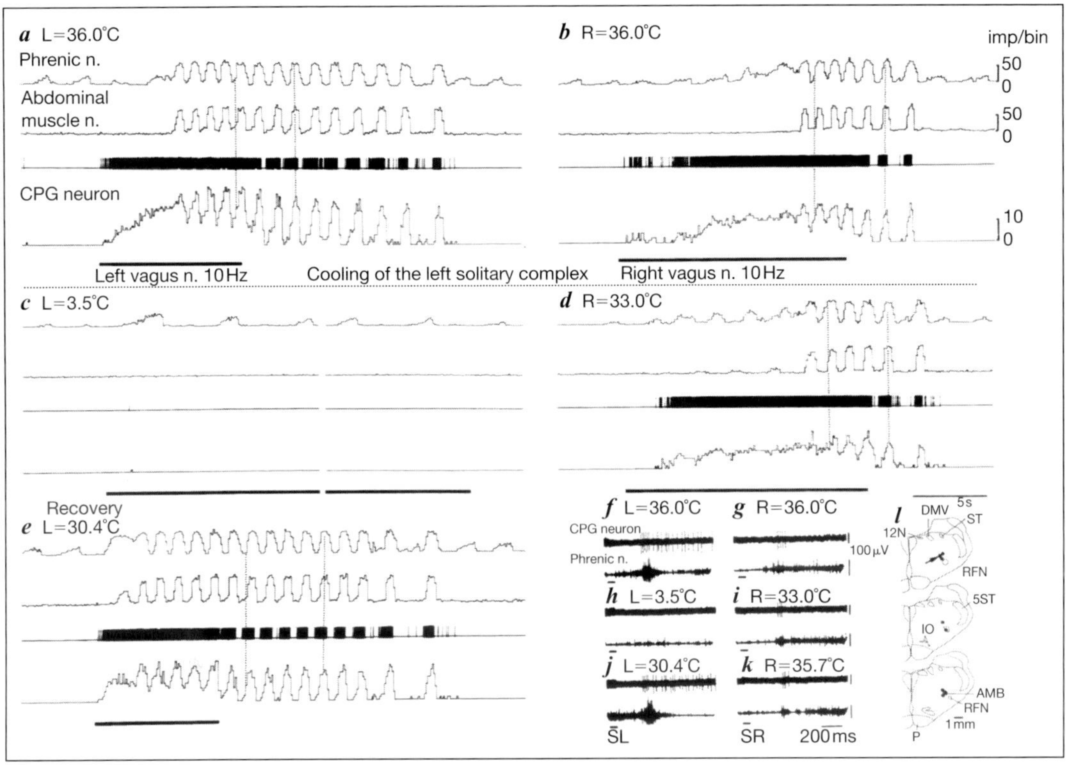

Fig. 10. Effects of cooling the mNTS on the firing of CPG SH-type neurons in response to vagal stimulation. Cooling probes were attached to the surface of the bilateral vagal triangles, but only the left probe was perfused with cooled alcohol. Temperatures of spaces between the cooling probes and the surfaces of the vagal triangles are shown. ***a–e*** Neuronal firings during emetic responses to 10-Hz stimulation of the left (***a***, ***c***, ***e***) and right (***b***, ***d***) vagus nerves. ***a***, ***b*** Control responses. ***c*** During cooling of the left mNTS, all emetic responses of the neuron and nerves to stimulation of the left vagus nerve were completely suppressed. ***d*** However, these emetic responses were still evoked by stimulation of the contralateral (right) vagus nerve. ***e*** The emetic responses to stimulation of the left vagus nerve reappeared when the temperature of the left mNTS had recovered. ***f–k*** Responses of a CPG neuron and the phrenic nerve to pulse-train stimulation of the left (***f***, ***h***, ***j***) and right (***g***, ***i***, ***k***) vagus nerves. ***f***, ***g*** Control responses before cooling. ***h***, ***i*** Responses during cooling. ***j***, ***k*** Responses after cooling. ***l*** Recording sites of 9 CPG SH-type neurons that showed similar effects of cooling of the mNTS. Thick arrow indicates the recording site of the CPG neuron shown in this figure.

effects of fourth ventricular administration of apomorphine and glutamate [22], which were shown to activate neurons in the area postrema [30]. Firing of the mNTS neuron shown in figure 11 gradually increased up to 50 impulses/s after a fourth ventricular application of glutamate, and an episode

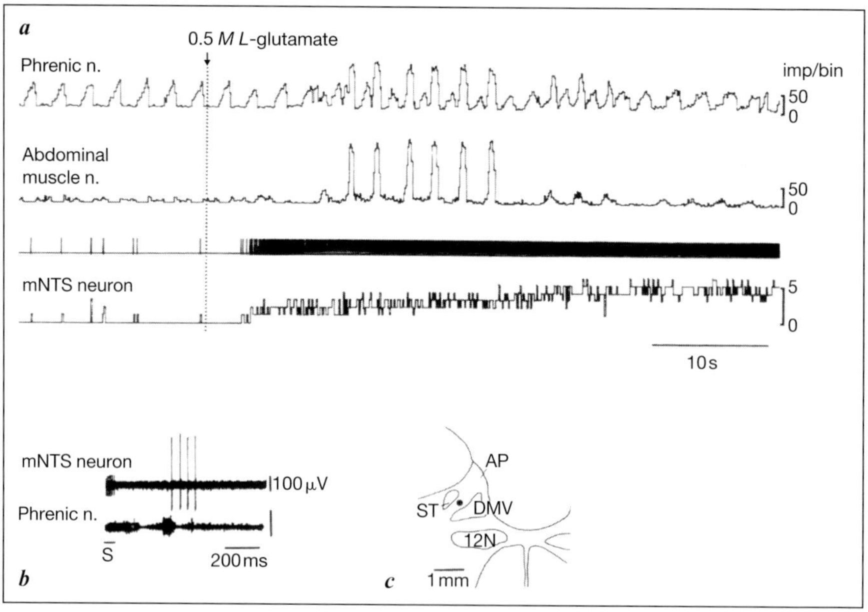

Fig. 11. Response of an mNTS neuron to the application of 0.5 *M L*-glutamate to the fourth ventricle. ***a*** Neuronal firings progressively increased after application, and retching was induced as firing progressed. ***b*** Response of this neuron to pulse-train vagal stimulation. ***c*** Recording site of this neuron.

of retching was induced as firing progressed. Similar enhancing effects of glutamate were observed in all 13 of the other neurons examined, while apomorphine enhanced firing selectively in 6 of the 10 mNTS neurons examined. On the other hand, it is well known that stimulation of the vestibular organ produces emesis, so-called motion sickness. Yates et al. [31] demonstrated that 8 of 31 neurons recorded from the solitary complex responded to stimulation of both vestibular and vagal nerves, and that 4 of these 8 neurons were located in the mNTS. These results strongly support the assumption that mNTS neurons comprise the final common afferent pathway that directly or indirectly mediates emetic activities originating from various sources, e.g., the abdominal viscera, the area postrema and vestibule, to the CPG for vomiting.

This assumption was further supported by our later experiments [32]. The number of firings in response to pulse-train vagal stimulation significantly increased in 6 CPG neurons after an intramuscular injection of apomorphine (0.3 mg/kg), as shown in figure 12. Moreover, spontaneous firing increased in 4 of the 6 CPG neurons.

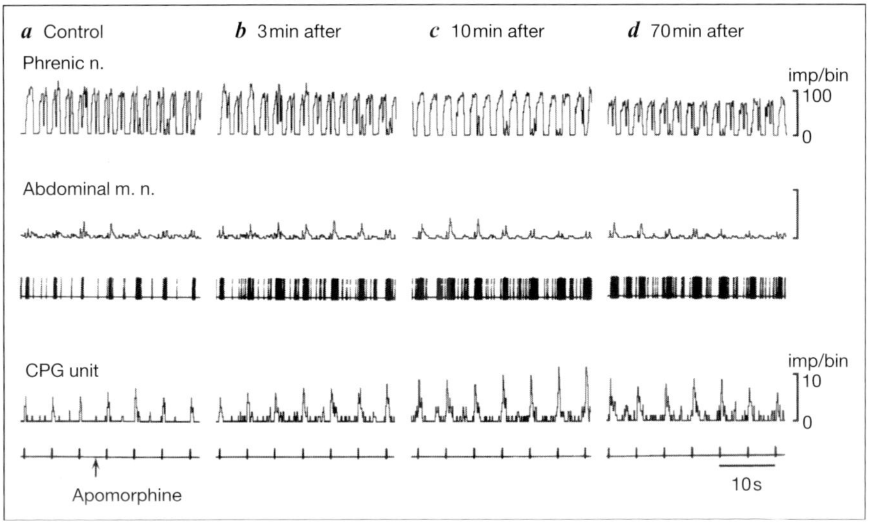

Fig. 12. Effects of apomorphine on the responses of a CPG neuron to pulse-train vagal stimulation. Apomorphine (0.3 mg/kg, i.m.) was administrated in ***a*** (arrow). ***b–d*** Responses at the indicated times after the administration of apomorphine.

Vomiting Activities of Medullar Respiratory Premotoneurons Projecting to the Spinal Cord

It is well established that respiratory motoneurons of the diaphragm and abdominal muscles are innervated by respiratory premotoneurons in the caudal medulla. Miller et al. [16] recorded firings of 27 expiratory premotoneurons from the ventral respiratory group (VRG) area caudal to the obex and observed firing patterns during fictive vomiting in paralyzed decerebrate cats. Nine of the 27 neurons produced bursts of higher frequency firings than their expiratory discharges synchronously with retching bursts of the phrenic and abdominal muscle nerves (SH-type firing). Koga [33] performed similar experiments in dogs and reported that 13 of 30 expiratory premotoneurons produced SH-type bursts during fictive retching. They concluded from these results that these expiratory premotoneurons contribute to induce vomiting contractions of the abdominal muscles.

In contrast to these expiratory premotoneurons, Miller et al. [34] reported that SH-type firings were found in only one of 51 inspiratory premotoneurons recorded from the dorsal respiratory group (DRG) area (from 0.2 mm caudal to 1.4 mm rostral to the obex) and the VRG area (from 2 mm caudal to 2.4 mm rostral to the obex). They concluded that inspiratory premotoneurons do not make a major contribution to activation of the diaphragm and external intercostal muscles during vomiting and that some other, as yet unidentified, pathway plays an important role in controlling the muscles during vomiting.

Koga [33] observed firing patterns of 39 inspiratory premotoneurons recorded from the VRG area 2 mm rostral to 3 mm caudal to the obex in decerebrate dogs. Fourteen of the 39 inspiratory premotoneurons produced SH-type firings during fictive retching. This result seems to be inconsistent with that of Miller et al. [34] mentioned above. Except for the difference in animal species, the most obvious difference in the experimental conditions seems to be artificial ventilation, i.e., end-tidal CO_2 was maintained within 3–5% in cats, but within 2–3.5% in dogs. To resolve this inconsistency, we observed vomiting activities of inspiratory premotoneurons in two groups of dogs, i.e., end-tidal CO_2 was kept lower than 3.5% in one group of 7 dogs and higher than 3.5% in another group of 9 dogs [35]. We recorded unitary activities from 75 and 139 inspiratory premotoneurons from the VRG area (2 mm rostral to 3 mm caudal to the obex) in the lower and higher groups, respectively. In both groups, about 40% (34/75, 57/139) of the inspiratory premotoneurons produced SH-type firings during fictive vomiting. Therefore, it may be concluded that inspiratory premotoneurons make a major contribution to vomiting contractions of the diaphragm, at least in dogs. This conclusion, however, does not exclude the participation of other neurons.

Soon after that study [34] Nonaka and Miller [36] found that 23 of 43 propriospinal inspiratory neurons in the upper cervical cord (C1-C3) produced SH-type firings during fictive vomiting. Subsequently, Miller and Yates [37] performed bilateral injections of kainic acid in the C1–C3 spinal segments to evaluate emetic functions of upper cervical inspiratory neurons, and reported that these procedures had no major effects on phrenic, intercostal or abdominal nerve activities during respiration, vomiting and coughing. Based on these results, they concluded that upper cervical inspiratory neurons are not essential for inducing vomiting contractions of the inspiratory muscles.

Next, Miller et al. [38] recorded firings of 4 inspiratory neurons from the medullary midline area, and reported that 3 of these 4 neurons exhibited SH-type firings during fictive vomiting and one of these 3 neurons had an axon projecting to the upper cervical cord. In another series of experiments in 5 cats, they performed 6–12 injections of neurotoxic kainic acid at 0.5- to 1-mm intervals along the midline 1–6 mm rostral to the obex, and reported that fictive vomiting was abolished after these injections in 4 cats, and was greatly attenuated in the remaining cat. Based on these results, they suggested that the lesion removed an important source of facilitatory input to the spinal respiratory motoneurons and/or the brainstem circuit that mediates vomiting.

Neuronal Mechanism Releasing Respiratory Premotoneurons from Respiratory Inputs during Retching

As mentioned above, about 40% of inspiratory [35] and 30% of expiratory premotoneurons [33] exhibited SH-type bursts during retching, 8% of inspiratory and 13% of expiratory premotoneurons produced BH-type bursts, and the remaining majority produced no or only low-frequency firings modulated with the retching rhythm in dogs. These results seem to show that respiratory activities disappeared during retching from all respiratory premotoneurons and were replaced to a greater or lesser extent with retching activities. This is also the case with expiratory and inspiratory premotoneurons of cats [16, 34]. Since respiratory premotoneurons are known to be driven from propriobulbar respiratory neurons in the respiratory rhythm generator area [39, 40], these results suggest that the respiratory rhythm generator is suppressed during retching. To evaluate this assumption, we observed the activities of inspiratory neurons in the reticular area adjacent to the semicompact part of the nucleus ambiguus [41]. These inspiratory neurons have been proposed to comprise the pre-Bötzinger complex (preBÖT) and are assumed to play a key role in the generation of respiratory rhythm [42].

Inspiratory activities disappeared during retching in all 12 pre-inspiratory neurons of the preBÖT [41]. The pre-inspiratory neuron was identified in cats by Connelly et al. [43], and Gray et al. [44] demonstrated that the pre-inspiratory neuron plays a key role in the genesis of respiratory rhythm. Therefore, the respiratory rhythm generator is thought to be suppressed during retching. Inspiratory firings were also suppressed during retching in all 12 constant inspiratory neurons and in all but 1 of 12 augmenting inspiratory neurons of the preBÖT [41]. These two types of inspiratory neurons are both excitatory and drive inspiratory premotoneurons [39]. These results suggest that the respiratory rhythm generator is suppressed during retching, and that respiratory premotoneurons are released from driving inputs from the respiratory rhythm generator.

The origin of this suppression was suggested by the results reported by Miller and co-workers [45, 46]. They observed vomiting activity of respiratory neurons, which are densely distributed in the reticular area ventrolateral to the RFN, which has been called the Bötzinger complex (BÖT). SH- and BH-type bursts were produced by 8 of 12 decrementing inspiratory neurons [45] and 11 of 20 augmenting expiratory neurons, respectively, during fictive vomiting in cats [46]. Similarly, Fukuda and Koga [21] reported that 3 and 4 of 10 decrementing expiratory neurons in the BÖT produced SH- and BH-type discharges, respectively, during fictive retching in dogs. Since all of these neurons in the BÖT are considered inhibitory neurons which produce widespread inhibitory effects on propriobulbar as well as bulbospinal respiratory neurons [39], they may contribute to the suppression of the respiratory rhythm generator and respiratory premotoneurons during vomiting.

Pathway Connecting the CPG to Respiratory Premotoneurons

If the vomiting activities of phrenic and abdominal muscle motoneurons are mediated by respiratory premotoneurons located in the VRG area caudal to the obex, these respiratory premotoneurons should be directly or indirectly driven from the CPG. Therefore, if the axons directly descend from the CPG, stimulation of the VRG area at the obex level should produce an antidromic spike in CPG neurons. We examined this assumption in 21 dogs, and found that 9 of 27 non-respiratory CPG SH-type neurons produced an antidromic spike in response to VRG stimulation [47]. Based on this result, we concluded that the vomiting activities of phrenic and abdominal muscle premotoneurons are mediated by the axons of CPG SH-type neurons which directly project to the caudal VRG.

When these experiments were performed, we believed that the vomiting reflex arc is closed, as shown in figure 1.

Neuronal Mechanisms for Switching Retching to Expulsion

Peripheral Mechanisms of Switching

The reader may be aware that retching was not followed by expulsion when vagal stimulation was used to induce fictive vomiting in decerebrate paralyzed dogs. We were concerned by this unexpected phenomenon for years. Therefore, we observed vomiting in decerebrate non-paralyzed dogs [48]. In experiments in 2 decerebrate dogs, vomiting was induced by gastric distention with air, and typical results are shown in figure 13. In this case, retching started just after the stomach was distended further by an additional injection of air. Each retch is represented by a negative pulse in the trace of intratracheal pressure (indicated by a filled triangle). Surprisingly, these negative pulses were not accompanied by any transient changes in the traces of tracheal O_2 and CO_2 that were comparable to the changes caused by tracheal air flow during respiration. This result indicates that tracheal air does not flow during the initial half of the retching phase (R1), as demonstrated by Gold and Hatcher [49]. These results are consistent with previous electrophysiological results demonstrating that the adductors of the glottis act concomitantly with each retch [21, 50–52]. Consequently, the partial pressures of arterial O_2 and CO_2 steadily increased and decreased, respectively, during the initial phase of retching, and reached their respective maximum and minimum values during the late retching phase (R2). Both the maximum and minimum values were maintained until episodes of expulsion, while actual ventilation occurred between retches in the late retching phase (R2) as indicated by rapid transient changes tracheal O_2 and CO_2.

These results indicated that hypoxia and/or hypercapnia that develop during retching induce a phase transition from retching to expulsion. If this assumption is valid, then interrupting artificial ventilation during fictive retching in paralyzed dogs may induce a phase transition from fictive retching to fictive expulsion.

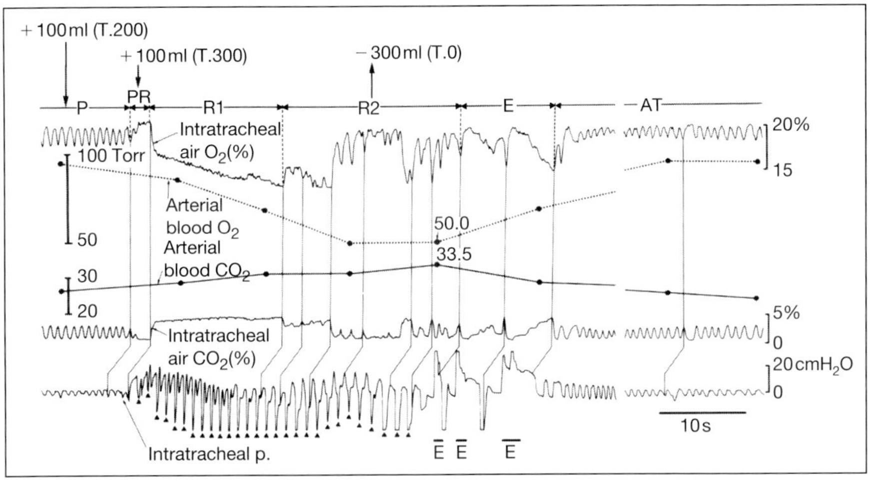

Fig. 13. Changes in intratracheal pressure and CO_2 and O_2 concentrations in tracheal air and arterial blood during actual vomiting in a non-paralyzed decerebrate dog. From top to bottom, traces represent tracheal air O_2 (TrO_2, vol%), arterial blood O_2 tension (PaO_2, Torr), arterial blood CO_2 tension ($PaCO_2$, Torr), tracheal CO_2 ($TrCO_2$, vol%) and intratracheal pressure. Each actual retch is represented as a negative pressure pulse on the trace of intratracheal pressure (▲) and an actual expulsion corresponds to a positive pressure pulse, which is indicated by a horizontal bar (E). Vomiting was induced by stomach distention with 3 injections of 100 ml of air at ↓. Total volumes of injected air are indicated in parentheses as T.200 = 200 ml, T.300 = 300 ml. All 300 ml of air was removed at ↑. Vomiting and preceding and subsequent respiratory changes were divided into the prodromal phase (P), preretching phase (PR), first retching phase (R1), second retching phase (R2), expulsion phase (E) and after-tachypnea phase (AT). Traces (12 s) during the AT phase were omitted.

Figure 14 shows an example of experiments that were performed in 5 decerebrate paralyzed dogs to examine this assumption. A chain of 21 fictive retches was induced by stimulation of vagal afferents at an end-tidal tracheal CO_2 of 3.4%, however, fictive expulsion did not occur (fig. 14a). In contrast, when artificial ventilation was discontinued 14 s before retching began, tracheal CO_2 reached 7.3% at the 12th fictive retch and 2 episodes of fictive expulsion were successively induced. We assumed from these results that the hypoxia and/or hypercapnia that develop during retching trigger the phase transition from retching to expulsion.

If this assumption is valid, arterial chemoreceptor afferents may participate in the phase transition. To examine this assumption, sinus nerve afferents were stimulated during fictive retching in 8 paralyzed decerebrate dogs, as shown in the example in figure 15. End-tidal tracheal CO_2 was maintained at 2.6% throughout the experiment. A long chain of fictive retches, without expulsion,

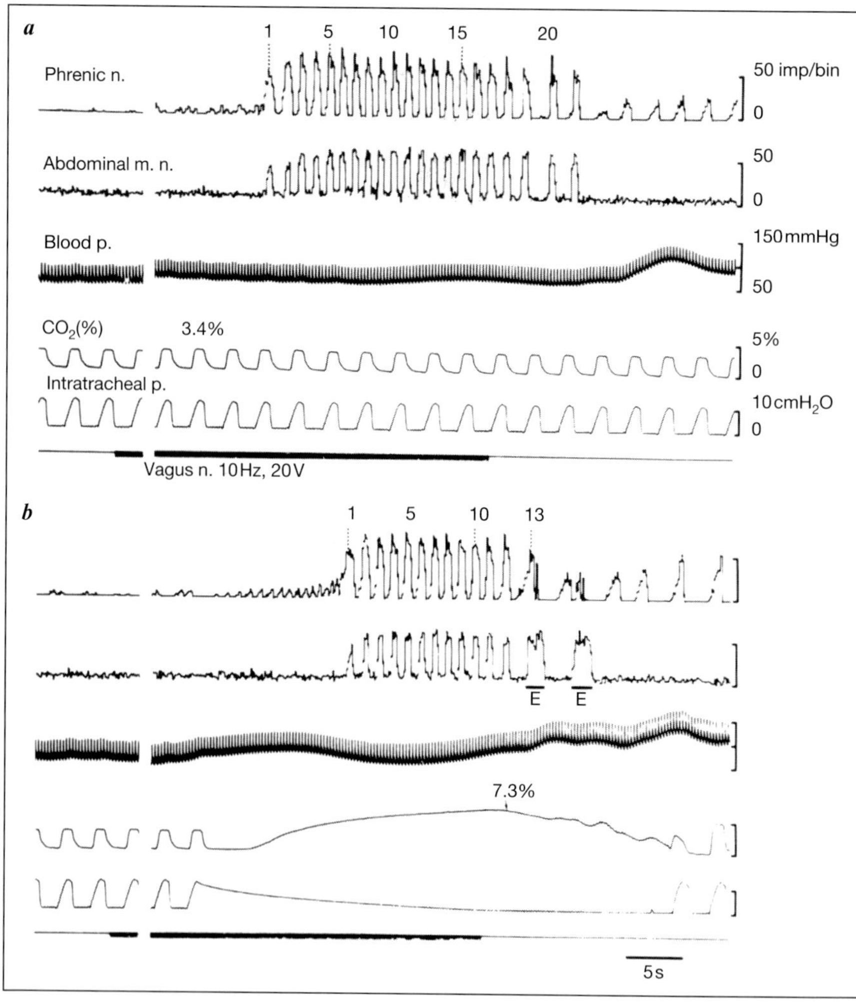

Fig. 14. ***a***, ***b*** Effects of interrupting artificial ventilation on fictive retching which had been induced by stimulating abdominal vagal afferents. From top to bottom, the traces show frequency histograms of the phrenic and abdominal muscle nerves, arterial blood pressure, CO_2 concentration in tracheal air (CO_2(%)), intratracheal pressure and downward pulses representing pulses for stimulating the vagus nerve. Artificial ventilation was discontinued during the period indicated by the intratracheal pressure trace in ***b***. $TrCO_2$ increased to 7.3% and two episodes of fictive expulsion (E) were induced.

was induced by vagal stimulation (fig. 15a). However, sinus nerve stimulation superimposed on the vagal stimulation just after the 20th retch induced a transition from fictive retching to fictive expulsion (fig. 15b). We concluded that the phase transition from retching to expulsion was induced by hypoxia and/or

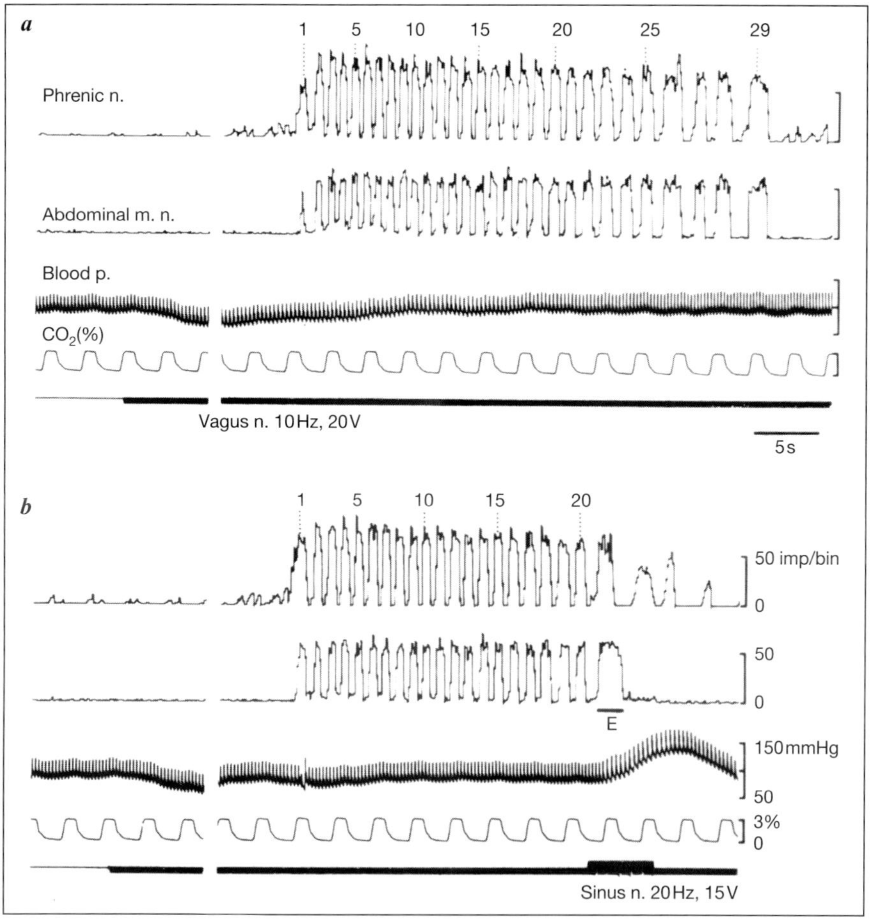

Fig. 15. Effects of stimulation of sinus nerve afferents on fictive retching. Fictive retching without fictive expulsion was induced by vagal stimulation at an end-tidal CO_2 of 2.6% (***a***). Fictive expulsion was induced by stimulation of left sinus nerve afferents which was superimposed on vagal afferent stimulation (***b***).

hypercapnia that developed during retching via, at least in part, arterial chemoreceptor afferents.

Central Neuronal Mechanisms for the Transition from Retching to Expulsion

When we learned that chemoreceptor afferents participate in the phase transition from retching to expulsion, we knew that CPG neurons exhibit appropriate firing patterns to generate retching, but did not know the firing

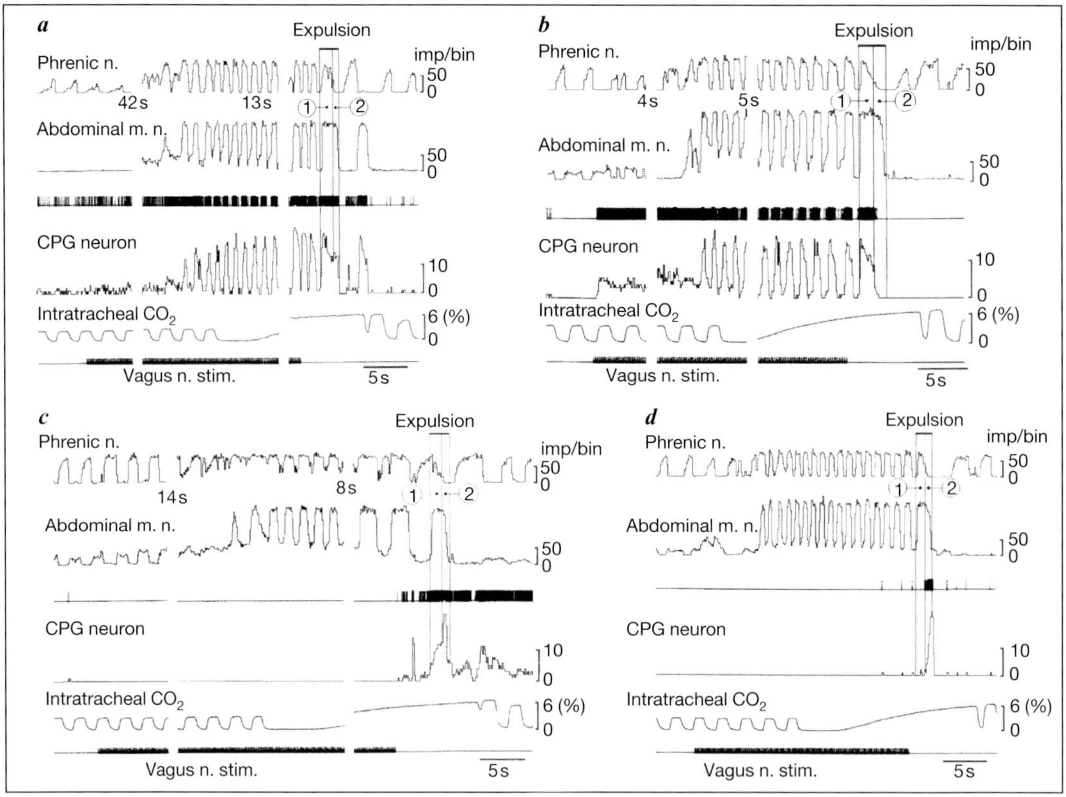

Fig. 16. Types of CPG neurons during fictive vomiting. From top to bottom, the traces in ***a–d*** represent frequency histograms of discharges of the phrenic and abdominal muscle nerves, rectified pulse of unitary firing of a CPG neuron and a frequency histogram of the unitary firing, CO_2% of tracheal air, and pulses for stimulating the vagus nerve. Fictive expulsion was induced by discontinuing artificial ventilation, as indicated in the tracheal CO_2 trace. ***a*** SH-type retching and abdominal m.-n. type expulsion bursts of a CPG neuron. ***b*** SH-type retching and phrenic n.-type expulsion burst of a CPG neuron. ***c*** Second-phase burst produced by a CPG neuron. ***d*** After-discharge produced by a CPG neuron.

patterns of these CPG neurons during expulsion. Since CPG neurons are assumed to play key roles in the transition from retching to expulsion, we recorded unitary firings from 84 non-respiratory neurons in the CPG area of 54 decerebrate paralyzed dogs, and found that these neurons produced the following four firing patterns with fictive expulsion induced by a discontinuation of artificial ventilation or sinus nerve stimulation [53]: (1) Thirteen of the 84 neurons produced the firing pattern shown in figure 16a. Since this pattern is assumed to be suitable for producing retching and expulsion activities of abdominal muscle motoneurons, we called CPG neurons of this type abdominal m.n.-type. (2) Twenty-two of the 84 neurons exhibited firing patterns similar to the example shown in figure 16b. Since this pattern seems to be suitable for inducing retching and expulsion activities of phrenic motoneurons, we called CPG neurons of this type phrenic n.-type. (3) Eight of the 84 neurons produced a vigorous burst at the second phase of expulsion, as shown in figure 16c. We thought that neurons of this type may play a key role in patterning expulsion firings of the phrenic n.-type and abdominal m.n.-type CPG neurons, since bursts of neurons of this type seem to be suitable for shortening expulsion bursts of phrenic n.-type CPG neurons and for prolonging expulsion bursts of abdominal m.n.-type CPG neurons during the second phase of expulsion. We called CPG neurons of this type second-phase burst-type. (4) Ten of the 84 neurons discharged a burst concomitantly with the end of an expulsion burst of the abdominal muscle nerve (fig. 16d). These neurons may contribute to terminate the expulsion bursts of abdominal m.n.-type CPG neurons, and we called these the after discharge-type. The remaining 31 neurons did not produce any firings at the transition or during expulsion. We also elucidated in later experiments that these four types of CPG neurons produce similar firing patterns during gagging induced by stimulation of pharyngolaryngeal afferents [54]. Based on these results, we concluded that vomiting motions of the diaphragm and abdominal muscles are patterned entirely in the CPG.

At that time, we were fortunately offered a selective non-peptide NK_1 receptor antagonist, GR205171 [3], by Glaxo-Wellcome Co., and began experiments to determine the site of the antiemetic action of this antagonist.

The Site of the Antiemetic Action of NK_1 Receptor Antagonists

Possibility That the Site Exists in the mNTS

Subcutaneous injection of resiniferatoxin, an ultra-potent capsaicin analogue, transiently induced emesis in *Suncus murinus* [55], and then blocked emesis induced by radiation and copper sulfate in the ferret and by motion, cisplatin, copper sulfate, nicotine and resiniferatoxin itself in *S. murinus* [56]. Vagotomy is known to reduce the emetic effects of these stimuli (see review by Naylor and Rudd [57]). Similarly, the application of capsaicin or resiniferatoxin to the fourth ventricle was shown to produce transient retching, and then simultaneously abolish retching and the firing of mNTS neurons in response to vagal stimulation [58].

Capsaicin is well known to release and then deplete substance P from central nerve terminals of nociceptive afferents in the spinal cord (see review by Holzer [59]). Similarly, capsaicin has also been shown to reduce substance P levels in the vagus nerve and medulla oblongata [60–62]. Furthermore, some vagal C afferents are known to contain immunoreactive substance P [63, 64]. These results show that capsaicin-sensitive vagal afferents have substance P as a transmitter.

Neurons of the solitary nucleus have been shown to have binding sites for substance P which are blocked by NK_1 receptor antagonist [7]. Tattersall et al. [6] demonstrated that the injection of NK_1 receptor antagonists in or near the solitary nucleus inhibits cisplatin-induced emesis in the ferret.

These findings suggest the possibility that substance P acts as an excitatory neurotransmitter in the synapse between emetic vagal afferents and mNTS neurons, which in turn drive the CPG for vomiting. To evaluate this possibility, we observed the effects of GR205171 on the activity of mNTS neurons and on retching induced by the stimulation of either abdominal vagal afferents or the mNTS in dogs [65].

Effects of Intravenous Injection of an NK_1 Receptor Antagonist, GR205171

The effects of GR205171 on fictive retching induced by stimulation of abdominal vagal afferents and by stimulation of the mNTS were observed in 23 and 4 dogs, respectively. Both types of retching were reversibly eliminated after an intravenous injection of GR205171 in all of the dogs with comparable latencies, as shown in figure 17. The elimination of retching in response to mNTS stimulation by GR205171 is consistent with the results of Tattersall et al. [6], and suggests that the site of the antiemetic action of NK_1 receptor antagonists is central.

Firings of 7 neurons in responses to pulse-train vagal stimulation were recorded from the mNTS area in 7 dogs, as shown in figure 18c. These neurons also fired during the application of 10-Hz vagal stimulation to induce retching (fig. 18a). All 7 neurons exhibited similar firing patterns, even after retching in response to vagal stimulation was abolished by an intravenous injection of GR205171 (fig. 18b).

These results are considered conclusive evidence to support the notion that the site of the antiemetic action of NK_1 antagonists exists downstream from the mNTS in the vomiting reflex arc (see fig. 1).

Zaman et al. [66] demonstrated that CP-99,994, an NK_1 receptor antagonist, abolished the emetic response induced by loperamide, an opiate receptor agonist, in ferrets, but did not have any significant effects on fos-like immunoreactivity in the solitary nucleus. If this NK_1 receptor antagonist blocked the receptors on mNTS neurons and eliminated the emetic response, fos-like immunoreactivity in mNTS neurons should be reduced, in contrast to their results. Therefore, they concluded that NK_1 receptor antagonists act at a site ‘deep’ in the solitary nucleus or elsewhere. Their conclusion is consistent with ours.

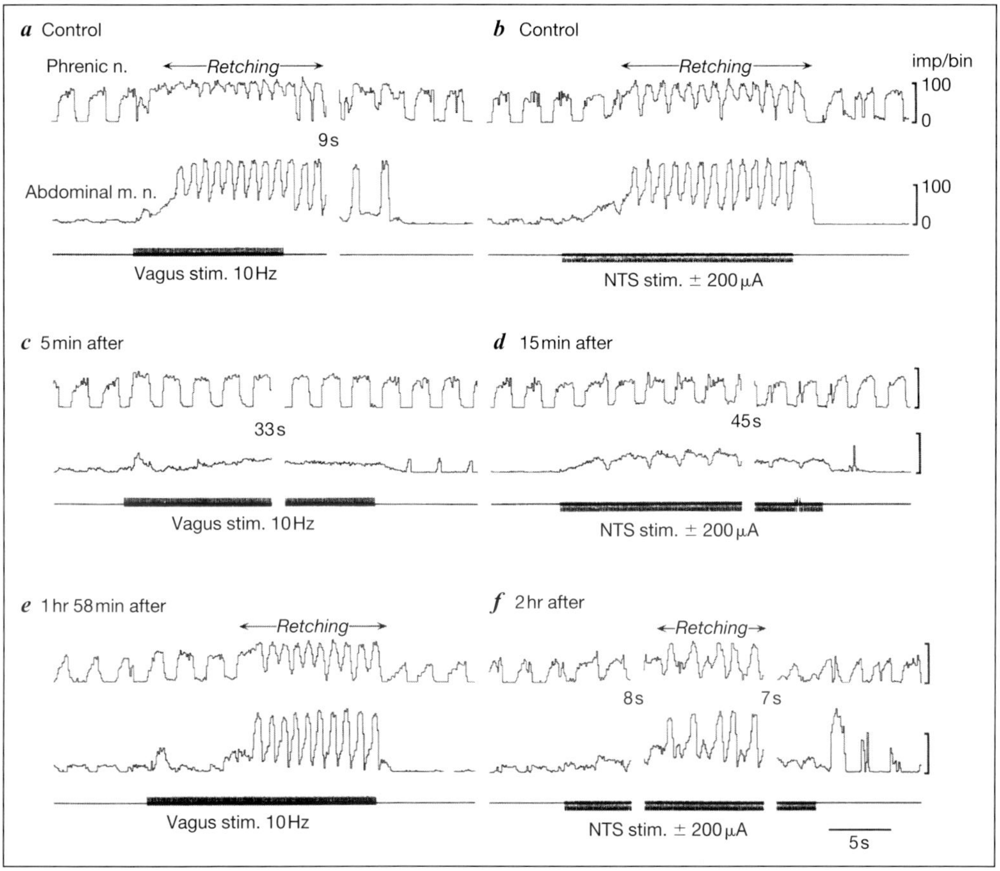

Fig. 17. Effects of GR205171 on retching responses to stimulation of abdominal vagal afferents (***a***, ***c***, ***e***) and the mNTS (***b***, ***d***, ***f***). ***a***, ***b*** Control retching in response to vagal stimulation and stimulation of the mNTS. ***c***, ***d*** Disappearance of retching responses. The records were obtained at the indicated number of minutes after the intravenous application of GR205171 (0.2 mg/kg). ***e***, ***f*** Recovery of retching responses. The records were obtained at the indicated number of minutes after the application of GR205171.

In addition, we recently found that the response of mNTS neurons to vagal stimulation disappeared concomitantly with fictive retching after a fourth ventricular application of NBQX, a glutamate non-NMDA receptor antagonist, in dogs [67]. Based on this result, we concluded that the activities of emetic vagal afferents are mainly mediated by glutamate and non-NMDA receptors on mNTS neurons.

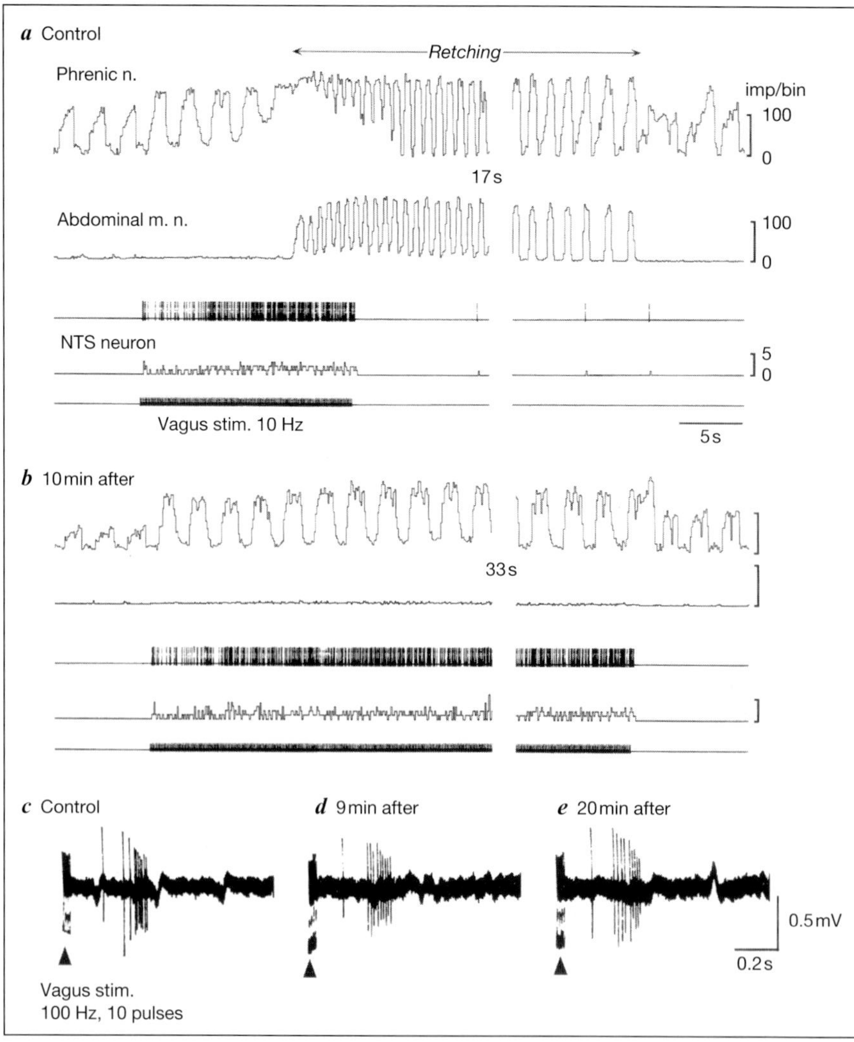

Fig. 18. Effects of GR205171 on responses of an mNTS neuron to vagal stimulation. ***a*** Control response of the mNTS neuron to vagal stimulation applied to induce retching. ***b*** Similar response exhibited by the mNTS neuron after retching in response to vagal stimulation was abolished by an intravenous application of GR205171 (0.1 mg/kg). ***c–e*** Raw photographs of an oscilloscope sweep. ***c*** Control response of the mNTS neurons to pulse-train vagal stimulation. ***d, e*** Similar responses obtained after the retching response was abolished by GR205171.

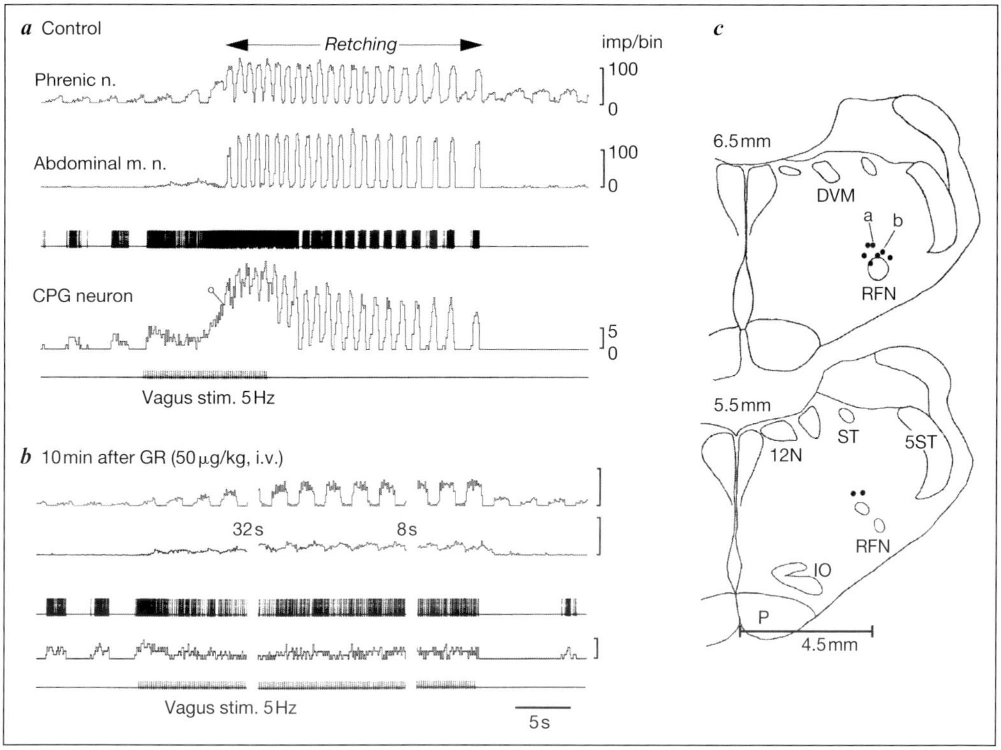

Fig. 19. Effects of GR205171 on the retching activities of a CPG SH-type neuron. ***a*** Control firing of the CPG neuron in response to 5-Hz vagal stimulation. ***b*** Firing induced at the indicated times after an intravenous injection of GR205171 (50 μg/kg). Note the disappearance of retching activities of the CPG neuron and of the phrenic and abdominal muscle nerves. Recording site of the neuron is shown in ***c*** (a). ***c*** Recording sites of 9 CPG SH-type neurons that showed similar effects of GR205171.

Effects of GR205171 on Retching Activities of CPG Neurons

Next, we examined the effects of an intravenous injection of GR205171 on retching firings of CPG neurons to ascertain whether the site of the antiemetic action of NK_1 receptor antagonists is upstream or downstream of the CPG [32]. From among many unitary firings recorded from the CPG area, one CPG SH-type neuron was selected in each of 9 dogs. The gradually increased firing in the prodromal phase and retching bursts in the 9 CPG neurons, as well as the retching bursts in the phrenic and abdominal muscle nerves, disappeared after an intravenous injection of GR205171 (fig. 19). However, even after the gradual increase and retching bursts in firings of CPG neurons were abolished by the application of GR205171, a transient increase in firings at the onset of vagal

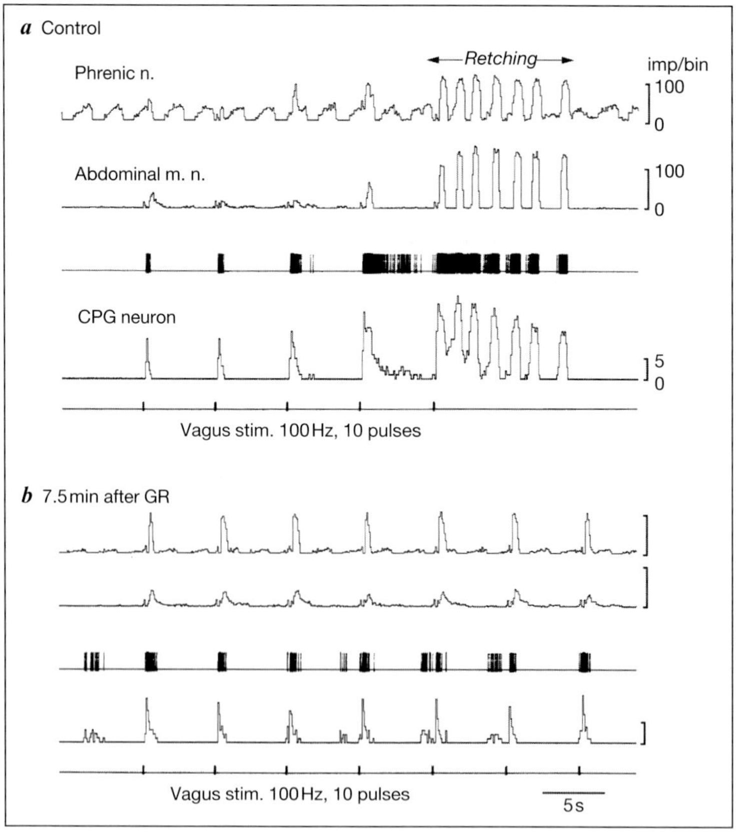

Fig. 20. Effects of GR205171 on the responses of a CPG SH-type neuron to pulse-train vagal stimulation. ***a*** Control: Note that the responses showed a vigorous 'wind-up' and finally developed into retching bursts. ***b*** Responses obtained 7.5 min after an intravenous injection of GR205171 (50 μg/kg). Note that the responses did not exhibit a 'wind-up'.

stimulation remained, and this was followed by low-frequency sustained firings in all 9 neurons (fig. 19b). These results showed that the responses of CPG neurons to vagal stimulation consisted of fast and slow components which are insensitive and sensitive, respectively, to NK_1 receptor antagonists. The recording sites of these 9 neurons are shown in figure 19c.

To elucidate the properties of both components further, responses to pulse-train vagal stimulation were examined in 6 of these 9 CPG neurons [32]. Responses of the CPG neurons were easily facilitated by the repetition of pulse-train vagal stimulation (wind-up), and finally developed into rhythmic retching bursts (fig. 20). Intravenous application of GR205171 abolished the 'wind-up' phenomenon in the responses and subsequent retching bursts. However, the CPG neurons discharged a burst in response to each pulse-train of vagal stimulation even after the application of GR205171. Thus, these bursts seem to correspond to the initial transient increase and the fast component. The bursts of the first component did not develop into rhythmical retching bursts after the application of GR205171. Therefore, the 'wind-up' property of the slow component is thought to be essential for generating neuronal retching activities, while the fast component, which may be mediated by a transmitter other than substance P, may not be essential.

These results clearly demonstrated that the site of the antiemetic action of NK_1 receptor antagonists is located in the CPG or along the pathway connecting the mNTS to the CPG.

Effects of Microinjections of GR205171 on Vomiting

To precisely determine the site of antiemetic action, we performed the microinjection of GR205171 into the left medulla oblongata in decerebrate paralyzed dogs [68]. The right medulla was preliminary transected about 2.5 mm rostral to the obex to eliminate the emetic function of that half. All 73 injection sites at which an aliquot(s) of GR205171 solution (0.1 or 1 mg/ml) was injected are shown in figure 21.

Injections in the Reticular Area Ventrolateral to the Caudal Part of the Solitary Complex

Since Tattersall et al. [6] demonstrated that the injection of an NK_1 receptor antagonist into the solitary nucleus or in its vicinity inhibits cisplatin-induced emesis in the ferret, we first performed injections in the medulla area ventrolateral to the solitary complex (fig. 21c). We performed 32 injections (0.1 or 1.0 mg/ml, 0.5–30 μl) at 23 sites in this area in 6 dogs. Fictive retching in response to vagal stimulation was still observed after each of these injections, although it was interrupted for 10–124 min after injections at 5 sites in 4 dogs.

These interruptions only appeared after larger-volume injections (5–30 μl) at points at which smaller-volume injections did not have any effects on retching. These characteristics of the interruptions suggest that they are caused by the mechanical effects of large-volume injections rather than any antagonistic activity of GR205171 at NK_1 receptors. Therefore, these results suggest that NK_1 receptors that mediate retching in response to vagal stimulation do not exist in the medullar area ventrolateral to the caudal part of the solitary complex.

All three of the previous studies that performed stimulation in this medullar area consistently reported that stimulation produced vomiting and/or

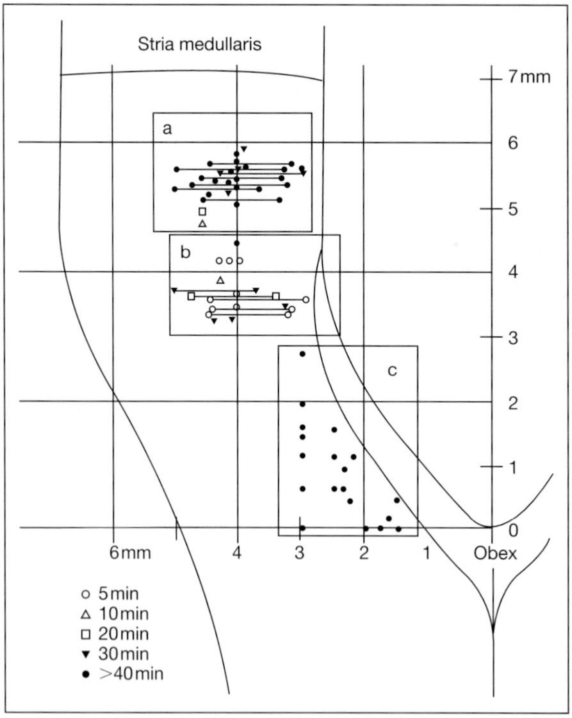

Fig. 21. Injection sites of GR205171 (0.1 or 1 mg/ml) are shown on a schematic representation of the dorsal view of the medulla oblongata in accordance with readings from the scale on the manipulator in which the injection micropipette was fixed. Symbols represent the number of minutes after the injection at which the disappearance of retching was first recognized, as shown in the lower left corner. When a site was injected repeatedly, the number of minutes after the first injection is shown. Paired injections are represented by two symbols connected by a horizontal line. ***a*** Injection sites in the area dorsal to the retrofacial nucleus. ***b*** Injection sites adjacent to the semicompact part of the nucleus ambigous. ***c*** Injection sites in the area ventrolateral to the caudal part of the solitary complex.

retching responses in cats and dogs [11, 14, 15]. These results suggest that cell bodies and/or axons that induce vomiting exist in this area. Wang and Borison [13] reported that destruction of this area by radiation suppressed vomiting responses to emetic drugs in dogs. Based on the results of their destruction and stimulation experiments, they suggested that the vomiting center exists in this medulla area. Miller et al. [19] performed the microinjection of kainic acid to produce the selective destruction of neurosoma in this area, and demonstrated that widespread destruction including the vomiting center does not abolish the vomiting response in cats. Radiation is now known to impair nerve fibers

[69, 70]. Therefore, these results in destruction and stimulation experiments are thought to show that the axons, but not the cell bodies themselves, that mediate the vomiting response exist in this area. This conclusion may be consistent with our conclusion that NK_1 receptors that mediate the retching response do not exist in this area.

Injections in the Reticular Area Dorsal to the RFN

Next, we performed the microinjection of GR205171 into the reticular area dorsal to the RFN, where we assumed that the CPG for vomiting exists, as mentioned above. We performed 16 single and 7 paired injections (0.1 or 1.0 mg/ml, 0.5 or 1 μl) in this area in 17 dogs (fig. 21a). In contrast to the injections in the area ventrolateral to the solitary complex, retching in response to vagal stimulation disappeared within 40 min after 5 of 16 single and 1 of 7 paired injections, while the response persisted in the majority of injections, as shown in fig. 21a.

After the observation periods in 9 of 16 single and 5 of 7 paired injections in this area, the same volume of pontamine sky blue solution was injected into the same injection points to estimate the diffusion area of GR205171. The areas stained by the injected dye are shown in figure 22.

Since the volume of GR205171 solution injected in this area was <1 μl in all cases, this disappearance is not thought to be caused by the mechanical damage of neural tissue. However, the latencies of the effects were much longer than the 5 min or less seen with the intravenous injection of GR205171. Therefore, we concluded that the CPG for vomiting is not the site of the antiemetic action of NK_1 receptor antagonists.

Among the 16 single injections, in 2 exceptional injections a retching response was eliminated after shorter latencies of 10 and 20 min. The injection sites in these 2 cases were caudal to the other sites (fig. 21a). These results suggest that the site of the antiemetic action of NK_1 receptor antagonists is located in a more caudal medullar part. We thought that the caudally adjacent medullar part is the reticular area around the semicompact part of the nucleus ambiguus, since our previous experiments had shown that stimulation of the reticular area effectively induces retching. Thus, we performed injections in the reticular area.

Injections in the Reticular Area Adjacent to the Semicompact Part of the Nucleus ambiguus

We performed 10 single and 5 paired injections (1 μl) of GR205171 solution (0.1 or 1 μg/ml) in this area. In contrast to the results in the other areas mentioned above, retching disappeared in all cases 5–30 min after injection (fig. 21b). After each injection, pontamine sky blue was then injected into the

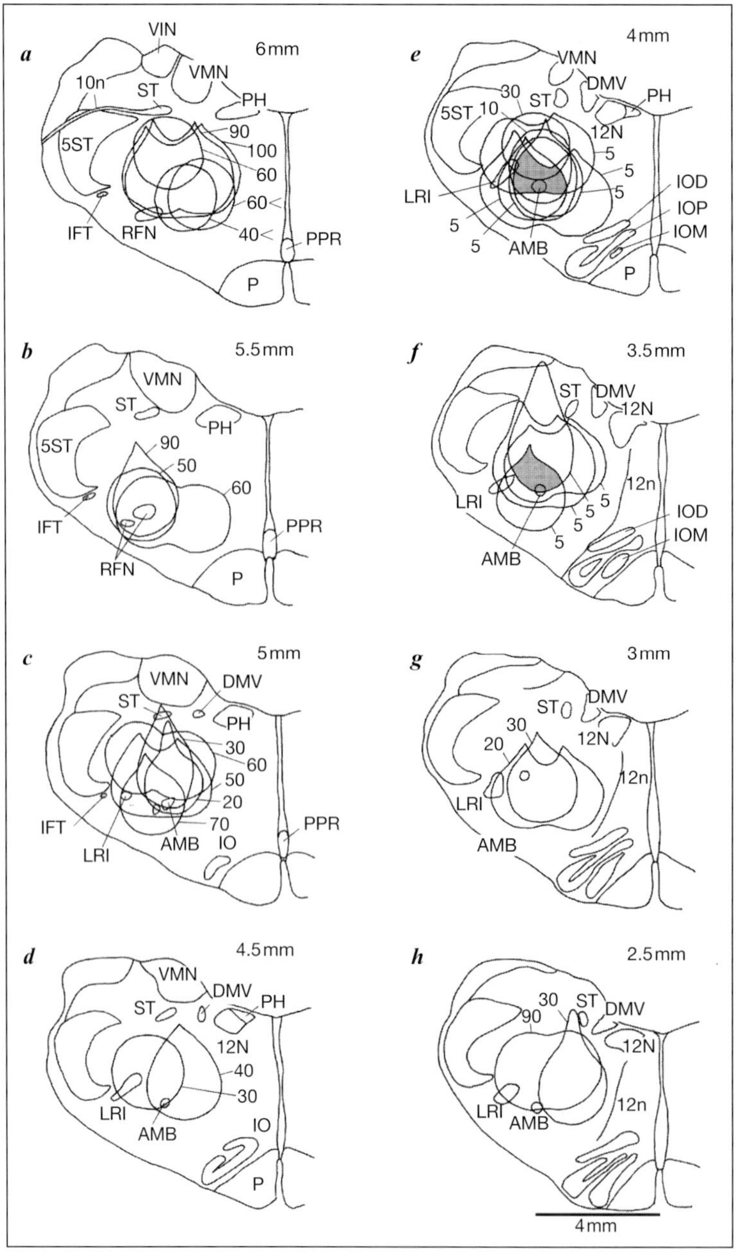
a
6mm
VIN
VMN
10n
ST
PH
5ST
90
100
60
60<
40<
IFT
RFN
PPR
P
b
5.5mm
VMN
ST
PH
5ST
90
50
60
IFT
RFN
PPR
P
c
5mm
VMN
DMV
ST
PH
30
60
50
20
70
IFT
LRI
AMB
IO
PPR
d
4.5mm
VMN
DMV
PH
ST
12N
40
30
LRI
AMB
IO
P
e
4mm
VMN
DMV
PH
30
5ST
10
ST
12N
5
5
5
LRI
5
5
5
AMB
IOD
IOP
IOM
P
f
3.5mm
ST
DMV
12N
12n
LRI
5
5
5
5
5
AMB
IOD
IOM
g
3mm
ST
DMV
30
20
12N
12n
LRI
AMB
h
2.5mm
30
ST
DMV
90
12N
12n
LRI
AMB
4mm

Table 1. Effects of 1-μl injections of various concentration solutions of GR205171 on retching response

Dose ng	Dogs, n	Effects of injection	
		disappeared[a]	continued[b]
10	2	2 (30, 30 min)	0
1.0	1	1 (5 min)	0
0.5	2	1 (20 min)	1 (70 min)
0.1	3	1 (20 min)	2 (60, 120 min)

[a,b]The number of dogs in which the retching response disappeared at the number of minutes indicated in the parentheses after the end of the injection and in which the retching response continued to appear throughout the observation period for the number of minutes indicated in the parentheses after the end of the injection, respectively.

same site to estimate the area for the diffusion of GR205171, and the areas stained by the dye are shown in figure 22.

After these injections of a concentrated solution (0.1 or 1 μg/ml) of GR205171, we performed 8 injections of diluted solutions into this area to define the threshold dose of the drug for abolition of the retching response in 7 dogs. The results are shown in table 1, and the effects of the injection of 1 μl of 1 μg/ml solution of GR205171 are shown in figure 24a–c. In this case, the retching response disappeared within 5 min after injection and reappeared 90 min later. Such recovery was also observed in another dog, i.e., the retching

Fig. 22. ***a–h*** Areas stained when pontamine sky blue was injected at the same site as GR205171 to estimate the area of the diffusion of GR205171. The stained area at the level at which the pipette track was recognized was transferred from the histological sections of each dog to these schematic sketches in accordance with landmarks, i.e., RFN, AMB, IOD, IOM, IOP, LRI, PPR, DMV, PH and 12N. The numeral attached to each stained area is the number of minutes after the injection at which the disappearance of the retching response was first recognized. The distance from the obex is shown above each schematic sketch. The shaded areas represent the medulla area commonly covered by the stained area at which an injection of GR205171 abolished a retching response within 5 min. 12n = Hypoglossal nerves; IOD = dorsal accessory nucleus of the inferior olive; IOM = medial accessory nucleus of the inferior olive; IOP = principal nucleus of the inferior olive; VIM = inferior vestibular nucleus; VMN = medial vestibular nucleus.

response disappeared 20 min after the injection (1 μl) of GR205171 (0.5 μg/ml) and reappeared 100 min later.

The Site of the Antiemetic Action of GR205171

The areas stained by pontamine sky blue, which was injected to estimate the area of the diffusion of GR205171, were distributed in the ventrolateral medulla from the level of the rostral part of the RFN to the rostral part of the nucleus ambiguus (fig. 22). Retching in response to vagal stimulation disappeared within 5 min after injection in the area adjacent to the semicompact part of the nucleus ambiguus (fig. 22e, f). This suppression was reproducible and its latency increased as the distance from the injection site to the semicompact part increased. Since the injection volume was <1 μl in all cases, this suppression is not thought to be due to the mechanical damage of neural tissue. All of the diffusion areas, in which retching disappeared within 5 min, commonly involved a medullar area dorsally adjacent to the semicompact part (fig. 22e, f). Suppression could be produced by the injection of 0.1 ng of GR205171. Since the threshold dose in the intravenous administration of GR205171 was 50 μg/kg in dogs [3, 65], 0.1 ng GR205171 may become subthreshold when it diffuses into >2 μg of medullar tissue. Therefore, the medullar area containing NK_1 receptor that is essential for inducing retching may not be much larger than 2 mm^3. Electrical stimulation of this medullar area has been shown to produce retching (see fig. 4). These results suggest that the site of the antiemetic action of NK_1 antagonists lies in a limited medullar area dorsally adjacent to the semicompact part of the nucleus ambiguus.

Possible Functions of the Site of the Antiemetic Action of GR205171

GR205171 injected into the area adjacent to the semicompact part of the nucleus ambiguus simultaneously suppressed the retching response and the maximum velocity of salivation attained during the prodromal phase of vomiting, as shown in figure 23. Similarly, augmented antral contractility during both the prodromal and retching phases had been shown to be suppressed along with retching by the intravenous administration of GR205171 in dogs [71].

These results suggest that the neurons in this medulla area with NK_1 receptors participate in the induction of both retching and autonomic prodromal signs. Therefore, we propose that this area be called the 'prodromal-sign center' of vomiting.

On the basis of many observations of gastrointestinal, cardiovascular and respiratory correlates of vomiting, Lang [72] proposed a hypothetical center which

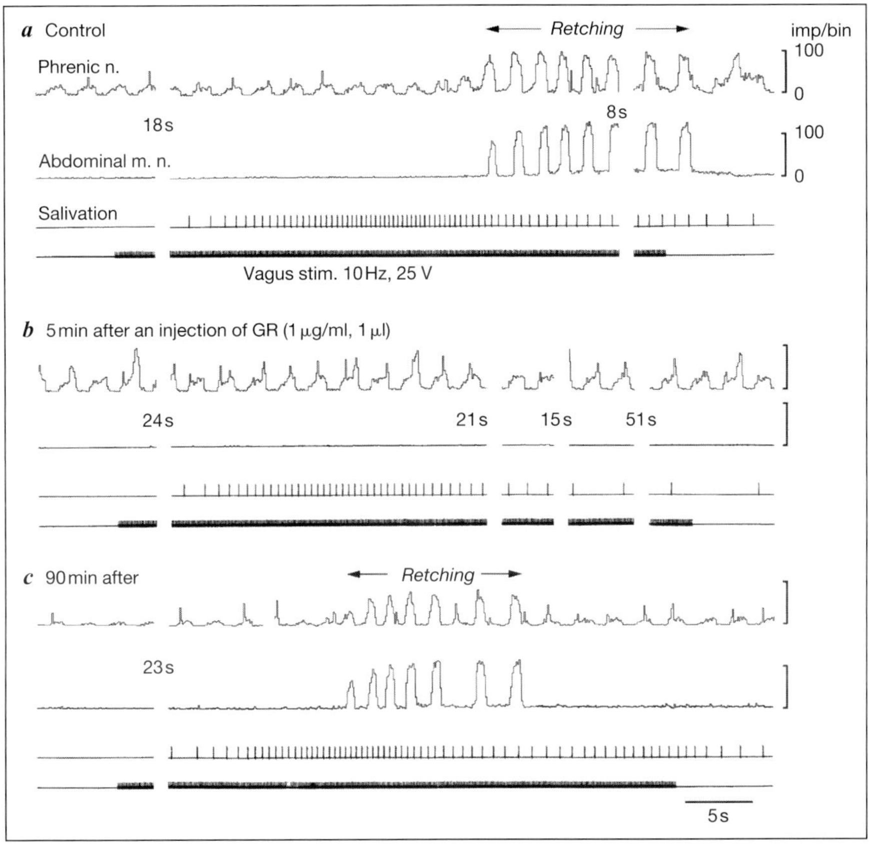

Fig. 23. Effects of the injection of smaller doses (0.1–10 ng) of GR205171 into the area adjacent to the semicompact part of the nucleus ambiguus on the retching response and salivation. ***a*** Control responses of retching and salivation. Salivation reached its maximum velocity before the onset of retching. ***b*** The retching response disappeared and the salivation velocity decreased 5 min after injection (1 μg/ml, 1 μl) of GR205171. ***c*** Both responses recovered 90 min after injection.

is activated by various emetic inputs and induces these correlates in parallel and somatomotor components of retching and expulsion sequentially. Furukawa and Okada [73] studied the perivomiting activity of parasympathetic postganglionic fibers to the submandibular gland and postulated a hypothetical center which they called 'the relay station of emetic afferents', which is activated by emetic inputs and in turn activates the salivary center and the CPG for vomiting, and then is

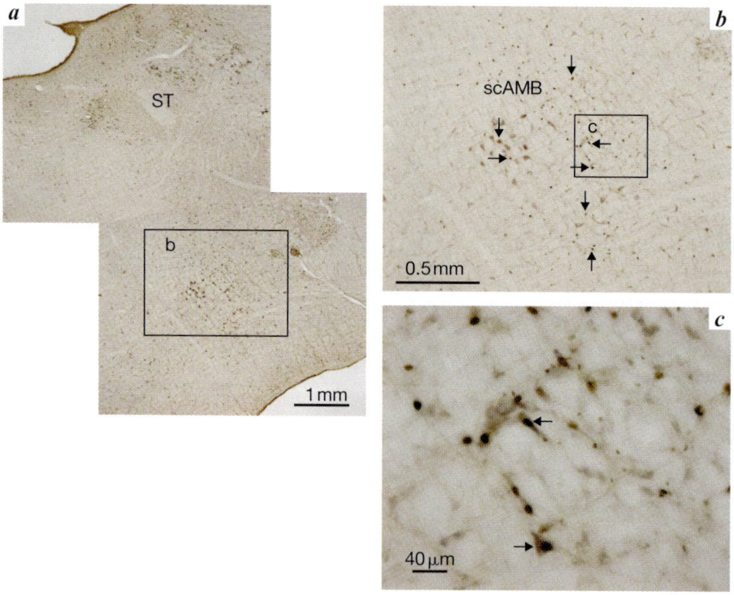

Fig. 24. C-fos- and NK_1 receptor-immunoreactive neurons in the prodromal-sign center area. ***a*** A section was obtained from a dog that had retched 10 times and was double-stained with antibodies to c-fos and NK_1 receptor. C-fos and NK_1 receptor immunoreactivity was realized by a nucleus stained black and a cell body stained brown, respectively. ***b***, ***c*** Higher-power magnification of area (b) in ***a*** and (c) in ***b***, respectively. The group of larger cells labeled scAMB is the semicompact part of the nucleus ambiguus. Arrows indicate cells that exhibited immunoreactivity for both c-fos and NK_1 receptor.

recurrently suppressed by the CPG. The prodromal-sign center in this study may be the neural tissue that comprises both of these hypothetical centers.

Immunohistochemical Identification of the Neurons Comprising the Prodromal-Sign Center

C-fos protein is well known to be expressed in neurons that have produced action potentials. Therefore, neurons of the prodromal-sign center are assumed to express c-fos protein and NK_1 receptors in dogs that have vomited repeatedly. Thus, we performed immunohistochemical staining of NK_1 receptors and c-fos protein in 4 dogs which had produced 300–400 retches during retching induced by 10 vagal stimulations at 5-min intervals [pers. unpubl. results]. A typical result is shown in figure 24. Fos-like immunoreactive neurons were distributed in the reticular area dorsolateral to the semicompact part of the nucleus ambiguus (fig. 24a, b) and neurons exhibiting both NK_1 receptor- and fos-like immunoreactivity were scattered in the nucleus and the reticular area in this preparation, as indicated by arrows (fig. 24b, c). Similar and more medial distributions of both immunoreactive neurons were recognized in other preparations.

Various respiratory neurons in the medullar area adjacent ventrolaterally to the semicompact part of the nucleus ambiguus are called the preBÖT and are hypothesized to play the central or key roles in the generation of respiratory rhythm as mentioned above. Recently, Gray et al. [44] demonstrated that rhythmogenic and other inspiratory neurons in the preBÖT express NK_1 receptor immunoreactivity. Consistently, NK_1 receptor-immunoreactive neurons were distributed in the medullar area ventrolateral to the semicompact part of the nucleus ambiguus in our preparations, and c-fos immunoreactivity coexists in some of these neurons. These neurons may be the inspiratory neurons in the preBÖT.

In our immunohistochemical preparations, another group of NK_1 receptor- and c-fos-immunoreactive neurons was distributed in the reticular area dorsal and dorsolateral to the nucleus ambiguus. The location and extent of this area may be consistent with the area that was commonly covered by the diffusion areas of GR205171 for injections by which retching was eliminated within 5 min. Therefore, these neurons are thought to comprise the prodromal-sign center.

Activities of Neurons in the Prodromal-Sign Center

The neurons comprising the prodromal-sign center are assumed to respond to vagal stimulation and produce firings appropriate to drive the CPG and a variety of autonomic activities in the prodromal phase of vomiting. Moreover, these neurons should exhibit a wind-up response to pulse-train vagal stimulation repeated at an appropriate frequency, since they should be activated via NK_1 receptors and the wind-up response of CPG neurons was suppressed by GR205171, as mentioned above (see fig. 20). To examine this assumption, we recorded unitary firings of 56 neurons in response to pulse-train vagal stimulation from the reticular area adjacent to the semicompact part of the nucleus ambiguus, and first examined their wind-up properties [74]. Only 11 of 56 neurons produced a wind-up response, as shown in figure 25a. Eight of the 11 neurons produced the firing pattern shown in figure 25b in response to the application of 10-Hz vagal stimulation to induce retching. The frequency of firing gradually increased during the prodromal phase and was close to maximal at the onset of retching. However, in contrast to CPG SH-type neurons, these neurons did not produce retching bursts. Firing was maintained at the maximum frequency during vagal stimulation and subsided after vagal stimulation was discontinued, and bursts that consisted of lower-frequency firings were produced synchronously with retching bursts of the phrenic and abdominal muscle nerves. The wind-up response and firings that progressed during 10-Hz vagal stimulation were suppressed by an intravenous application of GR205171 (fig. 25c, d).

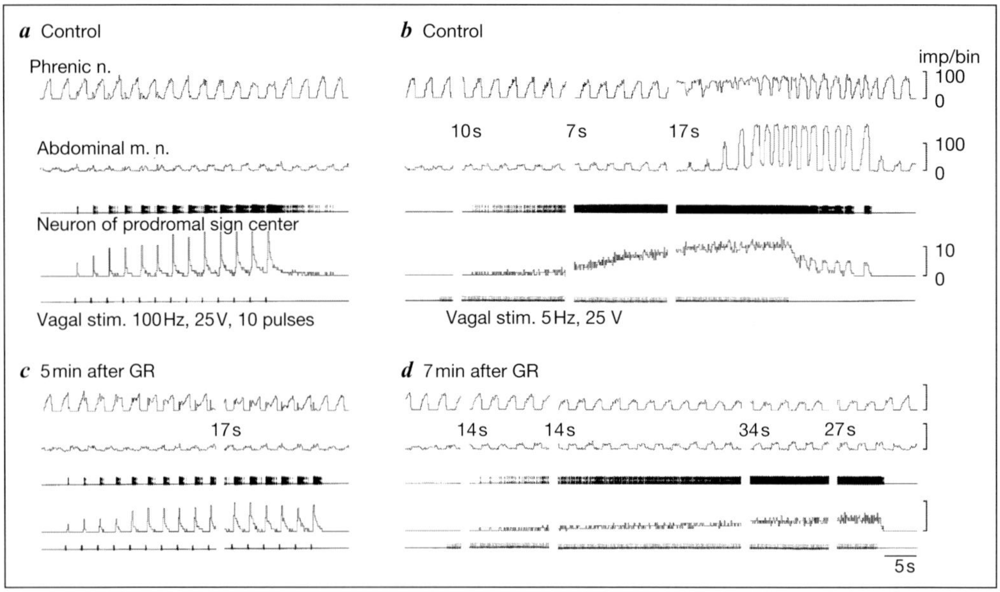

Fig. 25. Effects of GR205171 on the firing of a CPG-driving neuron in the prodromal-sign center in response to pulse-train (***a***, ***c***) and 5-Hz (***b***, ***d***) vagal stimulation. ***a***, ***b*** Control responses before intravenous injection of GR205171 (0.1 mg/kg). ***c***, ***d*** Responses obtained at the indicated number of minutes after injection.

The firings of neurons of this type during 10-Hz vagal stimulation and in the wind-up responses are very similar to those of CPG SH-type neurons with regard to their patterns and sensitivity to NK_1 receptor antagonist. Therefore, we thought that this type of neuron in the prodromal-sign center may drive CPG neurons and produce vomiting. Therefore, we called neurons of this type CPG-driving neurons.

The bursts produced synchronously with retching by CPG-driving neurons after the discontinuation of 5-Hz vagal stimulation suggest that CPG-driving neurons are activated by feedback inputs from CPG SH-type neurons, and that this positive-feedback circuit may contribute to the formation of gradually increasing firing of CPG-driving and CPG SH-type neurons.

Figure 26 shows the firing pattern exhibited by the 3 remaining neurons of the 11 neurons in response to the application of 10-Hz vagal stimulation to induce retching. Firing of neurons of this type gradually increased in frequency during the prodromal phase, similar to CPG-driving neurons, however, the firing decreased with the onset of retching (fig. 26a). This firing pattern is very similar to the temporal pattern in salivation, which developed during the prodromal phase and subsided with retching in decerebrate paralyzed dogs,

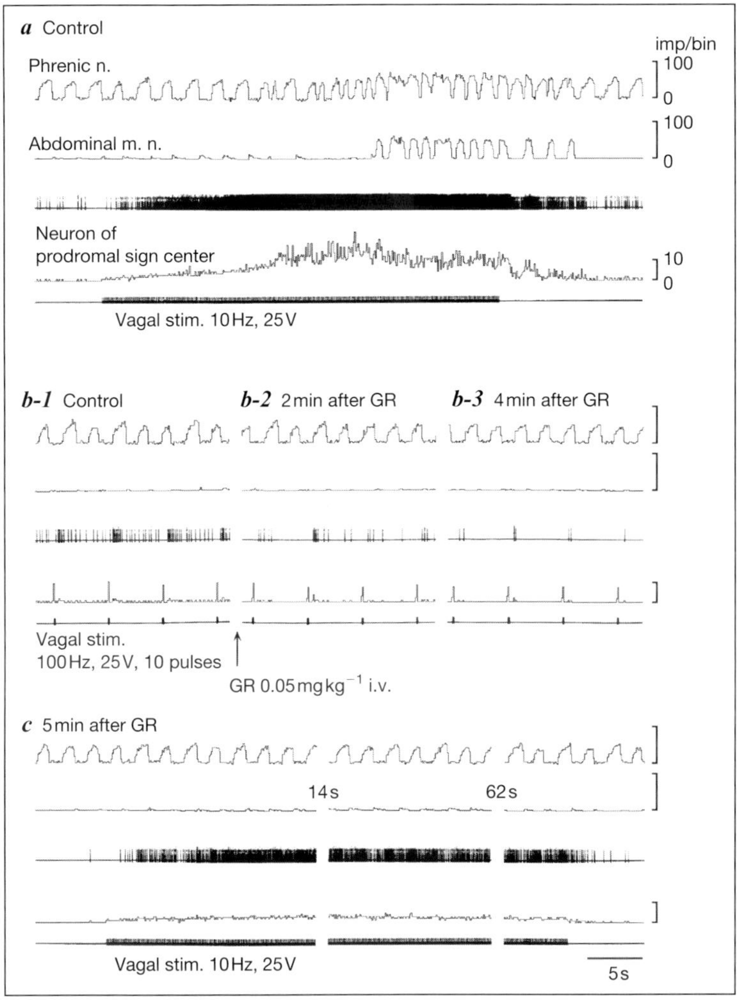

Fig. 26. Effects of GR205171 on the firing of a prodromal-sign neuron in the prodromal-sign center in response to 10-Hz (***a***, ***c***) and pulse-train (***b***) vagal stimulation. ***a***, ***b-1*** Control responses before intravenous injection of GR205171 (0.05 mg/kg). ***b-2***, ***b-3***, ***c*** Responses obtained at the indicated number of minutes after injection.

as shown in the examples in figures 7 and 24. Firings of neurons of this type in response to pulse-train and 10-Hz vagal stimulation were attenuated by an intravenous injection of GR205171 (fig. 26b, c). Since salivation produced with the retching response was suppressed by a microinjection of GR205171 in the prodromal-sign center area, we assumed that neurons of this type are

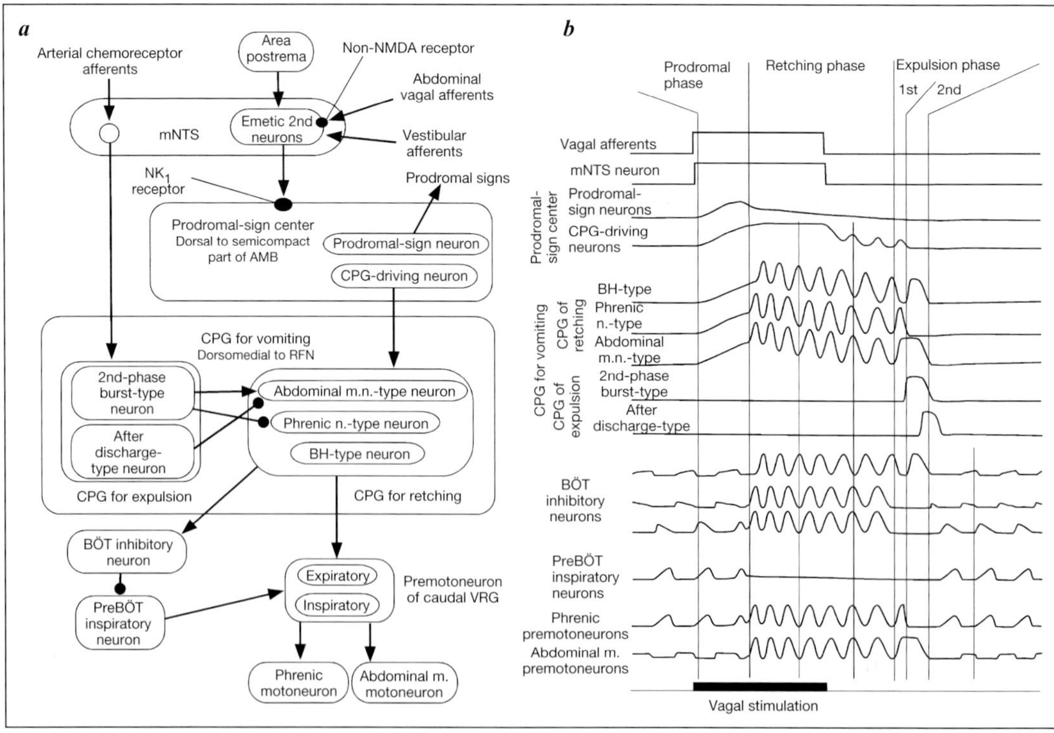

Fig. 27. Block diagram representing the central organization of emesis (***a***) and firing patterns of the neurons participating in the organization (***b***). Further explanations are listed in the Summary.

involved in prodromal signs of vomiting, and called such neurons prodromal-sign neurons.

Based on these results, we concluded that NK_1 receptor antagonists suppress prodromal signs and vomiting motions by blocking transmission from the final common pathway of various emetic afferents to the prodromal-sign center.

Summary

The above results suggest the following (fig. 27):

(1) Emetic vagal afferent activity is mediated by glutamate and non-NMDA receptors to the second-order neurons of the mNTS.

(2) Emetic inputs from the area postrema and the vestibular nerve also converge on the second-order neurons.

(3) Via NK_1 receptors, the second-order neurons activate the prodromal-sign center for vomiting, which is located in the reticular area dorsally adjacent to the semicompact part of the nucleus ambiguus. The prodromal-sign center consists of CPG-driving and prodromal-sign neurons.

(4) The prodromal-sign neurons produce an activity pattern that may be appropriate for inducing prodromal signs, e.g., salivation and gastric contraction.

(5) The CPG-driving neurons drive the CPG for retching, which is located in the reticular area dorsal to the RFN, and at least consist of SH- and BH-type neurons.

(6) The SH- and BH-type neurons produce vigorous rhythmic bursts concomitantly with retching bursts of the phrenic and abdominal muscle nerves and during the periods between retching bursts, respectively. Destruction of these neurons abolishes the retching response to vagal stimulation. Therefore, both types of neurons may generate retching rhythm by unknown processes.

(7) Most respiratory neurons in the reticular area ventrolateral to the RFN (Bötzinger complex, BÖT) produce SH- or BH-type retching bursts. These BÖT respiratory neurons are known to inhibit various respiratory neurons.

(8) Inspiratory neurons in the reticular area ventrolateral to the semicompact part of the nucleus ambiguus (pre-Bötzinger complex, preBÖT) are known to play an important role in the genesis of respiratory rhythm and to drive respiratory premotoneurons. Respiratory firings of most preBÖT inspiratory neurons are suppressed during retching, probably by BÖT SH- and BH-type respiratory neurons.

(9) One-third of the CPG SH-type neurons project to the ventrolateral reticular area (the ventral respiratory group, VRG) caudal to the obex, and may produce SH-type retching bursts in 40% of the inspiratory and 30% of the expiratory premotoneurons which are released from respiratory inputs from the respiratory rhythm generator.

(10) The SH-type retching bursts of the inspiratory and expiratory premotoneurons are sent to phrenic and abdominal muscle motoneurons, respectively, and produce retching motions.

(11) Pulmonary ventilation is almost completely suppressed during retching. This suppression may be caused by an absence of respiratory drive to respiratory motoneurons during retching and by contractions of the adductors of the glottis concomitant with retching bursts of the phrenic nerve.

(12) The interruption of pulmonary ventilation during retching causes hypercapnia and hypoxia, which activate at least arterial chemoreceptor afferents.

(13) Chemoreceptor afferents project through undefined pathways to the CPG area of retching, and drive the second-phase burst- and after discharge-type

neurons, which, respectively, produce vigorous bursts limited to the second phase of expulsion and at the end of expulsion bursts of the abdominal muscle nerve.

(14) The second-phase burst-type neurons may shorten the last retching burst of two-thirds of CPG SH-type neurons to form a phrenic n.-type expulsion burst, and prolong the burst of the remaining one-third to form an abdominal m.n.-type expulsion burst.

(15) After discharge-type neurons may terminate the expulsion burst of abdominal m.n.-type neurons, and may switch vomiting to respiration.

(16) The phrenic n.- and abdominal m.n.-type expulsion bursts of CPG SH-type neurons are sent to phrenic and abdominal muscle motoneurons via inspiratory and expiratory premotoneurons, respectively, and produce expulsive motion.

References

1 Bountra C, Bunce K, Dale T, Gardner C, Jordan C, Twissell D, Ward P: Anti-emetic profile of a non-peptide neurokinin NK_1 receptor antagonist, CP-99,994, in ferrets. Eur J Pharmacol 1993; 249:R3–R4.

2 Gardner CJ, Twissell DJ, Dale TJ, Gale JD, Jordan CC, Kilpatrick GJ, Bountra C, Ward P: The broad-spectrum anti-emetic activity of the novel non-peptide tachykinin NK_1 receptor antagonist GR203040. Br J Pharmacol 1995;116:3158–3163.

3 Gardner CJ, Armour DR, Beattie DT, Gale JD, Hawcock AB, Kilpatrick GJ, Twissell DJ, Ward P: GR205171: A novel antagonist with high affinity for the tachykinin NK_1 receptor, and potent broad-spectrum anti-emetic activity. Regul Pept 1996;27:45–53.

4 Rudd JA, Jordan CC, Naylor RJ: The action of the NK_1 tachykinin receptor antagonist, CP-99,994, in antagonizing the acute and delayed emesis induced by cisplatin in the ferret. Br J Pharmacol 1996;119:931–936.

5 Tattersall FD, Rycroft W, Hargreaves RJ, Hill RG: The tachykinin NK_1 receptor antagonist CP-99,994 attenuates cisplatin-induced emesis in the ferret. Eur J Pharmacol 1993;250: R5–R6.

6 Tattersall FD, Rycroft W, Francis B, Pearce D, Merchant K, MacLeod AM, Ladduwahetty T, Keown L, Swain C, Baker R, Cascieri M, Ber E, Metzger J, MacIntyre DE, Hill RG, Hargreaves RJ: Tachykinin NK_1 receptor antagonists act centrally to inhibit emesis induced by the chemotherapeutic agent cisplatin in ferrets. Neuropharmacology 1996;35:1121–1129.

7 Watson JW, Gonsalves SF, Fossa AA, McLean S, Seeger T, Obach S, Andrews PLR: The anti-emetic effects of CP-99,994 in the ferret and the dog: Role of the NK_1 receptor. Br J Pharmacol 1995;115:84–94.

8 Tattersall FD, Rycroft W, Hill RG, Hargreaves RJ: Enantioselective inhibition of apomorphine-induced emesis in the ferret by the neurokinin-1 receptor antagonist CP-99,994. Neuropharmacology 1994;33:259–260.

9 Gardner CJ, Twissell DJ, Gale JD, Kilpatrick GJ, Ward P: Effects of racemic CP-99,994, a tachykinin NK_1 receptor antagonist, on motion-induced emesis in *Suncus murinus*. Br J Pharmacol 1995;116:250.

10 Lucot JB, Obach RS, McLean S, Watson JW: The effect of CP-99994 on the responses to provocative motion in the cat. Br J Pharmacol 1997;120:116–120.

11 Borison HL, Wang SC: Functional localization of central coordinating mechanism for emesis in cat. J Neurophysiol 1949;12:305–313.

12 Wang SC, Borison HL: The vomiting center, a critical experimental analysis. Arch Neurol Psychiatry 1950;63:928–941.

13 Wang SC, Borison HL: The vomiting center: Its destruction by radon implantation in dog medulla oblongata. Am J Physiol 1951;164:520–526.
14 Miller AD, Wilson VJ: 'Vomiting center' reanalyzed: An electrical stimulation study. Brain Res 1983;270:154–158.
15 Fukuda H, Koga T: The Bötzinger complex as the pattern generator for retching and vomiting in the dog. Neurosci Res 1991;12:471–485.
16 Miller AD, Tan LK, Suzuki I: Control of abdominal and expiratory intercostal muscle activity during vomiting: Role of ventral respiratory group expiratory neurons. J Neurophysiol 1987;57: 1854–1866.
17 Ikeda M, Yamanaka Y: Electrical stimulation study on localization of the vomiting center (in Japanese). J Physiol Soc Jpn 1967;29:129–130.
18 Iwase Y, Ikeda M, Yoshikawa H: Induction of emesis by electrical stimulation of the surface of the medulla oblongata. J Physiol Soc Jpn 1967;29:712–713.
19 Miller AD, Nonaka S, Jakus J: Brain areas essential or non-essential for emesis. Brain Res 1994; 647:255–264.
20 Koga T, Qu R, Fukuda H: The central pattern generator for vomiting may exist in the reticular area dorsomedial to the retrofacial nucleus in dogs. Exp Brain Res 1998;118:139–147.
21 Fukuda H, Koga T: Non-respiratory neurons in the Bötzinger complex exhibiting appropriate firing patterns to generate the emetic act in dogs. Neurosci Res 1992;14:180–194.
22 Koga T, Fukuda H: Neurons in the nucleus of the solitary tract mediating inputs from emetic vagal afferents and the area postrema to the pattern generator for the emetic act in dogs. Neurosci Res 1992;14:166–179.
23 Benita M, Conde H: Effects of local cooling upon conduction and synaptic transmission. Brain Res 1972;36:133–151.
24 Reynolds DJ, Barber NA, Grahame-Smith DG, Leslie RA: Cisplatin-evoked induction of c-fos protein in the brainstem of the ferret: The effect of cervical vagotomy and the anti-emetic 5-HT_3 receptor antagonist granisetron (BRL 43694). Brain Res 1991;565:231–236.
25 Miller AD, Ruggiero DA: Emetic reflex arc revealed by expression of the immediate-early gene c-fos in the cat. J Neurosci 1994;14:871–888.
26 Boissonade FM, Sharkey KA, Davison JS: Fos expression in ferret dorsal vagal complex after peripheral emetic stimuli. Am J Physiol 1994;266:R1118–R1126.
27 Zaman S, Woods AJ, Watson JW, Reynolds DJ, Andrews PL: The effect of the NK_1 receptor antagonist CP-99,994 on emesis and c-fos protein induction by loperamide in the ferret. Neuropharmacology 2000;39:316–323.
28 Yamada Y, Tsukamoto G, Kobashi M, Sasaki A, Matsumura T: Abdominal vagi mediate c-Fos expression induced by X-ray irradiation in the nucleus tractus solitarii of the rat. Auton Neurosci 2000;83:29–36.
29 Ito H, Nishibayashi M, Kawabata K, Maeda S, Seki M, Ebukuro S: Immunohistochemical demonstration of c-fos protein in neurons of the medulla oblongata of the musk shrew (*Suncus murinus*) after veratrine administration. Exp Anim 2002;51:19–25.
30 Carpenter DO, Briggs DB, Strominger N: Responses of neurons of canine area postrema to neurotransmitters and peptides. Cell Mol Neurobiol 1983;3:113–126.
31 Yates BJ, Grelot L, Kerman IA, Balaban CD, Jakus J, Miller AD: Organization of vestibular inputs to nucleus tractus solitarius and adjacent structures in cat brain stem. Am J Physiol 1994;267: R974–R983.
32 Fukuda H, Koga T, Furukawa N, Nakamura E, Shiroshita Y: The tachykinin NK_1 receptor antagonist GR205171 abolishes the retching activity of neurons comprising the central pattern generator for vomiting in dogs. Neurosci Res 1999;33:25–32.
33 Koga T: Discharge patterns of bulbar respiratory neurons during retching and vomiting in decerebrate dogs. Jpn J Physiol 1991;41:233–249.
34 Miller AD, Nonaka S, Lakos SF, Tan LK: Diaphragmatic and external intercostal muscle control during vomiting: Behavior of inspiratory bulbospinal neurons. J Neurophysiol 1990;63: 31–36.
35 Koga T, Fukuda H: Bulbospinal augmenting inspiratory neurons may participate in contractions of the diaphragm during vomiting in decerebrate dogs. Neurosci Lett 1994;180:257–260.

36 Nonaka S, Miller AD: Behavior of upper cervical inspiratory propriospinal neurons during fictive vomiting. J Neurophysiol 1991;65:1492–1500.
37 Miller AD, Yates BJ: Evaluation of role of upper cervical inspiratory neurons in respiration, emesis and cough. Brain Res 1993;606:143–147.
38 Miller AD, Nonaka S, Jakus J, Yates BJ: Modulation of vomiting by the medullary midline. Brain Res 1996;737:51–58.
39 Ezure K: Synaptic connections between medullary respiratory neurons and considerations on the genesis of respiratory rhythm. Prog Neurobiol 1990;35:429–450.
40 Bianchi AL, Denavit-Saubie M, Champagnat J: Central control of breathing in mammals: Neuronal circuitry, membrane properties and neurotransmitters. Physiol Rev 1995;75:1–45.
41 Fukuda H, Koga T: Most inspiratory neurons in the pre-Bötzinger complex are suppressed during vomiting in dogs. Brain Res 1997;763:30–38.
42 Smith JC, Ellenberger HH, Ballanyi K, Richter DW, Feldman JL: Pre-Bötzinger complex: A brainstem region that may generate respiratory rhythm in mammals. Science 1991;254:726–729.
43 Connelly CA, Dobbins EG, Feldman JL: Pre-Bötzinger complex in cats: Respiratory neuronal discharge patterns. Brain Res 1992;590:337–340.
44 Gray PA, Rekling JC, Bocchiaro CM, Feldman JL: Modulation of respiratory frequency by peptidergic input to rhythmogenic neurons in the pre-Bötzinger complex. Science 1999;286:1566–1568.
45 Miller AD, Ezure K: Behavior of inhibitory and excitatory propriobulbar respiratory neurons during fictive vomiting. Brain Res 1992;578:168–176.
46 Miller AD, Nonaka S: Bötzinger expiratory neurons may inhibit phrenic motoneurons and medullary inspiratory neurons during vomiting. Brain Res 1990;521:352–354.
47 Koga T, Fukuda H: Descending pathway from the central pattern generator of vomiting. Neuroreport 1997;8:2587–2590.
48 Fukuda H, Koga T: Hypercapnia and hypoxia which develop during retching participate in the transition from retching to expulsion in dogs. Neurosci Res 1993;17:205–215.
49 Gold H, Hatcher RA: Studies on vomiting. J Pharmacol Exp Ther 1926;28:200–218.
50 Hukuhara, T, Okada H, Yamagami M: On the behavior of the respiratory muscles during vomiting. Acta Med Okayama 1957;11:117–125.
51 Tan LK, Miller AD: Innervation of periesophageal region of cat's diaphragm: Implication for studies of control of vomiting. Neurosci Lett 1986;68:339–344.
52 Grelot L, Barillot JC, Bianchi AL: Activity of respiratory-related oropharyngeal and laryngeal motoneurones during fictive vomiting in the decerebrate cat. Brain Res 1990;513:101–105.
53 Fukuda H, Koga T: Activation of peripheral and/or central chemoreceptors changes retching activities of Bötzinger complex neurons and induces expulsion in decerebrate dogs. Neurosci Res 1995;23:171–183.
54 Fukuda H, Koga T: Neuronal gagging activity patterns may be generated by neurons in the reticular area dorsomedial to the retrofacial nucleus in dogs. Exp Brain Res 1997;113:394–401.
55 Andrews P, Torii Y, Saito H, Matsuki N: The pharmacology of the emetic response to upper gastrointestinal tract stimulation in *Suncus murinus*. Eur J Pharmacol 1996;307:305–313.
56 Andrews PL, Okada F, Woods AJ, Hagiwara H, Kakaimoto S, Toyoda M, Matsuki N: The emetic and anti-emetic effects of the capsaicin analogue resiniferatoxin in *Suncus murinus*, the house musk shrew. Br J Pharmacol 2000;130:1247–1254.
57 Naylor RJ, Rudd JA: Pharmacology of ondansetron. Eur J Anaesthesiol 1992;9(suppl 6):3–10.
58 Shiroshita Y, Koga T, Fukuda H: Capsaicin in the fourth ventricle abolishes retching and transmission of emetic vagal afferents to solitary nucleus neurons. Eur J Pharmacol 1997;339:183–192.
59 Holzer P: Capsaicin: Selective toxicity for thin primary sensory neurons; in Herken H, Hucho F (eds): Selective Neurotoxicity. Berlin, Springer, 1992, pp 419–481.
60 Gamse R, Leeman SE, Holzer P, Lembeck F: Differential effects of capsaicin on the content of somatostatin, substance P and neurotensin in the nervous system of the rat. Naunyn Schmiedebergs Arch Pharmacol 1981;317:140–148.
61 Gamse R, Saria A, Lundberg JM, Theodorsson-Norheim E: Behavioral and neurochemical changes after intracisternal capsaicin treatment of the guinea pig. Neurosci Lett 1986;64:287–292.
62 South EH, Ritter RC: Capsaicin application to central or peripheral vagal fibers attenuates CCK satiety. Peptides 1988;9:601–612.

63 Helke CJ, Hill KM: Immunohistochemical study of neuropeptides in vagal and glossopharyngeal afferent neurons in the rat. Neuroscience 1988;26:539–551.
64 Thor KB, Hill KM, Harrod C, Helke CJ: Immunohistochemical and biochemical analysis of serotonin and substance P colocalization in the nucleus tractus solitarii and associated afferent ganglia of the rat. Synapse 1988;2:225–231.
65 Fukuda H, Koga T, Furukawa N, Nakamura E, Shiroshita Y: The tachykinin NK_1 receptor antagonist GR205171 prevents vagal stimulation-induced retching but not neuronal transmission from emetic vagal afferents to solitary nucleus neurons in dogs. Brain Res 1998;802:221–231.
66 Zaman S, Woods AJ, Watson JW, Reynolds DJ, Andrews PL: The effect of the NK_1 receptor antagonist CP-99,994 on emesis and c-fos protein induction by loperamide in the ferret. Neuropharmacology 2000;39:316–323.
67 Furukawa N, Hatano M, Fukuda H, Koga T: Non-N-methyl-*D*-aspartate receptors may mediate the transmission of emetic signals between visceral vagal afferents and the solitary nucleus in dogs. Neurosci Lett 1998;258:53–56.
68 Fukuda H, Nakamura E, Koga T, Furukawa N, Shiroshita Y: The site of the antiemetic action of tachykinin NK_1 receptor antagonists may exist in the medullary area adjacent to the semicompact part of the nucleus ambiguus. Brain Res 1999;818:439–449.
69 Powers BE, Beck ER, Gillette EL, Gould DH, LeCouter RA: Pathology of radiation injury to the canine spinal cord. Int J Radiat Oncol Biol Phys 1992;23:539–549.
70 Schultheiss TE, Kun LE, Ang KK, Stephens LC: Radiation response of the central nervous system. Int J Radiat Oncol Biol Phys 1995;31:1093–1112.
71 Furukawa N, Fukuda H, Hatano M, Koga T, Shiroshita Y: A neurokinin-1 receptor antagonist reduced hypersalivation and gastric contractility related to emesis in dogs. Am J Physiol 1998;275:G1193–G1201.
72 Lang IM: Digestive tract motor correlates of vomiting and nausea. Can J Physiol Pharmacol 1990;68:242–253.
73 Furukawa N, Okada H: Canine salivary secretion from the submaxillary glands before and during retching. Am J Physiol 1994;267:G810–G817.
74 Fukuda H, Koga T, Furukawa N, Nakamura E, Shiroshita Y: Firing patterns of neurons which may comprise the prodromal-sign center of vomiting in the reticular area dorsal to the semicompact part of the nucleus ambiguus. Jpn J Physiol 1999;49:S82.

Hiroyuki Fukuda
Department of Clinical Nutrition, Faculty of Medical Technology
Kawasaki University of Medical Welfare
Matsushima 288, Kurashiki 701-0193 (Japan)
Tel. +81 86 4621111, Fax +81 86 4633508, E-Mail hrfukuda@med.kawasaki-m.ac.jp

Donnerer J (ed): Antiemetic Therapy.
Basel, Karger, 2003, pp 78–97

Potential of Substance P Antagonists as Antiemetics

Pierre Diemunsch[a], *Laurent Grélot*[b]

[a]Service d'Anesthésie – Réanimation Chirurgicale, Hôpital de Hautepierre, Hôpitaux Universitaires de Strasbourg, Strasbourg et [b]UPRES EA 3285 – IFR Marey, Faculté des Sciences du Sport, Université de la Méditerranée, Aix-Marseille II, Marseille, France

An Overview of the Critical Concepts in Antiemetic Research

Vomiting (or emesis) has been from time immemorial a major concern in the practice of human medicine. In various ancient civilizations, the induction of vomiting with emetics was even used as a therapeutic tool [2]. At the present time, vomiting is viewed not as a therapy but more usually as a distressing side effect associated with various medical practices. Primarily, vomiting, the culminating sign of nausea, is a protective reflex occurring in a wide variety of vertebrates in response to the ingestion of a hazardous compound. This is clearly evidenced in the piglets by the bouts of vomiting induced by the intravenous or intraperitoneal administration of lipopolysaccharides, a component of the outer membrane of Gram-negative bacteria, which mimic the development of a septicemia or a bacterial infection in the gut [3]. However, in addition to this physiological response to the assimilation of bacterial toxins, vomiting can also occur in an extreme variety of circumstances which defy a simple description. In brief, emesis remains a critical problem during recovery from surgical procedures carried out under general anesthesia, in anticipation of anticancer cytotoxic therapy (i.e., psychological vomiting), and in other circumstances involving motion and vestibular disturbances (e.g., Ménière's disease). Lastly, vomiting can occur under natural circumstances where its benefits remain obscure (e.g., pregnancy sickness).

This chapter is based on the leading article published in *Drugs* in 2000 [1].

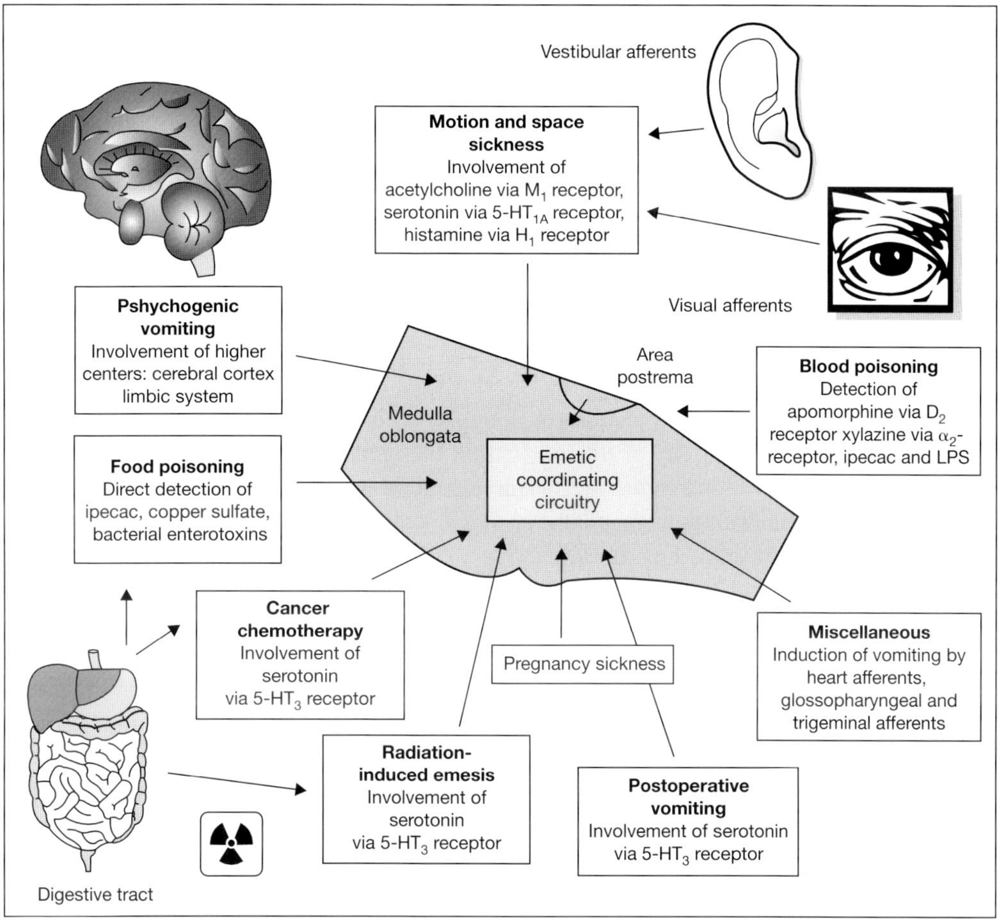

Fig. 1. Diagrammatic summary of different trigger inputs for vomiting. The emetic coordinating circuitry is located within the medulla oblongata of the brainstem. Area postrema is thought to contain a chemoreceptor trigger zone for vomiting. Neurotransmitters and receptor subtypes of major importance for eliciting vomiting are indicated for various inputs. D_2 = Dopamine type 2 receptor; H_1 = histamine type 1 receptor; M = muscarinic cholinergic, α_2 = α-adrenergic type 2 receptor; 5-HT = 5-hydroxytryptamine (i.e., serotonin). Adapted from Grélot and Miller [4].

The essential coordinating circuitry for producing the complex act of vomiting (i.e., the ill-localized 'vomiting center') is thought to be located within the medulla oblongata of the brainstem (fig. 1) [for review, see 4]. The numerous neurochemicals involved in that circuitry are not fully identified. The afferent systems triggering emesis release various neurotransmitters so that pharmacological agents exhibiting an effective antiemetic profile against one kind of vomiting can be ineffective against emesis induced by other stimuli. This is obvious in animal models of emesis, for which compounds acting as 5-HT_3 receptor antagonists exhibit potent antiemetic activity against acute chemotherapy-induced emesis but fail to block the emetic responses to other emetogens such as opioid and dopaminergic agonists, copper sulfate or motion. In humans, the introduction of selective 5-HT_3 receptor antagonists has incontestably represented a major advance in the control of acute emesis associated with antineoplastic cytotoxic therapy. However, there are still areas in emesis control where further improvement would be desirable, e.g., motion sickness and delayed cisplatin-induced emesis.

An attractive strategy to block emesis irrespective of its eliciting stimulus would be to treat patients (or animals) with a pharmacological agent able to depress the activity of neurons within the medullary emetic circuitry. Recently, chemicals acting as partial (buspirone and ipsaspirone) or full (8-OH-DPAT and SUN 8399) agonists of the 5-HT_{1A} receptor have shown broad-spectrum antiemetic activities in several species without marked adverse effects [for review, see 5]. Since tolerance to the antiemetic effects of 5-HT_{1A} receptor agonists did not develop rapidly, these compounds were expected to be clinically relevant. Unfortunately, most investigations in various animal models have shown that 5-HT_{1A} receptor agonists usually exhibit their weaker antiemetic properties against cisplatin-induced emesis, so that their clinical development rapidly appeared to be jeopardized. The pharmacological quest to make available a highly effective broad-spectrum antiemetic has led neuroscientists to investigate the role of neurotransmitter systems other than the serotonergic one and in particular the opioid system. Indeed, the neurotransmitter systems that opioid drugs modulate have been clearly implicated in emesis. In man, morphine and related analgesic drugs, both of which are poorly selective opioid receptor agonists, have the potential to increase the incidence of postoperative nausea and vomiting. However, compounds such as fentanyl or sufentanil activating mainly the μ subtype of opioid receptors have demonstrated a potent and broad-spectrum antiemetic activity in various animal species [for review, see 6]. Unfortunately, fentanyl enhances postoperative nausea and vomiting in human patients suggesting that species-related differences exist in the way opioid receptors modulate the emetic reflex. Since at the present time it is still difficult to dissociate pharmacologically the antiemetic properties of opioid receptor agonists from other unwanted side effects (e.g., respiratory depression), clinically accessible opioid drugs (agonists and antagonists) cannot be considered as promising antiemetics.

Recently, special attention has been focused on the role of neuropeptides, such as tachykinins, since they have been immunohistologically identified in the dorsal vagal complex of the ferret, an area regarded as essential in the elicitation of vomiting. The emetic action of the tachykinin substance P (SP) was described by Carpenter et al. [7] in 1984. Its putative role within the medullary emetic circuitry was first clearly pointed out by Andrews and Bhandari [8] in 1993. They demonstrated that resiniferatoxin, an ultra-potent capsaicin analogue, exhibits antiemetic properties in the ferret against both a centrally acting emetic chemical (i.e., loperamide) and two peripherally acting agents (i.e., radiation and copper sulfate). Andrews and Bhandari suggested that resiniferatoxin exerts its potent antiemetic activity by depleting SP at a central site in the emetic pathway. In such context, the development of potent and highly selective non-peptide NK_1 receptor antagonists, able to cross the blood-brain barrier to antagonize the central effects of SP, became crucial for providing powerful tools for investigation of the physiological role of SP in emesis. More generally, the development of these compounds was strongly demanded in several fields besides emesis, since the main indications foreseen for such drugs also included pain, migraine, rheumatoid arthritis, inflammatory bowel disease, asthma and chronic bronchitis.

The Tachykinins: Receptor Subtypes and Antagonists Relevant to Antiemetic Research

Tachykinins are members of a family of neuropeptides sharing the common C-terminal sequence Phe-Xaa-Gly-Leu-$MetNH_2$. In 1973, the term 'tachykinin' was coined by Ersparmer and Melchiorri to describe the rapid development of the contractile action produced by these peptides in smooth muscles. In mammals, the tachykinin family includes at least six chemicals among which SP, neurokinin A (NK_A) and neurokinin B (NK_B) are the most precisely characterized for their physiological effects. These peptides exert a plethora of biological activities through three G-protein-coupled receptor subtypes, identified as NK_1, NK_2 and NK_3 receptors [9]. According to the 'Montreal Nomenclature' [10], the NK_1 receptor is defined as the mediator of the biological activities encoded by the C-terminal sequence of tachykinins, for which SP is a more potent agonist than NK_A or NK_B. Since SP is believed to exert a key role within the central emetic circuitry, selective NK_1 receptor antagonists are expected to express potent antiemetic activity. A number of peptide-based NK_1 receptor antagonists with linear or cyclic sequences have been reported (e.g., spantide, L-668,169, GR82334, FR 113680, FK 224, etc.) but their inability to gain access to the central nervous system through the blood-brain barrier was though to represent a limitation to a putative clinical use for the control of emesis. In 1991, following a high throughput screening strategy, researchers at Pfizer Central Research (USA) disclosed the first non-peptide

NK_1 receptor antagonist: CP-96,345 ([(2S,3S)-*cis*-2-(diphenylmethyl)-N-[(2-methoxyphenyl)methyl]-1-azabicyclo[2,2,2]octan-3-amine]), and subsequently reported the series of piperidines exemplified by CP-99,994 ((2S,3S)-*cis*-3-(2-methoxybenzylamino)-2-phenylpiperidine)dihydrochloride) [11]. Succeeding intensive chemical and pharmacological research conducted in all the major 'drug companies' led to the disclosure of a wide variety of non-peptide NK_1 receptor antagonists belonging to different chemical classes, i.e., piperidines, perhydroisoindolones, quinuclidines, tryptophan derivatives and steroids [12]. The most recently synthesized compounds are highly selective, exhibiting nanomolar or subnanomolar affinities for human NK_1 receptors expressed in various cells.

When comparing the pharmacological effects of various NK_1 receptor antagonists, it is essential to keep in mind that species-related differences exist in the primary sequence of the NK_1 receptor protein [13]. These variations, which do not affect the agonist efficacy, determine dramatic species-related variations in the potency of non-peptide antagonists. For instance, the prototypical NK_1 receptor antagonist CP-96,345 binds with subnanomolar affinity to bovine brain, but it is 35-fold less active in displacing [^{3}H]-SP binding to rat brain. Therefore, the antiemetic efficiency of a given compound in an animal model is not conclusively predictive of its potentiality in humans. In addition, several factors can preclude a number of highly selective potent NK_1 receptor antagonists from being of clinical utility. Precisely, some of these pharmacological agents have been reported to bind without any enantio-selectivity with L-type Ca^{2+} channels irrespective of the species. For instance, CP-96,345 presents an equal affinity for Ca^{2+} channels and NK_1 receptors in the rat, so that many of the behavioral effects in that species might be due to the blockade of ion channels. Consequently, it is essential to be cautious in interpreting the results using a NK_1 receptor antagonist [14]. In addition, this implies that NK_1 compounds selected for clinical trials must exhibit the lowest 'non-specific' binding to Ca^{2+} channels to avoid severe cardiovascular adverse effects. Obviously, this point has been taken into account for chemicals administered during preliminary clinical trials, since CP-122,721 ([(+)-(2S,3S)-3-(2-methoxy-5-trifluoromethoxybenzyl)amino-2-phenylpiperidine]), a potent and non-competitive antagonist agent, exhibits a high affinity for human NK_1 receptors but a moderate one for Ca^{2+} channels [15]. Similarly, GR205171 ([2-methoxy-5-(5-trifluoromethyl-tetrazol-1-yl)-benzyl]-(2S-phenyl-piperidin-3S-yl)amine), another compound tested in human patients, has a subnanomolar affinity to human NK_1 receptors (expressed in CHO cells), and it is at least 1,000-fold selective with respect to non-tachykinin receptors and ions channels [16]. Finally, the affinity for the human NK_1 receptor of a third compound tested clinically: L-754,030 ([2-(R)-(1-(R)-(3,5-bis(trifluoromethyl) phenylethoxy)-3(S)-(4fluoro)phenyl-4-(3-oxo-1,2,4-triazol-5-yl)methylmorpholine]), is similar to that of CP-122,721 and that of GR205171, whereas its affinity for the Ca^{2+} channel is negligible (i.e., $IC_{50} > 1\ \mu M$ [17]). The final two requirements for the clinical development of a NK_1 receptor antagonist are the long-lasting efficacy and the oral biodisponibility of the compound. Thus, the poor orally active phenylpiperidine CP-99,994 was further chemically optimized but superseded in development by both CP-122,721 and GR205171.

Antiemetic Activity of NK_1 Receptor Antagonists in Animal Models

During the last 6 years, the antiemetic profile of 17 compounds have been evaluated and fully described to our knowledge in 26 publications. The emetic challenges were conducted in the ferret, house musk shrew (*S. murinus*), cat, dog, and more recently, the piglet, using 14 different emetogens (table 1). The experimental procedures in these numerous studies presented such marked differences concerning the choice of the animal species, the way to elicit vomiting (i.e., with chemicals, motion, X-irradiation, electrical stimulation of afferent pathways), and the nature, dose, route and timing of administration of the different NK_1 receptor antagonists, that a detailed description of the results would be tedious. However, the common conclusion brought forward in these studies was that NK_1 receptor antagonists displayed an unprecedentedly potent, and usually long-lasting, high antiemetic activity. This high level efficacy was observed irrespective of the route of administration (i.e., p.o., s.c., i.p., i.v., i.c.v.) with drugs able to penetrate the central nervous system.

A concise history of the major results leading to the clinical development of the NK_1 receptor antagonists as antiemetics is summarized below. The idea that these compounds could represent a new class of therapeutic agents for the treatment of emesis was first published by Bountra et al. [18] in 1993. They showed, in the ferret model, that an i.p. administration of 3 mg/kg of CP-99,994 (racemic) reduced by 84 and 96% (i.e., the lesser and major effects observed in this study) the total number of retches induced by morphine (0.5 mg/kg, s.c., 3-hour trial) and cyclophosphamide (200 mg/kg, i.p., 7-hour trial), respectively. Tattersall et al. [19] confirmed these results soon after, and demonstrated that the nearly complete control of the acute emetic response to cisplatin (10 mg/kg, i.p.) achieved in the ferret with (+) CP-99,994 (3 mg/kg, i.v.) resulted most likely from a stereo-specific blockade of NK_1 receptors, since CP-100,263 (i.e., the inactive enantiomer) was totally ineffective at the same dose. Subsequently, the optimized chemicals GR203040 [20], CP-122,721 [21] and then GR205171 [22] have proven more potent antiemetic potentialities than CP-99,994. In the

Table 1. Record of the NK_1 receptor antagonists which have proved potent antiemetic activities in animals against various emetogens

NK_1 receptor antagonists (route of administration)	Animal species	Emetogens	References
CP-99,994 (s.c., i.p., i.v.)	F, S, D, C	a + d-CDDP, $CuSO_4$, cyclophosphamide, ipecac, morphine, apomorphine, irradiation, nicotine, loperamide, ethanol, motion, elect X	18, 19, 25–27, 30, 32, 37, 59, 60
CP-122,721	F	a-CDDP, $CuSO_4$, ipecac, loperamide,	21
GR 203040 (s.c., i.v.)	F, S, D	a-CDDP, $CuSO_4$, cyclophosphamide, ipecac, morphine, irradiation	20, 37
GR 205171 (Vofopitant) (s.c., i.v.)	F, S, D, P	a + d-CDDP, irradiation, elect X, LPS	16, 23, 61
L-741,671 (i.v., i.c.v.)	F	a-CDDP	43
L-742,694 (i.v.)	F	a-CDDP	37
L-743,310 (i.c.v.)	F	a-CDDP	43
L-754,030 (MK-0869) (i.v., p.o.)	F	a + d-CDDP, morphine, apomorphine	17, 63
L-758,298 (i.v.)	F	a-CDDP	63
RP67580 (i.p.)		nicotine	59, 60
PD 154075 (Cl-1021; i.p.)	F	a + d-CDDP	28
RPR 100893 (Dapitant) (i.v.)	F	a-CDDP	37
HSP-117 (i.c.v.)	F	$CuSO_4$, morphine	44, 62
SR 140333 (Nolpitantium) (i.c.v.)	P	a-CDDP	Grélot et al., unpubl. data
Sendide (s.c.)	F	a-CDDP	45

F, S, D, C, and P: ferret, *S. murinus*, dog, cat and piglet, respectively; a + d-CDDP, acute and delayed cisplatin-induced vomiting; $CuSO_4$, copper sulfhate; elect X, electrical stimulation of the abdominal vagus nerves; LPS, lipopolysaccharides (bacterial endotoxins); s.c., subcutaneous; i.p., intraperitoneal; i.v., intravenous; i.c.v., intracerebroventricular; p.o., *per os*. [references in text and 59–63].

ferret, CP-122,721 (0.3 or 1 mg/kg, s.c.) abolished the emetic response to copper sulfate, loperamide, ipecac syrup and cisplatin. In fact, this chemical antagonized the acute emetic response to cisplatin during a 2-hour trial with an ID_{50} of 0.03 mg/kg. The long-lasting antiemetic effects of NK_1 receptor antagonists were first reported by Gardner et al. [20]. Indeed, GR205171 (0.3 mg/kg, s.c.) promptly abolished the cisplatin-induced emesis for a 4-hour period, and then minimal emesis occurred during the subsequent 20-hour period. A similar observation was made in the piglet, for which a single administration of GR205171 (1 mg/kg, i.v.) reduced by 91 and 86% the number of emetic events produced during the acute and delayed phases of cisplatin-induced emesis, respectively [23]. Moreover, a 1-mg/kg dose administered at the transition between the acute and delayed phases abolished the delayed emetic response to cisplatin for at least 44 h [21]. In that species, the long-lasting antiemetic effect of GR205171 was surprising, since the pharmacokinetic study revealed that GR205171 (1 mg/kg, i.v.) has a fairly short plasma half-life (3.4 ± 0.8 h). The ability to achieve a sustained blockade of central tachykinin NK_1 receptors in the absence of high plasma drug concentrations in vivo was also reported in a pain model (i.e. in the formalin paw test) in the gerbil with L-733,060 [24]. This might suggest that these two NK_1 receptor antagonists are rapidly distributed to their sites of action from where there are slowly eliminated. This property is advantageous since it strongly limits the occurrence of unwanted nonspecific effects in peripheral tissues (e.g., blockade of Ca^{2+} channels) associated with high plasma concentration of the drugs.

Several NK_1 receptor antagonists displayed a potent activity, in animal models, against vomiting elicited by some emetogens which are still difficult to control in human patients. Thus, CP-99,994, PD 154075 and GR205171 provided a satisfactory control of the delayed emetic response to cisplatin in both the piglet and ferret [21, 25–28]. The ultra-potent efficacy against both acute and delayed cisplatin-induced emesis has been clearly evidenced in the laboratory of one of the authors (L.G.). Comparison with results from our previously published and unpublished studies performed on more than 600 piglets demonstrated that GR205171 has the highest ratio of antiemetic activity/dose of any compound ever tested in our experimental model (i.e., cisplatin-induced emesis [29]). This is demonstrated clearly in figure 2. The clinical potential of NK_1 receptor antagonists can also be extended to provocative motion (CP-99,994 [23, 24, 30], GR203040 [18]), post-anesthesia-induced emesis (GR205171 [31]), and ethanol-induced vomiting (CP-99,994 [32]). Finally, in addition to the antiemetic effect, tachykinin NK_1 receptor antagonists may have potential in the treatment of drug-induced conditioned aversive behavior and nausea [21, 33].

Putative Site of Action of NK_1 Receptor Antagonists

As mentioned above, the putative involvement of SP within the central emetic circuitry was proposed by Andrews and Bhandari [8], on the basis of the emetic action of resiniferatoxin in ferrets. This was confirmed by Matsuki et al. [34] and

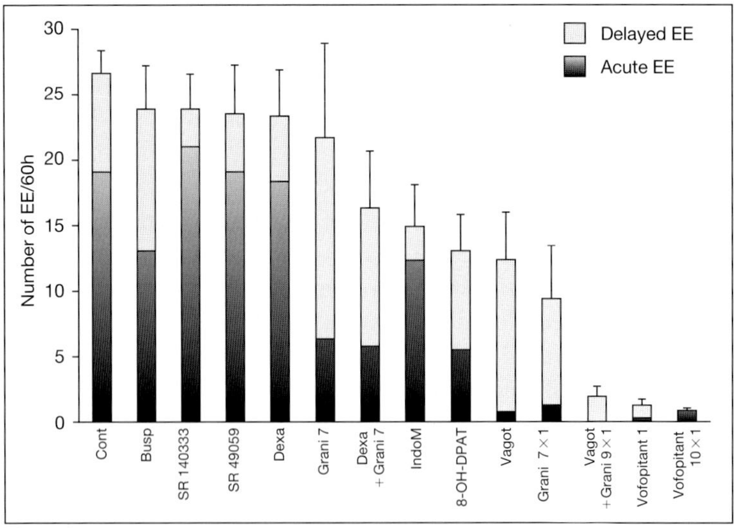

Fig. 2. Antiemetic properties of various pharmacological treatments and surgical procedures in piglets receiving a single high dose of cisplatin (CDDP, i.v., 5.5 mg/kg ≈ 125 mg/m^2), and then observed continuously for 60 h [details in 29]. EE, emetic events. Columns from left to right: Cont, control animals (n = 35); Busp, buspirone (i.e., a 5-HT_{1A} receptor agonist, 15 mg/kg 15 min prior to CDDP, n = 7); SR 140333, a selective tachykinin NK_1 receptor antagonist (3 mg/kg 15 min prior to CDDP, n = 8). SR 49059, a selective vasopressin V1a receptor antagonist (3 mg/kg 15 min prior to CDDP, n = 7). Dexa, dexamethasone (i.e., a corticosteroid, 20 mg 15 min prior to CDDP, and 10 mg 12 and 36 h after CDDP, n = 7); Grani 7, granisetron (i.e., a selective 5-HT_3 receptor antagonist, 7 mg/kg, n = 7); Dexa + Grani 7, association of dexamethasone and granisetron 7 (n = 7); IndoM, indomethacin (i.e., a cyclooxygenase inhibitor, 10 mg/kg 1 h prior to CDDP, and then 15 and 39 h after CDDP, n = 7); 8-OH-DPAT (i.e., a selective 5-HT_{1A} receptor agonist, 1 mg/kg 15 min prior to CDDP, n = 7); Vagot, bilateral cervical bivagotomy performed 3–4 days prior CDDP (n = 6). Grani 7 × 1, granisetron (1 mg/kg given every 5 h during the first 30 h post-CDDP, n = 7); Vagot + Grani 9 × 1, association of Vagot and granisetron (1 mg/kg given every 5 h from the 15th to 60th h post-CDDP, n = 6); Vofopitant 1, a selective tachykinin NK_1 receptor antagonist (GR 205171, 1 mg/kg 15 min prior to CDDP); Vofopitant 10 × 1 (GR 205171, 1 mg/kg given each 6 h throughout the 60-hour observation period). The bar above each box indicates SEM of the cumulative (acute + delayed) severity of the emetic crisis. The highest control of emesis was achieved by using the NK_1 receptor antagonist Vofopitant (GR 205171). Note that SR 140333 was totally ineffective probably due to poor penetration in the central nervous system. Results from Milano et al. [29], Grélot et al. [23, 64] and Girod et al. [65].

Shiroshita et al. [35], who demonstrated that the capsaicin analogue (s.c. in *S. murinus* and i.c.v. in dog) first induced transient emesis or retching, and then blocked these emetic responses to radiation and copper sulfate, and afferent vagal electrical stimulation, respectively. In a converging point of view, the broad-spectrum antiemetic profile of the NK_1 receptor antagonists suggests that they might act principally at central sites. This assertion has been conclusively supported by studies demonstrating that peptide-based potent NK_1 receptor antagonists (i.e., GR82334, sendide, spantide II and FK 888), unable to block vomiting when administered intravenously, appear much more effective when injected by an i.c.v. route [20, 36, 37]. Similarly, SR140333, a highly selective non-peptide compound, inactive at the dose of 3 mg/kg (i.v.) against the acute emetic response to cisplatin in both ferrets [35] and piglets, reduced by 90% this response in the latter species when applied centrally (1.5 mg, i.c.v. [Grélot et al., unpubl. data]).

The nucleus tractus solitarius (NTS) neurons lying ventrally to the area postrema in the so-called subnucleus gelatinosus are very strongly suspected to trigger the emetic act [2]. This medullary area is a converging site for projections arising from the area postrema, and the vestibular and vagal afferents [38]. NTS is a good candidate for the site of action of NK_1 receptor antagonist. Extensive SP-like immunoreactivity has been identified in this region and the tachykinins have been proposed as transmitters in vagal afferents [39–41]. Using in vitro autoradiography, Watson et al. [25, 26] showed that the high density [^{3}H]-SP binding in the NTS was displaced by CP-99,994. Similarly, recent PET studies in rhesus monkeys have demonstrated that peripherally administered ^{11}C-labelled GR205171 distributes into brain regions consistent with specific binding to NK_1 receptors [42]. Injection of 30 μg of CP-99,994, L-741,671 or L-743,310 into the vicinity of the NTS inhibited cisplatin-induced emesis in the ferret [43]. Moreover, the SP-induced discharge of action potentials of single NTS neuron recorded in slices of ferret brainstem is inhibited by HSP-117, an NK_1 receptor antagonist with potent antiemetic activity [44]. Altogether, these results suggest, but do not demonstrate, that NK_1 receptor antagonists exert their main antiemetic action by depressing the neural activity of NTS neurons, i.e., within the central emetic circuitry. However, a possible contribution from peripheral sites to this potent antiemetic effect should not be ignored. Indeed, injection of sendide (3 mg/kg, i.v.), a peptide-based drug, is active against cisplatin-induced emesis in the ferret likely through a gastrointestinal tract site of action [45]. The proposed mechanism underlying this effect might involve a blockade of the NK_1 receptors located on vagal terminals in the gut. This would decrease the intensity of the emetic afferent message to the medullary emetic circuitry [43]. In that view, the peripheral effect of NK_1 receptor antagonists might resemble that of the 5-HT_3 receptor antagonists on the serotonergic activation of vagal terminals. However, this hypothesis remains to be demonstrated since the possibility of a non-specific interaction of sendide on 5-HT_3 receptors or Ca^{2+} channels located on vagal terminals was not investigated.

In man as well as in animals, the numerous transmitters involved in the emetic process accounts for the incomplete efficacy of single-drug therapies for nausea and vomiting of various etiologies. Maybe due to their central role on a potential, final common pathway, NK_1 receptor antagonists have offered a broader spectrum antiemetic activity than 5-HT_3 receptor antagonists, dopamine receptor antagonists, anticholinergic agents, and corticosteroïds. It seems likely that, as was observed for pain management [46], combining medications from different classes may optimize the efficacy of NK_1 receptor antagonists for treatment of nausea and vomiting.

Data from the published clinical studies seem to confirm the usefulness of this class of drugs in man, in two types of indications: cancer chemotherapy-induced nausea and vomiting (CINV) and postoperative nausea and vomiting (PONV). Conversely, the NK_1 receptor antagonists were shown to be ineffective in motion-induced nausea, either alone or in combination with a 5-HT_3 receptor antagonist [47].

The five investigational drugs studied initially are: GR205171 (Glaxo-Wellcome), CP-122,721 (Pfizer), CJ-11,974 (Pfizer), L-754,030 (Merck) and its prodrug L-758,298. GR205171 is a potent and selective NK_1 receptor antagonist with high affinity for the human NK_1 receptor and potent antiemetic activity in various animal models of emesis. It is a high clearance compound (979–1,821 $ml \cdot min^{-1}$) with a large volume of distribution (412–888 l) and a moderately long elimination half-life of 5–8 h in man. CJ-11,974 is a selective NK_1 receptor antagonist with a K_i of 0.4 nm/l and which proved highly active in the ferret model of emesis. L-754,030, a trisubstituted morpholine acetal, is a selective NK_1 receptor antagonist also very active in animal models. L-754,030 has been studied in man directly and after administration of its prodrug L-758,298.

NK_1 Receptor Antagonists in Chemotherapy-Induced Nausea and Vomiting

Few studies have dealt with the prevention of acute and/or delayed CINV after high dose cisplatin in cancer patients (table 2).

Despite the small numbers of patients included, the design of the trials allowed comparison between arms consisting respectively of either a placebo, a NK_1 receptor antagonist, a 5-HT_3 antagonist, the association of a 5-HT_3 antagonist plus dexamethasone, or the association of a NK_1 receptor antagonist with either dexamethasone alone, or a 5-HT_3 antagonist plus dexamethasone.

In the study arms where a NK_1 receptor antagonist was *administered alone*, it proved either ineffective, or not superior to ondansetron for the control of

Table 2. NK_1 receptor antagonists for control of emesis: human studies

Authors	Type of study	Type of emesis	NK_1 receptor antagonist	Subjects, n	Associations	Outcomes
Fumoleau et al. [48]	MC, DB, R, P	Prevention of acute CINV after cisplatin ≥80 mg/m^2	GR205171 5 or 25 mg i.v.	4/16	None	Ineffective at 24 h
			GR205171 5 mg i.v.	7/16	Ondansetron 8 mg IV	No emesis: 5/7 at 24 h and no nausea: 2/7 at 24 h
			GR205171 25 mg i.v.	5/16	Ondansetron 8 mg IV	No emesis: 5/5 at 24 h and no nausea: 4/5 at 24 h
Diemunsch et al. [56, 58]	MC, DB, R, P, PC	Treatment of established PONV after gynecological surgery	GR205171 25 mg i.v.	36	None	GR205171 > to placebo for complete control of emesis and nausea
Kris et al. [50]	Open label, P	Prevention of acute and delayed CINV after cisplatin ≥80 mg/m^2	CP-122,721 50–200 mg PO	17	None (7/17)	15% no acute emesis and 86% no delayed emesis
					Ondansetron + dexamethasone (10/17)	100% no acute emesis and 80% no delayed emesis
Gesztesi et al. [54], *see also* Gesztesi et al. [55]	DB, R	Prevention of PONV after gynecological surgery	None	22/68	Ondansetron 4 mg IV	No differences for nausea scores but less emetic episodes in groups treated with CP-122,721
			CP-122,721 200 mg PO	22/68	None	
			CP-122,721 200 mg PO	24/68	Ondansetron 4 mg IV	
Hesketh et al. [57]	MC, DB, R, P, PC	Prevention of acute and delayed CINV after cisplatin ≥100 mg/m^2	CJ-11,974 100 mg PO twice a day, 5 days or placebo	61	Granisetron 10 μg/kg IV + dexamethasone 20 mg IV	No emesis on day 1: 85.7% ($p = 0.090$ vs. placebo) No emesis days 2–5: 67.8% ($p = 0.042$ vs. placebo)
Navari et al. [52]	MC, DB, R, PC	Prevention of acute and delayed CINV after cisplatin ≥70 mg/m^2	L-754,030 400 mg PO before cisplatin and 300 mg on days 2–5	54	Granisetron 10 μg/kg IV + dexamethasone 20 mg PO before cisplatin	No emesis on day 1: 93% ($p < 0.001$ vs. placebo) No emesis days 2–5: 82% ($p < 0.001$ vs. placebo)

Table 2. (continued)

Authors	Type of study	Type of emesis	NK_1 receptor antagonist	Subjects, n	Associations	Outcomes
			L-754,030 400 mg PO before cisplatin and placebo on days 2–5	54		No emesis on day1: 93% ($p < 0.001$ vs. placebo) No emesis days 2–5: 78% ($p < 0.001$ vs. placebo)
			None	51		No emesis on day 1: 67% No emesis days 2–5: 33%
Cocquyt et al. [49]	MC, DB, R	Prevention of acute and delayed CINV after cisplatin ≥50 mg/m^2	L-758,298: 60 or 100 mg i.v. before cisplatin	30	None	L-758,298 is almost as effective as ondansetron in acute emesis (day 1), and superior to ondansetron against delayed emesis (days 2–7)
			None	23	Ondansetron: 32 mg IV before cisplatin	
Campos et al. [53]	MC, DB, R	Prevention of acute and delayed CINV after cisplatin ≥70 mg/m^2	None	90	Granisetron 10 μg/kg IV + dexamethasone 20 mg PO before cisplatin + placebo on days 2–5	No emesis on day 1: 57% No emesis days 2–5: 29%
			L-754,030 (MK-0869): 400 mg PO before cisplatin + 300 mg PO on days 2–5	86	Granisetron 10 μg/kg IV + dexamethasone 20 mg PO before cisplatin	Best results with the three drugs: no emesis on day 1: 80% ($p < 0.1$ vs. no L-754,030); no emesis days 2–5: 63% ($p < 0.1$ vs. no L-754,030)
			L-754,030: 400 mg PO evening before + before cisplatin + 300 mg PO on days 2–5	89	Dexamethasone 20 mg PO before cisplatin	No emesis on day 1: 46% No emesis days 2–5: 51% ($p < 0.1$ vs. no L-754,030)
			L-754,030 (MK-0869): 400 mg PO before cisplatin + 300 mg PO on days 2–5	86	Dexamethasone 20 mg PO before cisplatin	No emesis on day 1: 43% No emesis days 2–5: 57% ($p < 0.1$ vs. no L-754,030)

This table summarizes the preliminary human studies of NK_1 receptor antagonists as antiemetics in man.

MC: multicenter; DB: double-blind; R: randomized; P: preliminary; PC: placebo-controlled; CINV: chemotherapy-induced nausea and vomiting; PONV: post-operative nausea and vomiting; IV: intravenous; PO: by mouth.

acute CINV after high doses of cisplatin. Fumoleau et al. [48] reported on the lack of efficacy of 5 or 25 mg GR205171 i.v. when given as a single antiemetic to prevent acute (24 h) CINV after cisplatin treatment ($\geq$80 mg/m^2). This study group consisted, however, of 4 patients only. Conversely, Cocquyt et al. [49] found that L-758,298, 60 or 100 mg i.v. was almost as effective as ondansetron 32 mg for the prevention of first-day CINV. The percentages of complete responders (no emetic episode and no escape medication) and major responders (1 or 2 emetic episodes and no escape medication) were respectively 37 and 17% with L-758,298 (failure rate: 47%), and 48 and 9% in the ondansetron group (failure rate: 44%). Although not favorable to L-758,298, these figures look more encouraging than those observed during the first 24 h in the short series of Fumoleau with GR205171. One possible explanation for this discrepancy may be the lower dose of cisplatin in the Van Belle series ($\geq$50 mg/m^2). In one early study by Kris et al. [50], CP-122,721 alone (50–200 mg single oral dose) allowed 15% of the patients to be free from acute emesis.

Except for these results in acute CINV, the NK_1 receptor antagonists have shown dramatic antiemetic activity in cisplatin-treated cancer patients. This is true for the prevention of acute CINV in association with a 5-HT_3 receptor antagonist or with a 5-HT_3 receptor antagonist plus dexamethasone, and also for the prevention of delayed CINV (days 2–5 or 7) either when used as a sole prophylactic drug or in combination with one of the previously mentioned associations.

In the Fumoleau study, GR205171 25 mg i.v. plus ondansetron 8 mg i.v. allowed complete control of acute emesis in all patients and absence of nausea in 4 out of 5. Acute emesis was also absent in 100% of patients receiving CP-122,721 with ondansetron plus dexamethasone [47]. In the work by Hesketh et al. [51], the rate of no acute emesis was increased from 66.8 to 85.7% when CJ-11,947 100 mg orally twice daily was associated with granisetron and dexamethasone. This difference, however, did not reach statistical significance. The well-designed three-arm study published by Navari et al. [52] showed that the association of L-754,030 with a preventive regimen of granisetron plus dexamethasone allowed a 93% no acute emesis rate which was statistically different from the 67% observed after the placebo plus the two conventional drugs.

As far as delayed emesis is concerned, a favorable profile of the NK_1 receptor antagonists has been shown for CP-122,721 and for L-758,298 when *used alone*, and for CP-122,721, CJ-11,947 and L-754,030 when used in *combination regimens*.

In the short Kris et al. [50] series, a single prophylactic dose of CP-122,721 allowed prevention of delayed vomiting in 6 out of 7 patients (86%) while the combination with a 5-HT_3 receptor antagonist and dexamethasone brought about this result in 8 out of 10 patients (80%).

L-758,298 alone proved significantly superior to ondansetron alone in the prevention of vomiting and nausea on days 2–7 after cisplatin administration [49].

In association with granisetron and dexamethasone, CJ-11,947 100 mg given orally twice daily during 5 days allowed 67.8% of the patients to remain with no emesis during days 2–5 ($p = 0.042$ when compared with the 36.6% observed after administration of a placebo twice a day instead of CJ-11,947) [51].

The study by Navari et al. [52] concerning L-754,030 confirmed the results already mentioned for acute CINV, for delayed emesis. Prevention of delayed emesis (days 2–5) was best achieved when L-754,030 rather than a placebo was administered either on day 1 or on days 1–5 with the association of granisetron and dexamethasone ($p < 0.001$). This regimen also brought significantly higher satisfaction scores when compared to the placebo ($p = 0.001$) and this result on a non-surrogate endpoint certainly deserves to be emphasized. The study suggests a benefit with continuation of L-754,030 treatment beyond the first day, through the entire chemotherapy cycle, but this needs to be investigated further.

Campos et al. [53] observed the same types of results in their study. The triple combination of oral L-754,030 with granisetron and dexamethasone proved more potent for *acute* CINV prevention, when compared to granisetron plus dexamethasone without NK_1 receptor antagonist. The combination of L-754,030 with dexamethasone showed comparable activity to the combination of granisetron and dexamethasone. As far as *delayed* CINV is concerned, L-754,030 showed superior efficacy when compared to granisetron (table 2).

NK_1 Receptor Antagonists in Postoperative Nausea and Vomiting

Comparing CP-122,721 200 mg orally to ondansetron 4 mg i.v. and to the combination of the two agents in the prevention of PONV, Gesztesi et al. [54] found no differences for postoperative nausea scores among the three groups but a significantly lower incidence of emetic episodes when CP-122,721 was part of the prophylactic regimen. The combination of CP-122,721 and ondansetron provided no additional benefit (table 2). The same group published additional data in 2000 [55] showing in a dose-ranging approach that oral CP-122,721 200 mg was more effective than oral CP-122,721 100 mg. The combination of CP-122,721 and ondansetron significantly prolonged the time to the administration of the first rescue antiemetic drug when compared with either drug alone, and prevented the occurrence of emesis in 98% of the patients. Nevertheless, patient satisfaction with the control of PONV after oral CP-122,721 200 mg prophylaxis was not different than after ondansetron 4 mg.

In a placebo-controlled treatment, in the setting of established PONV, Diemunsch et al. [56] showed GR205171 25 mg i.v. as a single agent to be superior to placebo for complete control of emesis and nausea. This benefit was maintained throughout the entire 24-hour study period. The proportion of patients requiring rescue medication during the 24-hour following drug administration was also less after treatment with GR205171 (61 vs. 83% after the placebo).

Safety

Safety of the NK_1 receptor antagonists in man has never been a concern in the clinical studies, and all the investigational drugs were well tolerated, with no drug-related toxicity. This was true for the clinically observed effects and for the measured laboratory parameters. No adverse events were reported that would preclude further studies of NK_1 receptor antagonists in man. One exception however has been reported consisting in a serious episode of dizziness possibly related to oral L-754,030 (400 mg) in the Campos study. Similarly, an increased incidence of mild or moderate headaches was observed after oral CP-122,721 (200 mg) in the Gesztesi dose-ranging study.

Despite the implication of SP in pain mechanisms, no obvious effects on pain threshold or on analgesia were observed in the human PONV studies. This is in opposition with the results of the study by Dionne et al. [57] showing that the NK_1 receptor antagonist CP-99,994 was effective in pain reduction after third molar extraction.

Other potential indications of the NK_1 receptor antagonists include asthma, anxiety, arthritis, migraine, schizophrenia, glaucoma as well as ocular hypotension, neural injury and stroke. It is so far unknown as to whether the doses required to treat CINV and PONV may provoke side effects related to this wide-spectrum activity.

Conclusion

Major improvement in the treatment of nausea and vomiting has been achieved with the advent of serotonin type 3 receptor antagonists. This class of drugs has become the gold standard in the management of both CINV and PONV [58], whereas motion sickness is still resistant to the setrons. Despite these advances, and although associations with other classes of antiemetics has further improved results, nausea and vomiting still remain a significant problem, notably in cancer chemotherapy and after surgery, where these symptoms can prove most distressing. The recent introduction of the NK_1 receptor antagonists seems promising firstly on a theoretical basis, since these drugs act on a target in the emesis mechanism which has not yet been exploited, secondly on a preclinical basis, since NK_1 receptor antagonists showed excellent results in various animal models of emesis, and finally if one considers the preliminary human data published so far. Interestingly, as in the case of the 5-HT_3 receptor antagonists, no major concern about safety has been raised after the initial human trials. Much work is still needed in order to consolidate these results and to answer questions concerning the optimal dose, the optimal schedule and duration of treatment, and the optimal antiemetic drug associations with the NK_1 receptor antagonists. Occurrence of other foreseeable effects of this class of drugs should also be controlled for, on large-scale trials.

Acknowledgement

The authors thank Heidi Cahen for her expertise in medical English translation.

References

1 Diemunsch P, Grélot L: Potential of substance P antagonists as anti-emetics. Drugs 2000;60: 533–546.
2 Bianchi AL, Grélot L: An overview of emesis; in Bianchi AL, Grélot L, Miller AD, King GL (eds): New Vistas on Mechanisms and Control of Emesis. Colloque INSERM/Libbey Eurotext, 1992, vol 223, pp 3–9.
3 Girod V, Bouvier M, Grélot L: Characterization of bacterial lipopolysaccharide-induced emesis in conscious piglets: Effects of bilateral cervical vagotomy, cyclooxygenase inhibitors and a 5-HT_3 receptor antagonist. Neuropharmacology 2000;39:2329–2335
4 Grélot L, Miller AD: Vomiting: Its in and outs. NIPS 1994;9:142–146.
5 Lucot JB: 5-HT_{1A} receptor agonists as anti-emetic; in Reynolds DJM, Andrew PLR, Davis CJ (eds): Serotonin and the Scientific Basis of Anti-Emetic Therapy. Oxford, Oxford Clinical Communications, 1995, pp 222–227.
6 Rudd JA, Naylor RJ: Opioid receptor involvement in emesis and anti-emesis; in Reynolds DJM, Andrew PLR, Davis CJ (eds): Serotonin and the Scientific Basis of Anti-Emetic Therapy. Oxford, Oxford Clinical Communications, 1995, pp 209–219.
7 Carpenter DO, Briggs DB, Strominger N: Peptide-induced emesis in dogs. Behav Brain Res 1984; 11:277–281.
8 Andrews PLR, Bhandari P: Resiniferatoxin, an ultrapotent capsaicin analogue, has anti-emetic properties in the ferret. Neuropharmacology 1993;32:799–806.
9 Maggi CA: The mammalian tachykinin receptors. Gen Pharmacol 1995;26:911–944.
10 Henry JL: Discussion of Nomenclature for TKs and Tachykin Receptor. Substance P and Neurokinins. New York, Springer, 1987, vol XVII.
11 McLean S, Ganong A, Seymour PA, et al: Pharmacology of CP-99,994: a non-peptide antagonist of the tachykinin NK-1 receptor. J Pharmacol Exp Ther 1993;267:472–479.
12 Quartara L, Maggi CA: The tachykinin NK_1 receptor. 1. Ligands and mechanisms of cellular activation. Neuropeptides 1997;31:537–563.
13 McLean S: Nonpeptide antagonists of the NK_1 tachykinin receptor. Med Res Rev 1996;16:297–317.
14 Rupniak NMJ, Boyce S, Williams AR, et al: Antinociceptive activity of NK_1 receptor antagonists: Nonspecific effects of racemic RP 67,580. Br J Pharmacol 1993;110:1607–1613.
15 McLean S, Ganong A, Seymour PA, et al: Characterization of CP-122,721: a nonpeptide antagonist of the neurokinin NK_1 receptor. J Pharmacol Exp Ther 1996;277:900–908.

16 Gardner CJ, Armour DR, Beattie DT, et al: A novel antagonist with high affinity for the tachykinin NK_1 receptor, and potent broad-spectrum anti-emetic activity. Regul Pept 1996;65:45–53.
17 Hale JJ, Mills SG, MacCoss M, et al: Structural optimization affording 2-(R)-(1-(R)-(3,5-bis(trifluoromethyl)phenylethoxy)-3(S)-(4fluoro)phenyl-4-(3-oxo-1,2,4-triazol-5-yl)methylmorpholine, a potent orally active, long-acting morpholine acetal human NK-1 receptor antagonist. J Med Chem 1998;41:4607–4614.
18 Bountra C, Bunce KT, Dale T, et al: Anti-emetic profile of a non-peptide, neurokinin NK_1 receptor anatagonist, CP-99,994, in ferrets. Eur J Pharmacol 1993;249:R3–R4.
19 Tattersall DF, Rycroft W, Hargreaves RJ, et al: The tachykinin NK_1 receptor antagonist CP-99,994 attenuates cisplatin-induced emesis in ferret. Eur J Pharmacol 1993;250:R5–R6.
20 Gardner CJ, Twissell DJ, Dale TJ, et al: The broad-spectrum anti-emetic activity of the novel non-peptide tachykinin NK_1 receptor, GR203040. Br J Pharmacol 1995;116:3158–3163.
21 Gonsalves SF, Watson JW, Ashton C: Broad-spectrum anti-emetic effects of CP-122,721, a tachykinin NK_1 receptor antagonist, in ferrets. Eur J Pharmacol 1996;305:181–185.
22 Gardner CJ, Bountra C, Bunce KT, et al: Anti-emetic activity of neurokinin NK_1 receptor antagonists is mediated centrally in the ferret. Br J Pharmacol 1994;112:516P.
23 Grélot L, Dapzol J, Estève E, et al: Potent inhibition of acute and delayed cisplatin-induced nausea and vomiting in piglets treated by GR205171, a novel highly selective NK_1 receptor antagonist. Br J Pharmacol 1998;124:1643–1650.
24 Rupniak NMJ, Carlson E, Boyce S, et al: Enantioselective inhibition of the formalin paw late phase by the NK_1 receptor antagonist L-733,060 in gerbils. Pain 1996;67:189–195.
25 Watson JW, Gonsalves SF, Fossa AA, et al: The anti-emetic effects of CP-99,994 in the ferret and the dog: Role of the NK_1 receptor. Br J Pharmacol 1995;115:84–94.
26 Watson JW, Nagahisa A, Lucot JB, et al: The tachykinins and emesis: Towards complete control? In Reynolds DJM, Andrew PLR, Davis CJ (eds): Serotonin and the Scientific Basis of Anti-Emetic Therapy. Oxford, Oxford Clinical Communications, 1995, pp 233–238.
27 Rudd JA, Jordan CC, Naylor RJ: The action of the NK_1 receptor antagonist, CP-99,994 in antagonizing the acute and delayed emesis induced by cisplatin in ferret. Br J Pharmacol 1996;119:931–936.
28 Singh L, Field MJ, Hughes J, et al: The tachykinin NK_1 receptor antagonist PD 154075 blocks cisplatin-induced delayed emesis in the ferret. Eur J Pharmacol 1997;321:209–216.
29 Milano S, Grélot L, Blower P, et al: The piglet as a suitable animal model for studying the delayed phase of chemotherapy-induced delayed emesis. J Pharmacol Exp Ther 1995;274:951–961.
30 Lucot JB, Obach RS, McLean S, et al: The effect of CP-99994 on the responses of provocative motion in the cat. Br J Pharmacol 1997;120:116–120.
31 Gardner C, Perren M: Inhibition of anaesthetic-induced emesis by a NK_1 or 5-HT_3 receptor antagonist in the house musk shrew, *Suncus murinus*. Neuropharmacology 1998;37:1643–1644.
32 Chen Y, Saito H, Matsuki N: Ethanol-induced emesis in the house musk shrew, *Suncus murinus*. Life Sci 1997;60:253–261.
33 McAllister KH, Pratt JA: GR205171 blocks apomorphine and amphetamine-induced conditioned taste aversions. Eur J Pharmacol 1998;353:141–148.
34 Matsuki N, Toyoda H, Saito H: Role of substance P in emesis. Folia Pharmacol Jpn 1996;108 (suppl 1):133–138.
35 Shiroshita Y, Koga T, Fukuda H: Capsaicin in fourth ventricle abolishes retching and transmission of emetic vagal afferents to solitary nucleus neurons. Eur J Pharmacol 1997;339:183–192.
36 Davidson JS, Oland L, Boissonade F: The effects of centrally injected NK_1 receptor antagonists on emesis in the ferret. Gastroenterology 1995;108:A589.
37 Rupniak NM, Tattersall FD, Williams AR, et al: In vitro and in vivo predictors of the anti-emetic activity of tachykinin NK_1 receptor antagonists. Eur J Pharmacol 1997;326:201–209.
38 Yates BJ, Grélot L, Kerman IA, et al: Organization of the vestibular inputs to nucleus tractus solitarius and adjacent structures in cat brainstem. Am J Physiol 1994;267:R974–R983.
39 Leslie RA: Neuroactive substances in the dorsal vagal complex of the medulla oblongata: Nucleus of the tractus solitarius, area postrema and dorsal motor nucleus of the vagus. Neurochem Int 1985;7:191–211.
40 Dockray GJ, Sharkey KA: Neurochemistry of visceral afferent neurones. Prog Brain Res 1986;67: 133–148.

41 Dockray GJ, Green T, Varro A: The afferent peptidergic innervation of the upper gastrointestinal tract; in Singer MV, Goebell H (eds): Nerves and GI Tract. Falk Symposium 50. Lancaster, Kluwer Academic, 1989, pp 105–122.
42 Fasth KJ, Bergstrom M, Kilpatrick G, et al: Brain uptake and receptor binding of two ^{11}C-labelled selective high affinity NK_1 antagonists, GR203040 and GR205171. J Label Comp Radiopharmceut 1997;40:665–667.
43 Tattersall FD, Rycroft W, Francis B, et al: Tachykinins NK_1 receptor antagonists act centrally to inhibit emesis induced by the chemotherapeutic agent cisplatin in ferrets. Neuropharmacology 1996;35:1121–1129.
44 Saito R, Suehiro Y, Ariumi H, et al: Anti-emetic effects of a novel NK-1 receptor antagonist HSP-117 in ferrets. Neurosci Lett 1998;254:169–172.
45 Minami M, Endo T, Kikuchi K, et al: Antiemetic effects of sendide, a peptide tachykinin NK_1 receptor antagonist, in the ferret. Eur J Pharmacol 1998;363:49–55.
46 Tsukasa S, Chikai S, Koichi TN, et al: Neurokinin receptor antagonists: Therapeutic potential in the treatment of pain syndromes. CNS Drugs 1997;8:436–447.
47 Reid K, Palmer JL, Wright RJ, et al: Comparison of the neurokinin-1 antagonist GR205171, alone and in combination with the 5-HT_3 antagonist ondansetron, hyoscine and placebo in the prevention of motion-induced nausea in man. Br J Clin Pharmacol 2000;50:61–64.
48 Fumoleau P, Graham E, Giovanni M, et al: Control of acute cisplatin-induced emesis and nausea with the NK_1 receptor antagonist GR205171 in combination with ondansetron. Proc Annu Meet Am Soc Clin Oncol 1998;17:58a, 225.
49 Cocquyt V, Van Belle S, Reinhardt RR, Decramer ML, O'Brien M, Schellens JH, Borms M, Verbeke L, Van Aelst F, De Smet M, Carides AD, Eldridge K, Gertz BJ: Comparison of L-758,298, a prodrug for the selective neurokinin-1 antagonist, L-754,030, with ondansetron for the prevention of cisplatin-induced emesis. Eur J Cancer 2001;37:823–825.
50 Kris MG, Radford JE, Pizzo BA, et al: Use of an NK_1 receptor antagonist to prevent delayed emesis after cisplatin. J Natl Cancer Inst 1997;89:817–818.
51 Hesketh PJ, Gralla RJ, Webb RT, et al: Randomized phase II study of the neurokinin-1 receptor antagonist CJ-11,974 in the control of cisplatin-induced emesis. J Clin Oncol 1999;17: 338–343.
52 Navari RM, Reinhardt RR, Gralla RJ, et al: Reduction of cisplatin-induced emesis by a selective neurokinin-1 receptor antagonist. N Engl J Med 1999;340:190–195.
53 Campos D, Pereira JR, Reinhardt RR, Carracedo C, Poli S, Vogel C, Martinez-Cedillo J, Erazo A, Wittreich J, Eriksson LO, Carides AD, Gertz BJ: Prevention of cisplatin-induced emesis by the oral neurokinin-1 antagonist, MK-869, in combination with granisetron and dexamethasone or with dexamethasone alone. J Clin Oncol 2001;19:1759–1767.
54 Gesztesi ZS, Song D, White PF: Comparison of a new NK_1 antagonist (CP122,721) to odanserton in the prevention of postoperative nausea and vomiting. Anesth Analg 1998;86(suppl 2):32.
55 Gesztesi Z, Scuderi PE, White PF, Wright W, Wender RH, D'Angelo R, Black S, Dalby PL, MacLean D: Substance P (neurokinin-1) antagonist prevents postoperative vomiting after abdominal hysterectomy procedures. Anesthesiology 2000;93:931–937.
56 Diemunsch P, Schoeffler P, Bryssine B, et al: Anti-emetic activity of the NK_1 receptor antagonist GR205171 in the treatment of established PONV following major gynaecological surgery. Br J Anaesth 1999;82:274–276.
57 Dionne RA, Max MB, Gordon SM, et al: The substance P receptor antagonist CP-99,994 reduces acute postoperative pain. Clin Pharmacol Ther 1998;64:562–568.
58 Diemunsch P, Korttila K, Kovac A: Current therapy for management of postoperative nausea and vomiting: The 5-HT_3 receptor antagonists. Ambul Surg 1999;7:111–122.
59 Tattersall FD, Rycroft W, Hill RG, et al: Enantiospecific inhibition of apomorphine-induced emesis in the ferret by the neurokinin-1 receptor antagonist CP-99,994. Neuropharmacology 1995;33: 259–260.
60 Tattersall FD, Rycroft W, Marmont N, et al: Enantiospecific inhibition of emesis induced by nicotine in the house musk shrew *(Suncus murinus)* by the neurokinin-1 receptor antagonist CP-99,994. Neuropharmacology 1995;34:1697–1699.

61 Girod V: Implication des mécanismes inflammatoires dans l'activation du réflexe émétique par le cisplatine et les lipopolysaccharides bactériens chez le porcelet; thèse de l'Université d'Aix-Marseille III, spécialité Neurosciences, 2002.
62 Saeki M, Sakai M, Saito R, Kubota H, Ariumi H, Takano Y, Yamatodani A, Kamiya H: Effects of HSP-117, a novel tachykinin NK receptor antagonist, on cisplatin-induced pica as a new evaluation of delayed emesis in rats. Jpn J Pharmacol 2001;86:359–362.
63 Tattersall FD, Rycroft W, Cumberbatch M, Mason G, Tye S, Williamson DJ, Hale JJ, Mills SG, Finke PE, MacCoss M, Sadowski S, Ber E, Cascieri M, Hill RG, MacIntyre DE, Hargreaves RJ: The novel NK_1 receptor antagonist MK-0869 (L-754,030) and its water-soluble phosphoryl prodrug, L-758,298, inhibit acute and delayed cisplatin-induced emesis in ferrets. Neuropharmacology 2000;39:652–663.
64 Grélot L, Milano S, Le Stunff H, et al: Repeated administration of the 5-HT_3 receptor antagonist granisetron reduces the incidence of delayed cisplatin-induced emesis in the piglet. J Pharmacol Exp Ther 1996;279:255–261.
65 Girod V, Dapzol J, Bouvier M, Grélot L: The COX inhibitors indomethacin and meloxicam exhibit anti-emetic activity against cisplatin-induced emesis in piglets. Neuropharmacology 2002;42: 428–436.

Prof. Pierre Diemunsch, MD
Service d'Anesthésie – Réanimation Chirurgicale
IRCAD, CHU, Hôpital de Hautepierre
Avenue Molière, F–67098 Strasbourg Cedex (France)
Tel. +33 3 88127078, Fax +33 3 88127074, E-Mail pierre.diemunsch@chru-strasbourg.fr

Donnerer J (ed): Antiemetic Therapy.
Basel, Karger, 2003, pp 98–112

Neuronal Mechanisms and Treatment of Motion Sickness

F. Schmäl, W. Stoll

Department of Otorhinolaryngology, Head and Neck Surgery,
University Hospital, Münster, Germany

Introduction

Strictly speaking, motion sickness is considered to be a physiological vertigo and thus is not a true sickness at all but a normal response to an abnormal situation. It is caused by certain kinds of motion and is induced during passive locomotion in vehicles, generated by unfamiliar body accelerations, to which the person has therefore not adapted, or by an intersensory conflict between vestibular and visual stimuli [1]. Motion sickness indiscriminately affects air, sea, road and space travelers. All individuals (humans and animals) possessing an intact vestibular apparatus can be made motion sick given the right quality and quantity of provocative stimulation, although there are wide and consistent individual differences in the degree of susceptibility [2, 3].

Cardinal signs of motion sickness are nausea, vomiting, pallor and cold sweating. Associated reactions include sighing, yawing, hyperventilation, flatulence, loss of body weight, headache and drowsiness. Because of the cardinal signs nausea and vomiting it seems to be necessary to describe the neuronal mechanisms and especially the therapy of motion sickness in a book, which presents all aspects of antiemetic therapy.

The Vestibular System

In humans a highly sophisticated mechanism for maintaining gaze (vestibulo-ocular reflex – VOR) and balance (vestibulospinal reflexes) during head and body movements has developed, which is dependent upon visual, vestibular and proprioceptive sensory information. The information is integrated in the central nervous system and is modulated by activity arising in the reticular formation, the extrapyramidal system, the cerebellum and the cerebral cortex.

Each vestibular labyrinth contains five vestibular receptors: two maculae of the otolith organs which can be stimulated by linear acceleration in horizontal (utricle) and vertical (saccule) direction and three cristae ampullares of the semicircular canals which detect angular accelerations in three different planes.

Neuronal Mechanism of Motion Sickness

For the past three decades, the sensory conflict theory, most extensively described by Reason and Brand [4], has provided a theoretical framework for the understanding of motion sickness. According to the theory, motion sickness results when the brain receives conflicting information about body motion from the visual and vestibular receptors and the proprioceptive system ('sensory mismatch').

Most sickness-provoking sensory conflicts can be attached to two different categories, namely (1) the conflict between visual and vestibular/proprioceptive signal, and (2) the conflict between canal and otolith signal. Furthermore, for every sensory conflict category, three subtypes of conflicts could be distinguished. From these two categories and three types of conflicts, we can derive six basic conflict types in which motion sickness might reasonably be expected to occur (table 1).

Conflict between Visual and Vestibular/Proprioceptive Signal

Type 1

Visual and vestibular receptors simultaneously signal motion, but of an uncorrelated or incompatible kind. One everyday example is the situation of a man who is standing on a sailing ship and is looking down at the motion of the waves. The same conflict occurred in a laboratory experiment in subjects wearing disturbing optical devices which reverse and invert the visual field. During this kind of experiment the vestibular perceived motion is contrary to the seen movement of the visual field. However, the degree of visual distortion necessary to produce symptoms does not need to be as extreme as this. A change in the prescription of spectacles is often sufficient to produce nausea during the early stage of wearing them. Another conflict situation occurs if a person is

Table 1. Six kinds of sensory rearrangements that can provoke motion sickness [4]

Type of conflict	Category 1: conflict between visual (A) and vestibular/proprioceptive signal (B)	Category 2: conflict between canal (A) and otolith (B) signal
Type 1		
Inputs A and B simultaneously receive contradictory or uncorrelated information	Watching waves over the side of a ship	Head movements made about the same axis other than that of the bodily rotation – cross-coupled angular acceleration
	Looking out of the side or rear windows of a moving vehicle Making head movements while wearing some optical device that disturbs vision	Low frequency oscillation between 0.1 and 0.3 Hz
Type 2		
Input A signals in the absence of the expected B signal	Cinema sickness Operating a fixed-base vehicle simulator with a moving visual display (simulator sickness)	Space motion sickness Caloric stimulation of the outer ear
	'Haunted-swing' type of fairground device	Positional alcoholic nystagmus associated with alcohol and heavy water
Type 3		
Input B signals in the absence of the expected A signal	Reading a map in a moving vehicle Riding in a vehicle without external visual reference Being swung in an enclosed cabin	Rotation about an earth horizontal axis Any rotation about an off-vertical axis Counter-rotation

looking out of the side window of a moving vehicle. In this case the perceived velocity is different to the seen velocity.

Type 2

The visual receptors perceive a relative motion of large portions of the visual field, of a kind normally associated with simultaneous vestibular stimulation signaling head and/or body movements, but where these latter are absent. Because in this setting a real body motion is missing, Schmäl and Stoll [5] create the terms *pseudo-kinetosis* or better *pseudo-motion sickness* to describe this kind of conflict. The following examples show situations which represent this kind of conflict:

Cinema sickness: Observers were readily made motion sick by watching a film shot from a car driving down a winding mountain road [6].

Simulator sickness: This form of motion sickness can be induced in the operators of fixed-base car or aircraft simulators where a moving visual display simulates the outside world as it would be viewed from a vehicle in motion.

Haunted swing: A swing was mounted in the center of a fully furnished room. When people took their seats on the swing it was apparently put into motion, but it was not the swing but the room which swung.

Type 3

This type of sensory conflict occurs in the presence of a vestibular stimulus while an expected correlated visual signal is absent. Situations which include such a conflict are reading a map in a moving vehicle, riding in a vehicle without external visual references and being swung in an enclosed cabin.

Conflict between Canal and Otolith Signal (Intralabyrinthine Conflict)

Type 1

This type of conflict occurs when canals and otoliths simultaneously signal contradictory information concerning the position and motion of the head. One typical example of this type of sensory conflict is the coriolis vestibular reaction (coriolis or cross-coupled stimulus) which occurs when a test subject, seated on a chair rotating at constant speed (e.g. in the horizontal plane), moves the head about the same axis other than that of rotation (e.g. forward and backwards).

Type 2

This kind of sensory conflict is characterized by the presence of a canal signal in the absence of an expected correlated signal from the otoliths. This conflict occurs during following situations:

Zero-gravity condition: On earth, every canal stimulation during head movements is combined with corresponding otolith stimulation. In case of zero-gravity condition in space when gravity is missing, no otolith signal occurs during canal stimulations in the frame of head movements.

Caloric stimulation of the horizontal semicircular canal: Even in an earth-based laboratory, applying a caloric stimulation to the horizontal semicircular canals can create a type 2 canal otolith conflict.

Type 3

During this setting, motion sickness is provoked by the presence of an otolithic signal in the absence of an expected back-up signal from the semicircular canals. This type of sensory conflict occurs only in the laboratory, namely during rotation (constant angular velocity!) about an earth-horizontal axis (barbecue rotation) and during counter-rotation.

Barbecue rotation: During this rotation with constant angular velocity that means without angular acceleration and thus without stimulation of the semicircular canals, the orientation of the otolith organs in relation to the gravity vector is permanently changing and consequently an otolith stimulation without canal stimulation occurs.

Counter-rotation: This stimulation can be performed with a device which consists of a secondary turntable mounted on a centrifuge of short radius. This secondary turntable was made to revolve at the same rate as the main centrifuge, but in the opposite direction. In this way, the test subject seated on the secondary turntable remained facing the same way since the counter-rotation of the secondary turntable cancelled out the rotation of the primary drive axis.

Some work groups [7–9] postulate that in some cases of motion sickness the conflict has its origin in the differences between the current received sensory information (visual and vestibular receptors get different information about head and body movements) and the stored experience (congruent visual and vestibular input). Pitman and Yolton [10] used for this store experience the term 'exposure history'.

Helling et al. [11] demonstrated in their experiments with fishes a different otolith mass between the right and left saccules. They assume that a misbalanced sensitivity of the statolith organs occurs but is totally compensated for by the vestibular system as long as physiological motion patterns take place. Decompensation leads to kinetosis under non-physiological motion patterns.

Diamond and Markham [12] found a significant correlation between the otolith asymmetry and the sensibility to space motion sickness in astronauts.

Motion Sickness Susceptibility

There are clearly wide individual differences in motion sickness susceptibility. To quantify this susceptibility it is possible to measure the time how long a test person can endure a sensory conflict, to analyze the strength of a motion sickness-provoking stimulus or to quantify the observed vegetative symptoms.

Different devices were developed to produce symptoms of motion sickness, e.g. apparatuses for barbecue rotation, off-vertical axis rotation and dynamic posturography with simultaneous presentation of incongruent visual stimuli [13]. However, most commonly, devices were used which are able to produce a coriolis- or cross-coupled stimulus. For example, a rotation chair (rotating about an earth vertical axis) which allows the test subject to perform simultaneously head movements in the frontal plane (up and down) (Lansberg test) [14, 15].

About 5–10% of all people are very susceptible to motion sickness, why all others only show a moderate susceptibility. Motion sickness susceptibility fluctuates with age [7]. Infants below the age of 2 years are generally immune to motion sickness but susceptibility seems to be at the highest level between the age of 2 and about 12 years. Beyond the age of 50, any kind of motion sickness is very rare.

Women appear to be more susceptible to motion sickness [16], especially during the time of menstruation [17] and during pregnancy. Thus, a relation to the female endocrine system was concluded. But in contrast, Cheung et al. [18] could not prove an influence of different phases of the menstrual cycle on subjective symptoms of motion sickness.

Because a benefit of placebo was observed in 45% of patients with motion sickness, there is evidence that psychological factors influence motion sickness susceptibility [19]. However, the most important aspect with regard to motion sickness susceptibility is the contents of the 'exposure history' which represents the stored experiences.

Busoni et al. [20] analyzed the impact of motion sickness on the incidence of vomiting after routine surgery in children (n = 420) who received general anesthesia and inguinal field block for common pediatric surgery. The children were randomly allocated into one of two groups (halothane or sevoflurane). In the postoperative period, the authors found that motion sickness-positive children vomit more than motion sickness-negative children, regardless of the inhalation anesthetic used. However, motion sickness-negative children displayed a higher incidence of vomiting when halothane was used rather than sevoflurane.

Pseudo-Kinetosis

As mentioned above, symptoms of motion sickness even occur when motion is signaled from the visual input in the absence of expected vestibular signals. These movements of the visual field without movement of the body have been reported in immobile people in wide-screen movie theaters (cinema sickness), in flight simulators that included a large moving visual display and during special kinds of computer games [21–23]. Because of the absence of acceleration stimuli on the vestibular organ, the term 'pseudo-kinetosis' was created [5].

Perhaps the earliest case of visually induced motion sickness was reported in 1894, when a huge swing was mounted in the center of a fully furnished room. When the customers took their seats on the swing it was apparently put into motion but in reality it was the room that swung. After a few minutes some people suffered from nausea and dizziness [24].

Because labyrinthine-defective subjects are immune to visual induced motion sickness, it must be suggested that the stimulation of vestibular centers is responsible for this phenomenon [7].

Normally, in the case of body movements, visual and vestibular receptors register the same information about body motion and thus the signals of both systems are congruent, but in people watching a film shot from a car driving down a winding mountain road, they were made motion sick because the motion signals of the visual system are incongruent to the absent signals of the vestibular system (body in rest).

Central Structures Involved in Motion Sickness

Kubo et al. [25] found in their experiments reciprocal connections between the vestibular nuclei and the hypothalamus. Even the hypophysis and the hypothalamus are involved in motion sickness because vasopressin neurons in the magnocellular-neurohypophyseal system are activated during motion-induced nausea [26] and during motion sickness-provoking stimuli an increasing histamine level could be proved [27].

McIntosh [19] postulated an emetic chemoreceptor trigger zone in the area postrema of the medulla oblongata, incriminated in producing motion sickness. In animal experiences the destruction of this cerebral region abolished the symptoms of motion sickness [28]. Supratentorial structures did not play an important role in the production of motion sickness because the removal of the cerebrum in animals did not change the motion sickness susceptibility [29].

In summary, the following structures appear to be vital links in the neural pathway responsible for motion sickness [10]: (a) vestibular apparatus (semicircular canals and otolith organs); (b) vestibulocochlear nerve; (c) vestibular nuclei in the brainstem; (d) nodulus and uvula of the cerebellum; (e) chemoreceptive trigger zone (medulla oblongata); (f) vomiting center (reticular formation); (g) hypothalamus and (h) the efferentes involved in the emetic response.

Prevention and Treatment of Motion Sickness

The best therapy for motion sickness is to escape the motion, but if this is not possible there are the following therapeutic options which are established in the prevention and/or treatment of motion sickness: (1) behavior measures, (2) adaptation and (3) drug treatment.

Behavior Measures

To prevent symptoms of motion sickness, head movements should be avoided by holding the head against the back of the seat [7]. Visual information that is in agreement with information from the vestibular and other sensory receptors suppress symptoms of motion sickness, whereas incongruent information of the visual and vestibular system promotes nausea and vomiting. Therefore, seasickness victims should be located on deck and asked to view the distant horizon. Furthermore, people who are very susceptible to motion sickness should choose seats at the windows during flights and when traveling by train. In a car, for example, it is important to maintain a forward-looking direction of gaze (just as the driver does most of the time) and to avoid glances to the side or rear that present the brain with uncorrelated visual information.

Because ethanol leads to a disturbed visual suppression of vestibular evoked eye movements, it is helpful not to drink alcohol to avoid the symptoms of motion sickness. Sleeping has a positive influence on the symptoms of motion sickness because it reduces the excitability of the vestibular system and thus minimizes the sensory conflict. Acupuncture at the P6 or Neiguan point to treat nausea and vomiting has been practiced in China for many years. More recently, acupressure at P6 has been used successfully to decrease the symptoms of pregnancy sickness and with mixed results [30–35] to decrease motion sickness. In this connection, Stern et al. [36] found that the Acuband worn on the wrist or forearm decreases the symptoms of motion sickness and the gastric activity that usually accompanies motion sickness.

Adaptation

It is well known that repeated or continued exposure to motion results in a declining motion sickness response in most individuals, and especially adaptation is one of the most effective therapies for motion sickness. While 'adaptation' means the decreasing response following continuous stimulation of a receptor system, the reduction of neuronal activity after repeated stimulation is called 'habituation'. For example, when at sea, in rough conditions, most people adapt within a few days [37], but when disembarking from a ship after more than 3 months the adaptation disappears and increased susceptibility is noted [2].

It is possible to distinguish three distinct stages in the temporal sequence of adaptive effect and after-effect: initial exposure effects, the effects of continued exposure and after-effects [4]. Furthermore, Reason and Brand [4] distinguished between 'sensory adaptation' (decreasing response following continuous stimulation of a receptor system) and 'protective adaptation' (adaptation to the sensory mismatch). The adaptation is normally highly specific to the particular stimulus conditions under which it was acquired. Thus, it is possible that sailors traveling on large ships may become sick when they are transferred to small boats [19].

It was found in helicopter-simulator studies that experienced instructors, who had presumably acquired an adaptive change from flying helicopters, were much more susceptible to sickness in the simulator than were the student pilots [7]. The same phenomenon was observed in people who often drive by car and then were tested in a car simulator. Presumably a very strong 'exposure history' seems to be responsible for this observation in trained people. A stimulus that is gradual in onset generates fewer symptoms and allows for more rapid adaptation than a stimulus that is abrupt in onset [38]. The longer the adaptation continues, the more frequently a special stimulus is given [4].

Helling and Westhofen [39] observed in professional seamen during their experiments at sea that at the beginning of the voyage there was a significantly lower gain in nystagmus in harmonic acceleration testing than in the inexperienced volunteers. During the voyage all professionals showed nearly constant gain values but all inexperienced individuals showed a decrease in gain only during the time of acute symptoms. This points to a central vestibular depression in adapted volunteers. In the absence of nausea induced by head or body movements, no adaptation occurs.

At least 5% of all humans with symptoms of motion sickness showed no signs of adaptation. Interestingly, active body movements favor rather an adaptation as passively induced movements during experimental induced visual disturbance by optical systems (inverting prisms) [40]. Therefore, an additional influence of the proprioceptive system must be proceeded here. The adaptation effects can also be explained by the sensory conflict theory. In situations which commonly produce sensory conflicts (sensory rearrangement) and motion sickness, our brain presumably stores appropriate traces, making the sensory conflict part of our 'exposure history'. Once this occurs there is no conflict between our expectations and the sensory information received and thus, after some time, no further symptoms of motion sickness occur.

In this exposure history the used movement sample is reprogrammed, i.e. it comes to a reorientation. In the absence of this now integrated conflict situation, symptoms of motion sickness occur once again. This effect is called 'mal de débarquement', 'landsickness or 'adaptive after-effect' [4]. The most typical examples of landsickness are found in persons after a long time on a ship, or the sickness in astronauts after returning to earth from a longer trip in space.

Drug Treatment

The first use of a drug was mentioned in the *Lancet* in 1869, where, in an anonymous letter to the editor, a combination of chloroform and tincture of belladonna was recommended for motion sickness. At least the sensory-mismatch theory led to three possible drug effects in patients with motion sickness: (1) reduction of the incongruent information; (2) faster update of the 'exposure history' and thus acceleration of adaptation processes, and (3) removal of vegetative symptoms.

Three kinds of neurotransmitters – histamine, acetylcholine and noradrenaline – play important roles in the neural processes of motion sickness, because antihistamines, scopolamine and amphetamine are effective in preventing motion sickness. Histamine H_1 receptors are involved in the development of the symptoms and signs of motion sickness, including emesis. On provocative motion stimuli, a neural mismatch signal activates the histaminergic neuron system in the hypothalamus, and the histaminergic descending impulse stimulates H_1 receptors in the emetic center of the brainstem. The histaminergic input to the emetic center through H_1 receptors is independent of dopamine D_2 receptors in the chemoreceptor trigger zone in the area postrema and serotonin 5-HT_3 receptors in the visceral afferent, which are also involved in the emetic reflex. Antihistamines block emetic H_1 receptors to prevent motion sickness. Scopolamine prevents motion sickness by modifying the neural store to reduce the neural mismatch signal and by facilitating the adaptation/habituation processes. The noradrenergic neuron system in the locus coeruleus is suppressed by the neural mismatch signal. Amphetamine antagonizes mismatch-induced suppression of noradrenergic neural transmission, resulting in preventing motion sickness [41]. It is assumed that all antimotion sickness drugs affect a hypothetical equilibrium between a central cholinergic and adrenergic system, which is influenced by movements [42].

The following drugs are useful for prevention and/or treatment of motion sickness:

Anticholinergic agents: Scopolamine, an acetylcholine antagonist, has long been effective for prophylaxis of motion sickness. During the past decades, transdermal scopolamine was developed to provide effective prophylaxis and consistent serum levels over an extended period (72 h) [43, 44]. The patch is placed over the postauricular skin, the site of highest skin permeability [38]. Effective protection is provided only if the patch is applied 8 h before exposure to motion. Its anticholinergic effects on the ciliary muscle of the eye lens, the salivary and sweat glands, and the heart cause side effects of scopolamine.

Klocker et al. [45] studied the effect of nasal administration of scopolamine in a double-blind trial. Scopolamine nasal spray was found to be an effective and safe treatment in motion sickness, with a fast onset of action within 30 min after administration.

Transdermal scopolamine is effective in preventing motion sickness for 72 h. However, by this route a prophylactic effect is obtained 6–8 h postapplication. By the oral route, scopolamine is effective within 0.5 h for a period of 6 h. Therefore, Nachum et al. [46] prefer the combination of transdermal and oral scopolamine (0.3 or 0.6 mg). This combination provides the required plasma levels to prevent seasickness, starting as early as 0.5 h posttreatment, with no significant adverse effects.

Sympathomimetics (catecholamine activators): These agents were mainly used during space flights. A 5- to 10-mg oral dose of dextroamphetamine has been shown to magnify the prophylactic effects of scopolamine and antihistamines. The drug appears to act centrally by stimulating either dopaminergic or noradrenergic pathways. Murray [44] concluded that a combination of scopolamine and dextroamphetamine seems to be the most effective antimotion sickness preparation. The most important side effect is the danger of addiction.

Antihistamines: The role of antihistamines in the treatment of motion sickness was discovered in 1949 [47]. A pregnant woman who was highly susceptible to motion sickness was given dimenhydrinate for urticaria. While taking this drug, she was immune to motion sickness. The ability of dimenhydrinate to both prevent and treat motion sickness likely stems from its antihistaminic and anticholinergic properties. Wood et al. [48] analyzed 15 different works with at least 5,184 patients and found an effectiveness of antihistamines in the treatment of motion sickness of 70%. The most common side effect was the sedation.

Weinstein and Stern [49] compared the two popular antihistamines dimenhydrinate (Dramamine) and cyclizine (Marezine) with regard to their antimotion sickness effect. They found that Marezine and Dramamine are similarly effective in preventing the overall subjective symptoms of motion sickness. While Dramamine's effectiveness may be related to its sedative properties, Marezine may work more directly on the stomach and thus be more effective in preventing gastric dysrhythmias and reports of gastrointestinal symptoms.

Neuroleptics: Phenothiazine was primarily used in the treatment of motion sickness, which had a stronger sedative effect compared to the antihistamines. The effect is probably based on an antidopamine influence in the chemoreceptive emetic trigger zone [50].

Ramanathan et al. [51] evaluated two intranasal dosage forms of promethazine in dogs for absorption and bioavailability relative to that of an equivalent intramuscular dose. They found that the intranasal application of promethazine offers great promise as an effective noninvasive alternative for treating space motion sickness due to its rapid absorption and bioavailability equivalent to the intramuscular dose. Intramuscular injections of promethazine in 25- or 50 mg dosages are commonly used to treat space motion sickness in astronauts. Cowings et al. [52] examined the effects of intramuscular injections of promethazine on performance, mood states and motion sickness in humans. Statistically significant decrements in performance were observed for both dosages of promethazine as compared with the placebo. They concluded that effective doses of promethazine currently used to counteract motion sickness in astronauts might significantly impair the task components of their operational performance.

Dopamine antagonists: The agent to mention here is metoclopramide, a centrally acting antidopaminergic drug. Although metoclopramide is an effective antiemetic agent that enhances gastric emptying and prevents cancer chemotherapy-induced emesis, some studies [53, 54] were unable to demonstrate any significant effects of this drug on motion sickness.

Serotonin (5-HT$_3$) receptor antagonist: The drugs ondansetron and granisetron are highly potent antiemetics. 5-HT$_3$ receptor antagonists inhibited the development of gastric tachyarrhythmia, but did not prevent the development of nausea and other symptoms of motion sickness. The antiemetics ondansetron and granisetron may act as gastric antidysrhythmics, but their ability to arrest the development of gastric tachyarrhythmia was not sufficient for the prevention of nausea [55].

Other drugs: In case of military activities, phenytoin in a dose of 1,200 mg/day was used. Furthermore, sailors reported some positive effects of cinnarizine (150 mg/day) to prevent motion sickness during sailing. Lee et al. [56] showed that the calcium antagonist flunarizine is a powerful peripherally acting labyrinthine suppressant, even with application in the prevention of motion sickness. The efficacy of ginger rhizome for the prevention of nausea, dizziness and vomiting as symptoms of motion sickness, as well as for postoperative vomiting and vomiting of pregnancy, has been well documented and proved beyond doubt in numerous high-quality clinical studies [57–59].

With regard to the side effects, Gordon et al. [60] assessed the influence of dimenhydrinate (100 mg), cinnarizine (50 mg) and transdermal scopolamine on the ability to perform simulated naval crew tasks. The effect of single doses of dimenhydrinate, cinnarizine and one transdermal scopolamine patch on psychomotor performance was evaluated. Dimenhydrinate significantly impaired decision reaction time and auditory digit span. Most of the subjects who took dimenhydrinate also reported a subjective decrease in well-being and general performance abilities. Cinnarizine and transdermal scopolamine did not affect performance abilities. Cinnarizine was free of significant side effects. Dry mouth was the only significant side effect of transdermal scopolamine.

These findings could be explained by the well-known sedative properties of dimenhydrinate and not by a specific effect on any particular cognitive or motor function. Our results suggest that dimenhydrinate (100 mg) adversely affects psychomotor function, whereas single doses of cinnarizine (50 mg) and transdermal scopolamine appear to be free of side effects on performance and seem to be a preferable anti-seasickness drug for use by a naval crew.

References

1 Brandt T, Daroff RB: The multisensory physiological and pathological vertigo syndromes. Ann Neurol 1980;7:195–203.
2 Oosterveld WJ: Motion sickness. J Travel Med 1995;2:182–185.
3 Wilson WD: Travel sickness in cattle. Vet Rec 1997;140:76.
4 Reason JT, Brand JJ: Motion Sickness. London, Academic Press, 1975.
5 Schmäl F, Stoll W: Kinetosen. HNO 2000;48:346–356.
6 Parker DM: A psychophysiological test for motion-sickness susceptibility. J Gen Psychol 1971; 85:87–92.
7 Money KE: Motion sickness. Physiol Rev 1970;50:1–39.
8 Oman CM: A heuristic mathematical model for the dynamics of sensory conflict and motion sickness. Acta Otolaryngol Suppl 1982;392:1–44.
9 Reason JT: Motion sickness adaptation: A neural mismatch model. J R Soc Med 1978;71:819–829.
10 Pitman JR, Yolton RL: Etiology and treatment of motion sickness: A review. J Am Optom Assoc 1983;54:31–38.
11 Helling K, Hausmann S, Flottmann T, Scherer H: Individual differences in susceptibility to motion sickness (in German). HNO 1997;45:210–215
12 Diamond SG, Markham CH: Validating the hypothesis of otolith asymmetry as a cause of space motion sickness. Ann NY Acad Sci 1992;656:725–731.
13 Nashner LM, Peters JF: Dynamic posturography in the diagnosis and management of dizziness and balance disorders. Neurol Clin 1990;8:331–349.
14 Scherer H, Frohlich G: Reactions to coriolis stimulations and postrotatory ENG response. A study on pilot candidates and pilots. Acta Otolaryngol 1972;74:113–117.
15 Scherer H, Helling K, Hausmann S, Clarke AH: On the origin of interindividual susceptibility to motion sickness. Acta Otolaryngol 1997;117:149–153.
16 Jokerst MD, Gatto M, Fazio R, Gianaros PJ, Stern RM, Koch KL: Effects of gender of subjects and experimenter on susceptibility to motion sickness. Aviat Space Environ Med 1999;70:962–965.
17 Grunfeld E, Gresty MA: Relationship between motion sickness, migraine and menstruation in crew members of a ‘round-the-world’ yacht race. Brain Res Bull 1998;47:433–436.
18 Cheung B, Heskin R, Hofer K, Gagnon M: The menstrual cycle and susceptibility to coriolis-induced sickness. J Vestib Res 2001;11:129–136.
19 McIntosh IB: Motion sickness – Questions and answers. J Travel Med 1998;5:89–91.
20 Busoni P, Sarti A, Crescioli M, Agostino MR, Sestini G, Banti S: Motion sickness and postoperative vomiting in children. Paediatr Anaesth 2002;12:65–68.
21 Dichgans J, Brandt T: Visual-vestibular interaction in self-motion perception and postural control; in Teuber L, Held R, Leibowitz HW (eds): Handbook of Sensory Physiology. Berlin, Springer, 1976, vol 5.
22 Fischer AJ, Oosterveld WJ: Motion sickness (in German). HNO 1979;27:285–291.
23 Yardley L: Motion sickness susceptibility and the utilisation of visual and otolithic information for orientation. Eur Arch Otorhinolaryngol 1990;247:300–304.
24 Wood R: The ‘haunted swing’ illusion. Psychol Rev 1895;2:277–278.
25 Kubo T, Matsunaga T, Matano S: Correlation between vestibular nuclei and the hypothalamus in the rat. Int J Equilib Res 1974;4:28–36.

26 Koch KL, Summy-Long J, Bingaman S, Sperry N, Stern RM: Vasopressin and oxytocin responses to illusory self-motion and nausea in man. J Clin Endocrinol Metab 1990;71:1269–1275.
27 Takeda N, Morita M, Kubo T, et al: Histaminergic mechanism of motion sickness. Neurochemical and neuropharmacological studies in rats. Acta Otolaryngol 1986;101:416–421.
28 Wang SC, Chinn H: Experimental motion sickness in dogs: Functional importance of chemoreceptive trigger zone. Am J Physiol 1954;186:111–116.
29 Nicholson AN, Pascoe PA, Spencer MB, Benson AJ: Jet lag and motion sickness. Br Med Bull 1993;49:285–304.
30 Barsoum G, Perry EP, Fraser IA: Postoperative nausea is relieved by acupressure. J R Soc Med 1990;83:86–89.
31 Bertolucci LE, DiDario B: Efficacy of a portable acustimulation device in controlling seasickness. Aviat Space Environ Med 1995;66:1155–1158.
32 Bruce DG, Golding JF, Hockenhull N, Pethybridge RJ: Acupressure and motion sickness. Aviat Space Environ Med 1990;61:361–365.
33 O'Brien B, Relyea MJ, Taerum T: Efficacy of P6 acupressure in the treatment of nausea and vomiting during pregnancy. Am J Obstet Gynecol 1996;174:708–715.
34 Dundee JW, Sourial FB, Ghaly RG, Bell PF: P6 acupressure reduces morning sickness. J R Soc Med 1988;81:456–457.
35 Hu S, Stritzel R, Chandler A, Stern RM: P6 acupressure reduces symptoms of vection-induced motion sickness. Aviat Space Environ Med 1995;66:631–634.
36 Stern RM, Jokerst MD, Muth ER, Hollis C: Acupressure relieves the symptoms of motion sickness and reduces abnormal gastric activity. Altern Ther Health Med 2001;7:91–94.
37 Groen J: Adaptation. Pract Otorhinolaryngol 1957;19:524.
38 Ruckenstein MJ, Harrison RV: Motion sickness. Helping patients tolerate the ups and downs. Postgrad Med 1991;89:139–144.
39 Helling K, Westhofen M: Experimental studies of motion sickness on board of a research ship (in German). HNO 1994;42:214–219.
40 Held R: Exposure history as a factor in maintaining stability of perception and co-ordination. J Nerv Ment Dis 1961;132:26–32.
41 Takeda N, Morita M, Horii A, Nishiike S, Kitahara T, Uno A: Neural mechanisms of motion sickness. J Med Invest 2001;48:44–59.
42 Wood CD, Graybiel A: A theory of motion sickness based on pharmacological reactions. Clin Pharmacol Ther 1970;11:621–629.
43 Becker G, Goossens H, Seemann K, Souchon F, Weitz T: Prevention of motion sickness with a transdermal therapeutic system containing scopolamine. A randomized, comparative double-blind study in the German Federal Navy (in German). Dtsch Med Wochenschr 1984;109:1881–1885.
44 Murray JB: Psychophysiological aspects of motion sickness. Percept Mot Skills 1997;85: 1163–1167.
45 Klocker N, Hanschke W, Toussaint S, Verse T: Scopolamine nasal spray in motion sickness: A randomised, controlled and crossover study for the comparison of two scopolamine nasal sprays with oral dimenhydrinate and placebo. Eur J Pharm Sci 2001;13:227–232.
46 Nachum Z, Shahal B, Shupak A, et al: Scopolamine bioavailability in combined oral and transdermal delivery. J Pharmacol Exp Ther 2001;296:121–123.
47 Gray L, Carliner P: The prevention and treatment of motion sickness. Science 1949;109:359.
48 Wood CD, Kennedy RE, Graybiel A, Trumbull R, Wherry RJ: Clinical effectiveness of anti-motion sickness drugs. Computer review of the literature. JAMA 1966;198:1155–1158.
49 Weinstein SE, Stern RM: Comparison of Marezine and Dramamine in preventing symptoms of motion sickness. Aviat Space Environ Med 1997;68:890–894.
50 Stoot J: Mechanism and treatment of motions sickness; in Davis C, Lake Bakaar G, Grahame-Smith D (eds): Nausea and Vomiting: Mechanisms and Treatment. Berlin, Springer, 1986.
51 Ramanathan R, Geary RS, Bourne DW, Putcha L: Bioavailability of intranasal promethazine dosage forms in dogs. Pharmacol Res 1998;38:35–39.
52 Cowings PS, Toscano WB, DeRoshia C, Miller NE: Promethazine as a motion sickness treatment: Impact on human performance and mood states. Aviat Space Environ Med 2000;71: 1013–1022.

53 Kohl RL: Failure of metoclopramide to control emesis or nausea due to stressful angular or linear acceleration. Aviat Space Environ Med 1987;58:125–131.
54 Oman CM, Lichtenberg BK, Money KE, McCoy RK: MIT/Canadian vestibular experiments on the Spacelab-1 mission. 4. Space motion sickness: symptoms, stimuli and predictability. Exp Brain Res 1986;64:316–334.
55 Levine ME, Chillas JC, Stern RM, Knox GW: The effects of serotonin ($5\text{-}HT_3$) receptor antagonists on gastric tachyarrhythmia and the symptoms of motion sickness. Aviat Space Environ Med 2000;71:1111–1114.
56 Lee JA, Watson LA, Boothby G: Calcium antagonists in the prevention of motion sickness. Aviat Space Environ Med 1986;57:45–48.
57 Grontved A, Brask T, Kambskard J, Hentzer E: Ginger root against seasickness. A controlled trial on the open sea. Acta Otolaryngol 1988;105:45–49.
58 Holtmann S, Clarke AH, Scherer H, Hohn M: The anti-motion sickness mechanism of ginger. A comparative study with placebo and dimenhydrinate. Acta Otolaryngol 1989;108:168–174.
59 Mowrey DB, Clayson DE: Motion sickness, ginger, and psychophysics. Lancet 1982;i:655–657.
60 Gordon CR, Gonen A, Nachum Z, Doweck I, Spitzer O, Shupak A: The effects of dimenhydrinate, cinnarizine and transdermal scopolamine on performance. J Psychopharmacol 2001;15:167–172.

Priv.-Doz. Dr. med. Frank Schmäl
Hals-Nasen-Ohrenklinik des Universitätsklinikums Münster
Kardinal-von-Galen-Ring 10
D–48149 Münster (Germany)
Tel. +49 251 8356801, Fax +49 251 8356812, E-Mail schmael.hno@uni-muenster.de

Donnerer J (ed): Antiemetic Therapy.
Basel, Karger, 2003, pp 113–120

Management of Opioid-Induced Nausea and Emesis

Rajender R. Aparasu[a], *Anuradha Aparasu*[b]

[a] College of Pharmacy, South Dakota State University, Brookings, S. Dak. and
[b] School of Medicine, University of South Dakota, Sioux Falls, S. Dak., USA

Introduction

Opioid analgesics such as morphine and meperidine are commonly used in the management of surgical and non-surgical pain. Although opioids are effective in relieving pain, nausea and emesis are troublesome side effects of opioid therapy. Often these symptoms can be a barrier to optimal pain management in patients receiving opioid therapy. Studies suggest that over 60% of patients receiving opioids experience nausea and emesis [1, 2]. Emesis is less frequent than nausea in patients taking opioids. The incidence of opioid-induced nausea and emesis varies with the type of opioid, dose, route of administration and duration of therapy [3–5]. The type of surgery and patient characteristics also influence opioid-induced nausea and emesis [1, 2, 5, 6].

In general, nausea and emesis are more frequent in the initial period of opioid therapy. These symptoms are mild and often discomforting for relatively short periods of time [6]. Most patients develop tolerance to these side effects over the course of time. However, studies suggest that nausea and vomiting associated with opioid therapy have a negative effect on functional outcomes and patient satisfaction [6]. In addition, intensity, duration and severity of nausea are positively associated with functional limitations such as the ability to concentrate and eat. Overall, nausea and emesis can influence patient outcomes and may limit usefulness of opioid therapy.

Pathophysiology

Complex central and peripheral mechanisms are involved in opioid-induced nausea and emesis. Opioids produce nausea and vomiting by stimulating dopamine release in the chemoreceptor trigger zone (CTZ) of area postrema of the medulla [7–10]. The CTZ activates the vomiting center in the reticular formation of the medulla, which in turn stimulates the vagus and splanchnic nerves resulting in nausea and vomiting.

Morphine and related opioids also increase vestibular sensitivity [7]. This increased stimulation of the vestibular apparatus causes nausea and emesis. In addition, the vestibular apparatus stimulates the vomiting center [8]. This can explain the higher incidence of opioid-induced nausea and emesis in ambulatory patients than in hospitalized patients [7].

Opioids also decrease intestinal motility causing constipation [11]. This can also result in nausea and vomiting. The cortex also influences the vomiting center via unclear mechanisms [9]. Through this input, patients with prior emetic experience with opioid therapy may have nausea even at the sight of the hospital.

Management

Pharmacotherapeutic approaches to manage nausea and emesis can be grouped into risk reduction, prevention and treatment. Tramer [12, 13] formulated these strategies as a rational approach to control postoperative nausea and vomiting. Although pathophysiology of nausea and emesis associated with opioids and surgery are somewhat different, the conceptual approaches for management of these undesired consequences are the same.

For patients receiving opioids, antiemetic therapy should be based on past medical history and present treatment needs. If possible, the risk of nausea and emesis should be reduced in patients receiving opioid therapy. If necessary, prophylactic therapy should be used to prevent nausea and emesis. In general, antiemetic treatment should be used after the onset of symptoms since the symptoms as well as the tolerance level vary from patient to patient.

Risk Reduction

The risk for nausea and emesis in patients receiving opioid therapy can be minimized. This can include avoidance of concomitant drugs that cause nausea and vomiting (e.g., amphotericin) [10]. Postoperatively, three interventions have been proven to be effective in controlling nausea and vomiting [13]. Use of propofol has been effective in reducing postoperative emesis in high-risk patients and in patients having outpatient surgeries [14]. Omitting nitrous oxide as a general anesthetic can prevent the risk of postoperative emesis [15].

Also, omitting antagonists of neuromuscular blockade during surgery can lessen postoperative nausea and vomiting [16].

Prevention

A number of antiemetic agents were examined for prophylactic effect in patients receiving opioid therapy. These agents can be grouped as anticholinergics (e.g., scopolamine), antihistamines (e.g., promethazine), butyrophenones (e.g., droperidol), corticosteroids (e.g., dexamethasone), substituted benzamides (e.g., metoclopramide), and serotonin receptor antagonists (e.g., ondansetron) [8, 11].

The activity of antiemetic agents varies and involves multiple mechanisms [8–11]. The antiemetic effects of anticholinergics and antihistamines are primarily due to their anticholinergic activity. Antihistamines are active at the vestibular apparatus and the vomiting center, whereas anticholinergics inhibit acetylcholine activity directly at the vomiting center.

Phenothiazines, butyrophenones and substituted benzamides are all dopamine D_2 receptor antagonists. These agents inhibit dopamine receptors in the CTZ and thereby prevent further sequelae. In addition, metoclopramide, a substituted benzamide, also has partial agonistic action on enteric postsynaptic neurons and thereby increases the motility of the stomach and small intestine. The inhibition of D_2 receptors also leads to extrapyramidal symptoms such as dystonia, parkinsonism, akathisia and tardive dyskinesia.

Antiemetic mechanism of corticosteroids is unclear [8, 11]. They probably inhibit prostaglandin synthesis in the hypothalamus. They also increase patient's acceptance of opioid therapy by improving their appetite and providing a sense of well-being. Serotonin receptor antagonists have been extensively studied in recent years for postoperative nausea and vomiting. Agents like ondansetron, granisetron and dolasetron inhibit 5-HT_3 in the CTZ and the vomiting center, one of the receptors that mediate the signaling in the vomiting center. They also antagonize vomiting signals in the afferent pathways from the stomach and small intestine. Serotonin receptor antagonists do not cause extrapyramidal effects, as they do not inhibit dopamine D_2 receptors.

Over the years, several studies were conducted involving a number of antiemetic agents to assess their prophylactic effect on opioid-induced nausea and emesis [1, 2]. Although examination of each of these studies can be informative, pooled quantitative analysis of these studies can be more useful and practical. Meta-analyses and systematic review are tools that can aid in understanding effectiveness of these agents by combining results from these studies. Both are statistical analytical tools that involve calculation of pooled effectiveness measures based on the data from several studies.

Hirayama et al. [2] conducted a meta-analysis of studies examining antiemetic agents for prophylaxis of opioid-induced nausea and emesis. Studies published from 1966 to 2000 and involving five antiemetic agents for postoperative opioid therapy were included. The agents examined were droperidol, metoclopramide, dexamethasone, propofol and ondansetron. According to their analysis, dexamethasone, droperidol and metoclopramide are effective in that order for prevention of opioid-induced nausea and emesis. Highest significant decrease (odds ratio 0.23, 95% confidence interval 0.15–0.35) in the incidence of nausea and emesis was observed with dexamethasone. The odds ratio and confidence interval for droperidol (dose range 1.25–10 mg) and metoclopramide (dose range 10–80 mg) were 0.27 (95% confidence interval 0.21–0.34) and 0.48 (95% confidence interval 0.30–0.75), respectively. The odds ratio for ondansetron was 0.40 but was not statistically significant. The findings suggest that dexamethasone 1.25–10 mg is the most effective agent and can reduce the incidence of nausea and vomiting from 66–80% to 16–50%.

Tramer and Walder [1] conducted a systematic review of prophylactic antiemetic agents for patient-controlled analgesia. Studies investigating seven different antiemetic agents were examined, namely droperidol, ondansetron, scopolamine, tropisetron, metoclopramide, propofol and promethazine. These studies were published from 1966 to 1998. According to the study, droperidol was the most frequently reported antiemetic agent for patient-controlled analgesia. Droperidol 0.5–11 mg/day was significantly more effective than placebo in preventing opioid-induced nausea and emesis. The numbers needed to treat for preventing nausea and emesis were 2.7 and 3.1, respectively. This suggests that 30% of the patients receiving opioids will benefit from droperidol. There was no dose response relationship for efficacy. However, adverse effects were dose-dependent with an increase in adverse effects like drowsiness occurring at doses >4 mg/day.

According to Tramer and Walder [1], serotonin receptor antagonists like ondansetron and tropisetron were the second most reported medications for patient-controlled analgesia. They were effective for emesis with little or no evidence of antinausea effect. The number needed to treat was approximately 5, thus suggesting that 20% of the patients receiving opioids will benefit from serotonin receptor antagonists. The effects of clonidine and promethazine were promising but were based on limited patients. Agents like scopolamine and propofol were not effective for opioid-induced nausea and emesis.

Several other agents such as prochlorperazine, naloxone and nalmefene were not included in the above meta-analysis studies. Initial clinical trials involving these agents were promising [17–19]. Prochlorperazine, a phenothiazine, has been widely used as an antiemetic agent but its use for opioid-induced nausea and emesis has to be further studied. Naloxone and nalmefene,

Table 1. Antiemetic agents for the management of opioid-induced nausea and emesis

Agents	Mechanism	Dose/day, mg	Prophylaxis	Treatment	Side effects
Droperidol	Blocks D_2 receptors in CTZ	1.25–10	+++	?	Oversedation, extrapyramidal symptoms
Dexamethasone	Inhibits hypothalamic prostaglandin synthesis	0.5–11	+++	?	Wound infection, delayed wound healing
Metoclopramide	Blocks D_2 and 5-HT_3 receptors	10–80	++	+?	Extrapyramidal symptoms
Ondansetron	Blocks 5-HT_3 in CTZ and vomiting center	4–16	+?	++	Headache, constipation

D_2 = Dopamine; 5-HT_3 = 5-hydroxytryptamine.

opioid antagonists, may have a place for the management of opioid-induced nausea and emesis; however, more research is needed to establish their role.

In summary, research suggests that dexamethasone and droperidol are the most effective agents to prevent opioid-induced nausea and emesis (table 1). Metoclopramide is also effective as prophylactic therapy for opioid-induced nausea and emesis. Serotonin receptor antagonists, especially ondansetron and tropisetron, are promising for opioid-induced nausea and emesis but further investigations are needed to establish their prophylactic effect. Although dexamethasone, droperidol and metoclopramide are effective, the adverse effects profile of these agents should be considered in choosing antiemetic therapy. Dexamethasone can cause wound infection and delay wound healing, whereas droperidol can cause oversedation. Extrapyramidal symptoms and parkinsonism are some of the undesirable effects of metoclopramide.

Treatment

Although there is extensive literature on prophylactic antiemetic therapy, there are very few studies investigating antiemetic agents for the treatment of opioid-induced nausea and emesis. In a recent systematic review, Kazemi-Kjellberg et al. [20] reported that only serotonin receptor antagonists were tested adequately for the treatment of postoperative nausea and vomiting. The data on other antiemetic agents for postoperative nausea and vomiting were also very limited. Although several antiemetic agents are available for the treatment [8–10], our literature review revealed that very few agents were adequately investigated for the treatment of opioid-induced nausea and emesis [21–24].

Only two antiemetic agents, ondansetron and metoclopramide, were studied using randomized clinical trials for the treatment of opioid-induced nausea and emesis.

In a study involving non-surgical patients, ondansetron 8 and 16 mg were effective in controlling opioid-induced nausea and emesis [21]. Complete control of emesis was achieved in 62 and 69% of patients receiving ondansetron 8 and 16 mg respectively when compared with 46% in the placebo group. In addition, patients receiving ondansetron 16 mg also had reduced nausea; the 8-mg dose did not achieve statistical significance. Also, patients receiving both 8 and 16 mg were more satisfied with their antiemetic therapy when compared to patients receiving placebo. In another study involving cancer patients, efficacy measures for both ondansetron 24 mg and metoclopramide 10 mg were not statistically significant when compared to placebo [22]. However, the study was limited to a very small number of patients.

In a comparative trial involving surgical patients, ondansetron at doses 8 and 16 mg was significantly effective than metoclopramide 10 mg for nausea and vomiting in postsurgical patients receiving opioid analgesia [23]. Complete control of emesis with 8 and 16 mg of ondansetron was achieved in 63 and 61%, respectively. In the metoclopramide group, emesis control was 48%. Both doses were statistically significant in controlling nausea when compared to metoclopramide. In another study, surgical patients receiving opioid therapy were treated with 4 and 16 mg of ondansetron for opioid-induced nausea and vomiting [24]. Significant control of emesis was achieved with both doses of ondansetron when compared to placebo. Nausea and patient satisfaction scores were also better for 16 mg group when compared to placebo.

In summary, several agents are used for the treatment of opioid-induced nausea and emesis. However, the efficacy data based on the clinical trials for these agents is lacking. Only two agents were adequately studied for opioid-induced nausea and emesis (table 1). Research suggests that ondansetron appears to be an effective agent to treat opioid-induced nausea and emesis in both surgical and non-surgical patients. However, further research is needed to establish the use of other agents, especially metoclopramide, for the management of opioid-induced nausea and emesis.

Conclusions

Nausea and emesis are common and troublesome side effects of opioid therapy. These symptoms can be a barrier to optimal patient outcomes in both surgical and non-surgical patients. There are several approaches for risk reduction, prevention and treatment of opioid-induced nausea and emesis. Unlike postoperative nausea and vomiting, routine use of antiemetic agents to prevent opioid-induced nausea and emesis may not be necessary as the incidence of nausea and vomiting with opioid therapy is variable and less frequent.

If possible, the risk of nausea and emesis should be reduced in patients receiving opioid therapy. This can include avoidance of medications that can increase the risk. Antiemetic therapy should be used for prophylaxis in surgical patients receiving opioid therapy since there is a high incidence of nausea and emesis in postsurgical patients. Several antiemetic agents were examined for prophylactic therapy. The studies strongly support the use dexamethasone and droperidol for prophylaxis of opioid-induced nausea and emesis. Metoclopramide is also effective for opioid-induced nausea and emesis but use of ondansetron as prophylactic therapy is not supported.

In most non-surgical patients receiving opioids, antiemetic agents should be used after the onset of nausea. Although several agents are being used, only ondansetron has been proven to be effective in the treatment of opioid-induced nausea and emesis in both surgical and non-surgical patients. Most of the research in the area of opioid-induced nausea and emesis has focused on prophylactic therapy, especially in surgical patients. Research on the treatment of opioid-induced nausea and emesis is very limited. More research is needed to examine the use of other antiemetics for the treatment of opioid-induced nausea and emesis.

References

1 Tramer MR, Walder B: Efficacy and adverse effects of prophylactic antiemetics during patient-controlled analgesia therapy: A quantitative systematic review. Anesth Analg 1999;88:1354–1361.

2 Hirayama T, Ishii F, Yago K, Ogata H: Evaluation of the effective drugs for the prevention of nausea and vomiting induced by morphine used for postoperative pain: A quantitative systematic review. Yakugaku Zasshi 2001;121:179–185.

3 Robinson SL, Fell D: Nausea and vomiting with use of a patient-controlled analgesia system. Anaesthesia 1991;46:580–582.

4 Woodhouse A, Mather LE: The effect of duration of dose delivery with patient-controlled analgesia on the incidence of nausea and vomiting after hysterectomy. Br J Clin Pharmacol 1998;45:57–62.

5 Zun LS, Downey LV, Gossman W, Rosenbaumdagger J, Sussman G: Gender differences in narcotic-induced emesis in the emergency department. Am J Emerg Med 2002;20:151–154.

6 Aparasu R, McCoy RA, Weber C, Mair D, Parasuraman TV: Opioid-induced emesis among hospitalized non-surgical patients: Effect on pain and quality of life. J Pain Symptom Manage 1999; 18:280–288.

7 Reissine T, Pasternak G: Opioid analgesics and antagonits; in Hardman JG, Limbird LE (eds): Goodman & Gliman's The Pharmacological Basis of Therapeutics. New York, McGraw-Hill, 1996, chapt 23, pp 521–555.

8 Clayton BD, Frye CB: Nausea and vomiting; in Herfindal ET, Gourley DR (eds): Clinical Pharmacy and Therapeutics, ed 7. Philadelphia, Williams & Wilkins, 2000, chapt 26, pp 553–569.

9 Lindley C: Nausea and vomiting; in Koda-Kimble MA, Yong LY (eds): Applied Therapeutics, ed 7. Philadelphia, Lippincott Williams & Wilkins, 2001, chapt 6, pp 1–17.

10 Taylor T, Holland EG: Nausea and vomiting; in Dipero JT, Talbert, Yee GC, Matzke GR, Wells BG, Posey LM (eds): Pharmacotherapy: A Pathophysiology Approach. Stamford, Appleton & Lange, 1997, chapt 35, pp 751–765.
11 Brunton LL: Agents affecting gastrointestinal water flux and motility; emesis and antiemetics; bile acids and pancreatic enzymes; in Hardman JG, Limbird LE (eds): Goodman & Gliman's The Pharmacological Basis of Therapeutics. New York, McGraw-Hill, 1996, chapt 38, pp 917–949.
12 Tramer MR: A rational approach to the control of postoperative nausea and vomiting: Evidence from systematic reviews. I. Efficacy and harm of antiemetic interventions, and methodological issues. Acta Anaesthesiol Scand 2001;45:4–13.
13 Tramer MR: A rational approach to the control of postoperative nausea and vomiting: Evidence from systematic reviews. II. Recommendations for prevention and treatment, and research agenda. Acta Anaesthesiol Scand 2001;45:14–19.
14 Tramer M, Moore A, McQuay H: Propofol anaesthesia and postoperative nausea and vomiting: Quantitative systematic review of randomized controlled studies. Br J Anaesth 1997;78:247–255.
15 Tramer M, Moore A, McQuay H: Omitting nitrous oxide in general anaesthesia: Meta-analysis of intraoperative awareness and postoperative emesis in randomized controlled trials. Br J Anaesth 1996;76:186–193.
16 Tramer MR, Fuchs-Buder T: Omitting antagonism of neuromuscular block: Effect on postoperative nausea and vomiting and risk of residual paralysis. A systematic review. Br J Anaesth 1999; 82:379–386.
17 Williams PI, Smith M: An assessment of prochlorperazine buccal for the prevention of nausea and vomiting during intravenous patient-controlled analgesia with morphine following abdominal hysterectomy. Eur J Anaesthesiol 1999;16:638–645.
18 Joshi GP, Duffy L, Chehade J, Wesevich J, Gajraj N, Johnson ER: Effects of prophylactic nalmefene on the incidence of morphine-related side effects in patients receiving intravenous patient-controlled analgesia. Anesthesiology 1999;90:1007–1011
19 Choi JH, Lee J, Choi JH, Bishop MJ: Epidural naloxone reduces pruritus and nausea without affecting analgesia by epidural morphine in bupivacaine. Can J Anaesth 2000;47:33–37.
20 Kazemi-Kjellberg F, Henzi I, Tramer MR: Treatment of established postoperative nausea and vomiting: A quantitative systematic review. BMC Anesthesiol 2001;1:2.
21 Sussman G, Shurman J, Creed MR, Larsen LS, Ferrer-Brechner T, Noll D, Allegra J, Montgomery R, Schreck D, Grafstein E, Ramalanjaona G, Patel V, Ducharme J, Ortenwall P, Foster E, Ames M: Intravenous ondansetron for the control of opioid-induced nausea and vomiting. International S3AA3013 Study Group. Clin Ther 1999;21:1216–1227.
22 Hardy J, Daly S, McQuade B, Albertsson M, Chimontsi-Kypriou V, Stathopoulos P, Curtis P: A double-blind, randomised, parallel-group, multinational, multicentre study comparing a single dose of ondansetron 24 mg p.o. with placebo and metoclopramide 10 mg t.d.s. p.o. in the treatment of opioid-induced nausea and emesis in cancer patients. Support Care Cancer 2002;10:231–236.
23 Chung F, Lane R, Spraggs C, McQuade B, Jacka M, Luttropp HH, Alahuta S, Rocherieux S, Roy M, Duvaldestin P, Curtis P: Ondansetron is more effective than metoclopramide for the treatment of opioid-induced emesis in post-surgical adult patients. Ondansetron OIE Post-Surgical Study Group. Eur J Anaesthesiol 1999;16:669–677.
24 Rung GW, Claybon L, Hord A, Patel C, Kallgren M, Koppel J, Benedetti C, Creed M, Asgharian A, Bryson J: Intravenous ondansetron for postsurgical opioid-induced nausea and vomiting. S3A-255 Study Group. Anesth Analg 1997;84:832–838.

Rajender R. Aparasu, PhD
College of Pharmacy – Box 2202 C, 1 Administration Lane
South Dakota State University, Brookings, SD 57007 (USA)
Tel. +1 605 6886646, Fax +1 605 6886232, E-Mail Rajender_Aparasu@sdstate.edu

Donnerer J (ed): Antiemetic Therapy.
Basel, Karger, 2003, pp 121–160

Prevention and Treatment of Postoperative Nausea and Vomiting

Anthony L. Kovac

Department of Anesthesiology, University of Kansas Medical Center, Kansas City, Kans., USA

Introduction

Postoperative nausea and vomiting (PONV) continues to be a common side effect of surgery and anesthesia. With the change in emphasis from inpatient to outpatient care, and the possibility of delayed discharge or unexpected hospital admission, PONV has been called the 'big little problem' [1]. PONV affects the economics of medical care, as well as the degree of patients' satisfaction, comfort and quality of life. PONV is often of greater concern to patients than postoperative pain [2].

There is continuing interest in the prevention and treatment of PONV because of: (1) an increase in ambulatory and office-based anesthesia; (2) new anesthesia techniques and medications that help patients bypass the post-anesthesia care unit (PACU); (3) the importance of postoperative care and avoiding the postoperative complications of pain, nausea and vomiting; (4) introduction of new antiemetics; (5) use of old and new antiemetic medications and techniques, for combination and multimodal therapy, and (6) relative ineffectiveness of the currently used antiemetics as monotherapy for PONV.

Although the efficacy of antiemetic therapy for prevention and treatment of PONV has been frequently studied, it is not well understood. The best approach for optimal prevention and treatment of PONV is not always evident. This chapter will review: (1) the anatomy, neurophysiology and baseline risk factors of PONV; (2) antiemetic medications in common use; (3) side effects of antiemetic medications, and (4) comparison and use of antiemetics and techniques alone, combined, or as multimodal therapy for prevention and treatment of PONV.

Incidence of PONV

Considering all types of patient populations and surgical procedures, it is estimated that PONV may have an incidence as high as 70–80% among certain high-risk patients and surgeries. An overall estimate of PONV is approximately 20–30% of all adult surgical patients. Infants have approximately a 5% incidence of postoperative vomiting (POV), which increases in children older than 3 years to an incidence of approximately 40%, peaking at puberty. During the first 2 h in the PACU, the incidence of nausea and vomiting are estimated to occur in 20 and 5% of patients, respectively. For the following 2–24 postoperative hours, nausea and vomiting are estimated to occur in 50 and 25% of patients, respectively [3]. Although rare, severe, intractable nausea and vomiting is one of the leading causes of unanticipated hospital admission and is estimated to occur in approximately 0.18% of all postsurgical patients [4]. However, even patients with no PONV in the PACU may experience PONV following discharge home and the initiation of opioid pain medications. In a post-discharge survey conducted up to 5 days postoperatively with patients who did not experience PONV in the PACU, Carroll et al. [5] determined that more than 35% of patients who had no PONV in the PACU, experienced PONV following discharge. This PONV can slow a patient's return to normal daily activities and affect patient satisfaction.

Mechanism for Nausea and Vomiting

Vomiting is the expulsion of gastrointestinal (GI) contents via the mouth. Retching is labored, spasmodic, rhythmic contractions of the respiratory muscles (diaphragm, chest, abdominal wall), that occurs with movement of the stomach and esophagus without vomiting. While retching and vomiting are objective patient responses, nausea is subjective and is an unpleasant sensation associated with the urge to vomit [6].

Peripheral and central nervous system (CNS) mechanisms for nausea and vomiting were proposed by Borison and Wang [7, 8]. The peripheral mechanism involves GI stimuli of the vagus nerve. The CNS mechanism involves stimulation of multiple emetogenic receptors in the area postrema, chemoreceptor trigger zone (CTZ), nucleus of the solitary tract, and vomiting center (see figure 1 in chapter 1).

The CNS neuroemetic receptors that are involved with PONV include dopamine D_2, opioid, muscarinic, cholinergic, histamine and serotonin (5-hydroxytryptamine, 5-HT_3) receptors [9]. The area postrema contains 5-HT_3, opioid and dopamine D_2 receptors [10–12]. In the nucleus of the solitary tract are enkephalin, muscarine and histamine receptors [9, 13, 14]. Perioperative stimuli cause the release of these CNS emetogenic chemicals, initiating the vomiting reflex.

The physiology of PONV involves peripheral stimulation via cranial nerve (CN) VIII (acoustic-vestibular), CN IX (glossopharyngeal), CN X (vagus), and the GI reflex [7, 9, 11, 15]. Afferent input to the area postrema occurs via the glossopharyngeal and vagal nerves [10, 11]. The CNS areas associated with vasomotor activity, balance and respiration are located near the vomiting center. Stimulation and release of emetogenic chemicals from the CNS emetic centers in turn stimulate the respiratory, vasomotor and salivatory centers. This causes a response of the stomach, esophagus, diaphragm and abdominal muscles [6], resulting in physiological reactions, such as, salivation, sweating, tachycardia, tachypnea, cardiac dysrhythmias, dizziness and motion sickness that are frequently observed with PONV [6, 16]. Blockade of the central receptors and the peripheral reflex is hypothesized to be the mechanism of action of the currently used antiemetics [15].

With multiple CNS receptor sites available to cause PONV, single drug antiemetic therapy has not been 100% effective for all patients and all types of surgical procedures. Compared to chemotherapy-induced nausea and vomiting (CINV), the etiology of PONV is more complex, multifactorial, and involves patient-, medical- and surgical-related risk factors. One of the goals of antiemetic therapy in order to effectively prevent and/or treat PONV is to determine the efficacy and safety of antiemetic interactions as well as to decrease the patients' baseline risk of developing PONV [17, 18].

PONV Risk Factors (table 1)

Medical-Related Risk Factors

Patients with a history of motion sickness may have PONV due to stimulation of the acoustic-vestibular nerve (CN VIII) secondary to endolymph movement in the semicircular canals [19]. Metabolic causes of nausea and vomiting include diabetes, uremia, electrolyte imbalance (sodium, potassium), chemotherapy, radiation therapy and the hormonal variations in estrogen or progesterone that occur during pregnancy (hyperemesis gravidarum) [6, 20]. Intracranial causes of nausea and vomiting occur secondary to increased intracranial pressure causing direct CNS pressure and stimulation of the vomiting center [2, 19, 20]. Sensory stimulation also may occur secondary to inflammation of the airway, posterior pharynx, abdomen, GI tract, kidneys, bladder, testes or cervix, initiating the nausea and vomiting reflex [15, 20–23].

Anesthesia-Related Risk Factors

Opioid use in the pre-, intra-, or postoperative periods increases the baseline risk for PONV by stimulating opioid receptors in the area postrema [24–26].

Table 1. PONV risk factors

Patient-related factors	
Females > 3 × males	
Prior history of motion sickness or PONV	
Non-smoking history	
Pediatric patient: 3–16 years	
Concomitant medical problems (diabetes, bowel obstruction, etc.)	
State of fluid hydration (hypovolemia)	
Anesthesia-related factors	
Inhalation anesthetics	
Nitrous oxide	
Opioid analgesics	
Surgery-related factors (type/area of surgery)	
Laparoscopy	Shoulder
Mastoid-inner ear	Breast
Intra-abdominal	Testicle/scrotum
Strabismus repair	
Tonsillectomy	
Oral, plastic, ENT procedures (swallowing of blood)	
Postanesthesia care unit-related factors	
Patient movement (vestibular changes)	
Hypovolemia (orthostatic hypotension)	
Pain	

Postoperative patient movement causes changes of endolymph in the inner ear, increasing the incidence of opioid-induced emesis [23–25].

Ether and cyclopropane were highly emetogenic inhalation agents that had a PONV risk as high as 75–80% [6, 26]. While inhalation anesthetics can cause PONV in the early 0- to 2-hour postoperative period, there appears to be no difference in the incidence of PONV risk between desflurane and sevoflurane or between these agents and isoflurane [27, 28]. Nitrous oxide (N_2O) has been shown to increase PONV risk by direct stimulation of the vomiting center and sympathetic nervous system [29–32]. Peripheral N_2O stimulation occurs by the distention of air containing spaces of the middle ear, GI tract and gallbladder [33]. An increased incidence of PONV was determined in patients who received anesthesia with N_2O versus anesthesia without N_2O in a meta-analysis of N_2O anesthesia studies [17, 29].

Intravenous (IV) hypnotics, such as propofol [34–37], methohexital [36] and thiopentone [35], have less of an incidence of PONV, compared to ketamine [38, 39] or etomidate [40–42]. Reversal of muscle relaxants with an anti-cholinesterase, such as neostigmine, has been shown to cause an increase in the incidence of PONV due to the muscarinic effects of these drugs that increase GI motility [43].

Substituting glycopyrrolate for atropine does not affect GI motility. This suggests that when anticholinesterases and muscarinic cholinergic antagonists are given in the usual ratios, PONV may not be affected [6, 44]. Tramèr and Fuchs-Buder [45] determined that the crucial neostigmine dose causing PONV was 2.5 mg. There was no evidence that smaller doses would have any emetogenic effect and omitting reversal of neuromuscular block increased the risk of residual muscle paralysis [17, 45].

Regional anesthesia alone has a lower incidence of PONV compared to general anesthesia [6, 46]. However, regional anesthesia such as spinal or epidural causing hypotension secondary to sympathetic blockade can cause nausea, retching and/or emesis with an incidence of approximately 10–20% [47, 48]. There is an increased incidence of nausea and vomiting when a sympathetic block was achieved above the tenth thoracic (T_{10}) dermatome [48]. Nausea and vomiting also may occur during intra-abdominal GI manipulation under regional anesthesia due to a direct tactile effect, decreased cerebral blood flow (secondary to hypotension), increased GI atony, and vagal stimulation [48].

Postoperative pain can be a cause of PONV. Use of IV opiates has been shown to both relieve and cause nausea in patients who have pain with nausea. Opioid analgesia and nausea can be reversed with naloxone, resulting in a return of pain with nausea [6, 49].

In the PACU, pain, opioids, patient movement, hemodynamic stability, hypovolemia, orthostatic hypotension and the initiation of oral intake increase a patient's risk for developing PONV [50–54]. Patient movement and early ambulation in the PACU increases baseline PONV risk due to stimulation of the vestibular nerve causing motion sickness. Orthostatic changes may cause hypotension and thereby decrease cerebral perfusion and blood flow to the vomiting center [19, 52, 55]. Orthostatic hypotension can occur secondary to dehydration caused by an aggressive preoperative bowel preparation, blood loss or inadequate perioperative IV fluid replacement [6, 50]. Perioperative IV fluid hydration with at least 20 ml/kg of crystalloid has been determined by Suntheringham et al. [51] to decrease the possibility of postoperative nausea. Intravenous fluid administration should maintain urine output between 0.5 to 1.0 ml/kg/h.

Patient-Related Risk Factors

Patient-related PONV risk factors may include age, weight, gender, nonsmoking history, past history of PONV or motion sickness and/or exposure to emetogenic drugs, pain, concomitant medical problems, state of fluid hydration, orthostatic hypotension and CNS pathology [6, 16, 54–61].

The use of evidence-based medicine has helped define the patient-related baseline risk factors for PONV. Systematic reviews and meta-analyses have yielded important conclusions from the analysis of multiple randomized controlled trials with large numbers of patients. Tramèr [17] has used meta-analysis and the concepts of number needed to treat (NNT) and number needed to harm (NNH) as tools that aid the clinical practitioner to easily compare and analyze the degree of efficacy and adverse event rates, respectively, of different medications (fig. 1). Tramèr uses as an example that if a perfect response is defined as 100%, then a 20% response gives an NNT of 5 (100% divided by 20%) and 5 patients need to receive a prophylactic antiemetic for one to not have PONV who would have done so had they received no treatment at all or a placebo. Similarly, a NNH of 36 refers to the fact that 36 patients would have to receive the medication for one patient to show an adverse event.

The baseline PONV risk of patients can be estimated from previous studies and meta-analyses. There is a threefold increased PONV incidence in patients with a history of PONV or motion sickness [59–61]. Female patients have a two to three times greater PONV incidence than males [6, 22, 23]. In adults, there is a correlation between increasing age and decreasing incidence of PONV, with a lower incidence of PONV in geriatric patients [6, 52, 54].

PONV studies in pediatric patients are limited to vomiting (objective data) and not nausea (subjective response). One of the main parental postoperative

Fig. 1. Number-needed-to-treat (NNT) of antiemetics used for PONV and number-needed-to-harm (NNH) of antiemetics used for PONV. ***A*** The endpoint is prevention of nausea or vomiting, within 6 h after surgery ('early' efficacy) or within 24 h after surgery ('late' efficacy). Thus, for each intervention, antinausea and antivomiting efficacy can be interpreted separately, as well as short-term and long-term efficacy. Symbols are numbers-needed-to-treat to prevent nausea or vomiting. Areas of symbols are plotted proportional to the number of analyzed patients. Horizontal bars are 95% confidence intervals. The upper boundary of the 95% confidence interval around the number-needed-to-treat places the treatment in the least favorable light. If this upper limit lies within what would be considered to be the minimal clinically relevant effect (for instance, a number-needed-to-treat of 5 to prevent PONV), the result indicates a definitely useful treatment. ***B*** The number-needed-to-harm is the number of patients needed to be treated with the intervention for one to show an adverse reaction, who would not have shown this reaction had they not received the intervention. Symbol areas are fixed, and no confidence intervals are shown. The reason is that some numbers-needed-to-harm are based on a limited number of patients who showed the adverse drug reaction. Yet these numbers-needed-to-harm may be clinically relevant. Statistical significance was arbitrarily set at $p < 0.05$. Black symbols represent adverse drug reactions which happened statistically significantly more often with the intervention. White symbols indicate absence of statistical significance. Printed with permission from Tramèr [17].

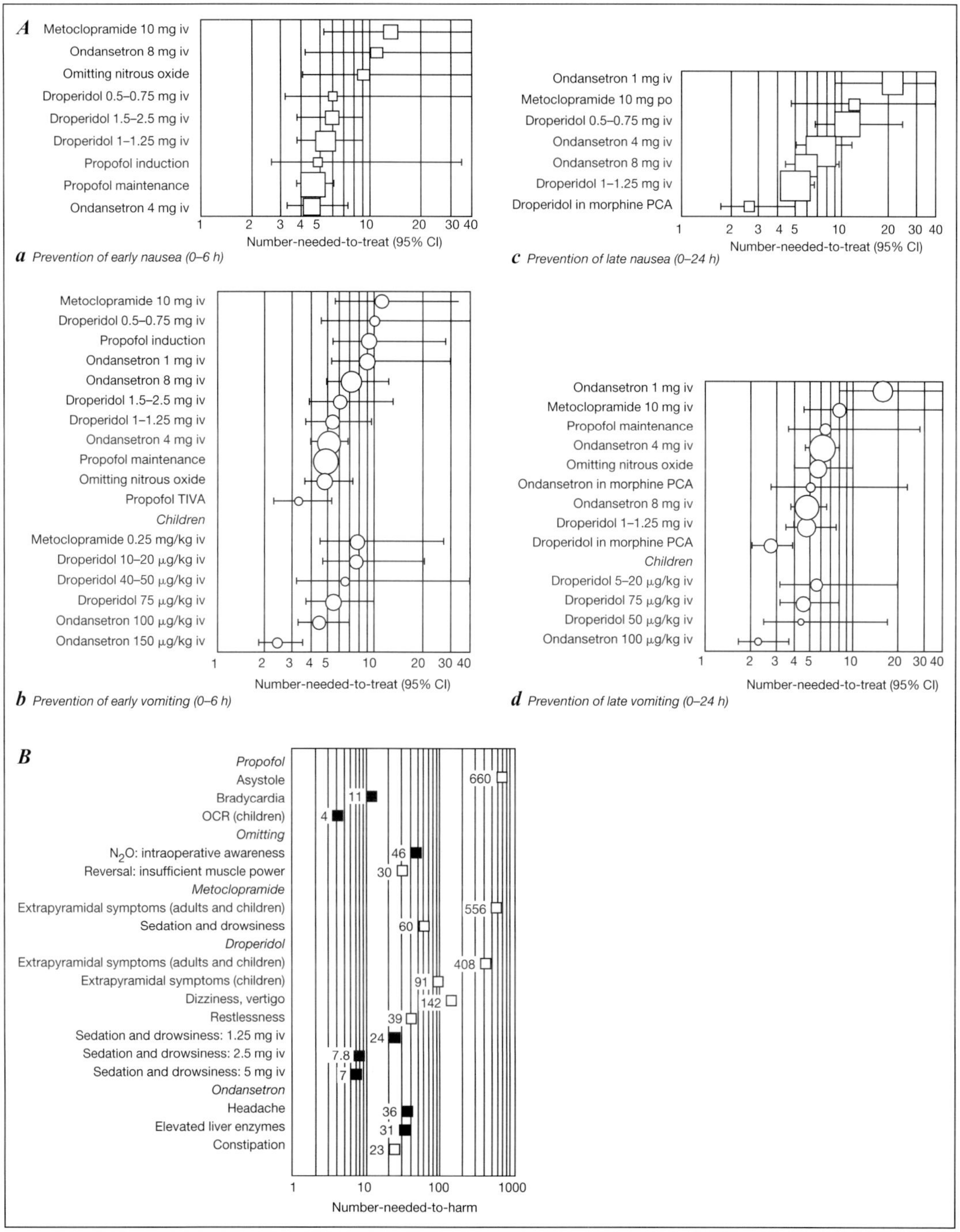
A
Metoclopramide 10 mg iv
Ondansetron 8 mg iv
Omitting nitrous oxide
Droperidol 0.5–0.75 mg iv
Droperidol 1.5–2.5 mg iv
Droperidol 1–1.25 mg iv
Propofol induction
Propofol maintenance
Ondansetron 4 mg iv
1 2 3 4 5 10 20 30 40
Number-needed-to-treat (95% CI)
a Prevention of early nausea (0–6 h)
Ondansetron 1 mg iv
Metoclopramide 10 mg po
Droperidol 0.5–0.75 mg iv
Ondansetron 4 mg iv
Ondansetron 8 mg iv
Droperidol 1–1.25 mg iv
Droperidol in morphine PCA
1 2 3 4 5 10 20 30 40
Number-needed-to-treat (95% CI)
c Prevention of late nausea (0–24 h)
Metoclopramide 10 mg iv
Droperidol 0.5–0.75 mg iv
Propofol induction
Ondansetron 1 mg iv
Ondansetron 8 mg iv
Droperidol 1.5–2.5 mg iv
Droperidol 1–1.25 mg iv
Ondansetron 4 mg iv
Propofol maintenance
Omitting nitrous oxide
Propofol TIVA
Children
Metoclopramide 0.25 mg/kg iv
Droperidol 10–20 μg/kg iv
Droperidol 40–50 μg/kg iv
Droperidol 75 μg/kg iv
Ondansetron 100 μg/kg iv
Ondansetron 150 μg/kg iv
1 2 3 4 5 10 20 30 40
Number-needed-to-treat (95% CI)
b Prevention of early vomiting (0–6 h)
Ondansetron 1 mg iv
Metoclopramide 10 mg iv
Propofol maintenance
Ondansetron 4 mg iv
Omitting nitrous oxide
Ondansetron in morphine PCA
Ondansetron 8 mg iv
Droperidol 1–1.25 mg iv
Droperidol in morphine PCA
Children
Droperidol 5–20 μg/kg iv
Droperidol 75 μg/kg iv
Droperidol 50 μg/kg iv
Ondansetron 100 μg/kg iv
1 2 3 4 5 10 20 30 40
Number-needed-to-treat (95% CI)
d Prevention of late vomiting (0–24 h)
B
Propofol
Asystole 660
Bradycardia 11
OCR (children) 4
Omitting
N2O: intraoperative awareness 46
Reversal: insufficient muscle power 30
Metoclopramide
Extrapyramidal symptoms (adults and children) 556
Sedation and drowsiness 60
Droperidol
Extrapyramidal symptoms (adults and children) 408
Extrapyramidal symptoms (children) 91
Dizziness, vertigo 142
Restlessness 39
Sedation and drowsiness: 1.25 mg iv 24
Sedation and drowsiness: 2.5 mg iv 7.8
Sedation and drowsiness: 5 mg iv 7
Ondansetron
Headache 36
Elevated liver enzymes 31
Constipation 23
1 10 100 1000
Number-needed-to-harm
1

complaints and the leading cause of readmission of children is postoperative vomiting (POV) [6, 56, 57]. Before puberty, there are no differences in the POV incidence between boys and girls. The POV incidence in children decreases after puberty. As the incidence of POV in children is two times that of adults, more children than adults will need POV prophylaxis. However, overall, the POV baseline risk factors in children are the same as adults [62, 63].

Anxiety can cause PONV due to hyperventilation, air swallowing and α_1-adrenergic mechanisms that increase plasma epinephrine and norepinephrine levels [21, 52]. Obesity is controversial as a risk factor, but there appears to be a positive correlation between body weight and postoperative emesis [6]. This increase in PONV may be due to increased drug deposition in adipose cells, increased residual gastric volume, or increased esophageal reflux, as well as gallbladder and GI disease in obese patients [6, 64]. In addition, obese patients may have more PONV secondary to an overall lower total mg/kg dose of antiemetic, which is achieved when a fixed dose is administered, especially to patients weighing more than 80 kg. Many antiemetic studies have been conducted in adult patients who weighed between 40 and 80 kg. Non-smoking history increases PONV, as patients with a strong smoking history have less PONV possibly secondary to sensitization to nicotine and other carcinogen toxins in smoke. Tobacco smoke is thought to induce the liver CYP1A2 P_{450} enzyme. Use of opioid analgesics increases PONV risk secondary to stimulation of CNS opioid neuroreceptors [6, 23].

Surgery-Related Risk Factors

There is a higher risk of PONV in adults following eye, oral, plastic, ear, nose, throat (ENT), dental, head and neck, gynecologic, obstetric, laparoscopic, shoulder, varicose vein stripping, breast and abdominal procedures (table 1) [6, 16, 22, 23, 25, 65–68]. Oral, plastic or ENT procedures with an increased occurrence of swallowed blood increase PONV risk, as blood is a very strong emetogenic stimulus. Sinclair et al. [61] studied 18,000 ambulatory surgery patients and found that patients undergoing gynecologic laparoscopy, dental surgery, orthopedic shoulder operations, strabismus surgery, breast augmentation and varicose vein stripping operations had an increased PONV risk by more than 15%. In children, there is an increased incidence of POV with specific operations, which include adenotonsillectomy, penile surgery, orchiopexy, strabismus repair and hernia repair [16, 56, 57].

Duration of surgery is a risk factor. Sinclair et al. [61] estimated that each 30-min increase in surgical time increased the risk of PONV by approximately 60%. Therefore, if the PONV risk in a patient is 10%, after 30 min, the patient's risk is increased to 16%; after 60 min, the risk is increased to 22%, and so on.

PONV Risk Scores

Routine prophylaxis for PONV is neither necessary nor cost-effective for all patients or all surgical procedures, as not all patients require prophylactic antiemetics. Determining the underlying baseline PONV risk as low, medium, high or extremely high is important for each specific patient population and surgical procedure to help determine whether or not to choose prophylactic antiemetic therapy, and if so, what therapy to choose. Low PONV risk patients may not benefit from prophylaxis and instead be at risk from the harmful side effects of antiemetic medications. Tramèr [18] concluded that there is a finite risk of adverse drug reactions with most antiemetic interventions. This risk is illustrated by the concept of NNH.

When analyzing randomized, controlled trials, a placebo control group is necessary in antiemetic studies to determine the underlying baseline PONV risk of the patient population being studied [17]. A placebo group with a high baseline PONV incidence indicates that the study population is at high risk for PONV. Conversely, a placebo group with a low baseline PONV incidence indicates that the study group represents a population with a low PONV risk. No antiemetic prophylaxis should be administered to patients at low risk for PONV. Instead, antiemetic prophylaxis should be administered to patients at moderate to extremely high risk for PONV [62].

PONV risk scores and treatment algorithms have been proposed to help determine baseline PONV risk [59, 59a, 60, 69]. The data of Koivuranta et al. [59a] was combined with that of Apfel et al. [60] to develop a simplifed PONV risk score. This is a very useful, simple and easy-to-remember PONV risk scoring system, which indicated four baseline PONV risk factors: (1) female gender; (2) history of motion sickness or PONV; (3) non-smoking history, and (4) use of postoperative opioids. When a total of 0, 1, 2, 3 or 4 of these risk factors were present, the baseline risk of PONV was predicted to be approximately 10, 20, 40, 60 and 80%, respectively (table 2).

PONV Therapy Algorithms

Using the estimated baseline risk for PONV as a starting point, and via an algorithm, Watcha [69] recommended the type of antiemetic medication to be used as therapy for PONV prophylaxis and treatment (fig. 2). Low risk was defined as <10%, mild to moderate risk as 10–30%, high risk as 30–60%, and extremely high risk as >60%. In addition to the patient-related PONV risk factors by Apfel et al. [60], Gan [59] used a PONV prevention/treatment algorithm which included both patient and surgical risk factors (fig. 3). Based on their PONV

Table 2. Guide to determine PONV risk – simplified risk score for predicting PONV [adapted from 60]

Risk factors	Total number of risk factors present	PONV, % incidence	PONV risk
	0	10	Low
Female gender	1	21	Mild
Hx PONV and/or motion sickness	2	39	Moderate
Non-smoker	3	61	High
Postoperative opioids	4	79	Extremely high

Risk factors are additive. ↑ PONV incidence with ↑ total number of risk factors.

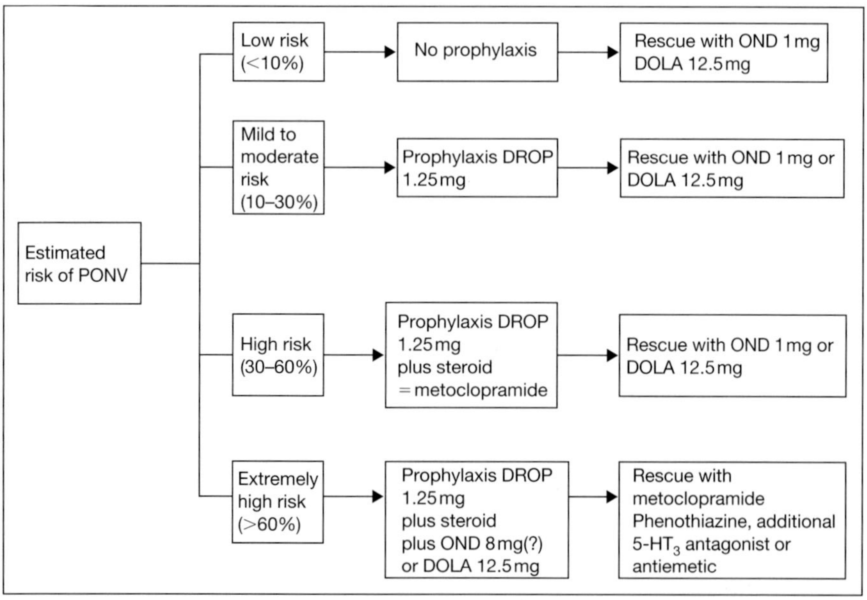

Fig. 2. The cost-effective management of PONV flow diagram by Watcha [69]. Printed with permission. Guidelines for the prophylaxis and therapy of PONV. A low, mild, moderate, high and extremely high risk for PONV can be determined by the presence of none, one, two, three or four of the following factors, respectively: (1) female gender; (2) non-smoker status; (3) previous PONV or motion sickness; (4) opioid use from table 2 above. DOLA = Dolasetron; DROP = droperidol; OND = ondansetron; PONV = postoperative nausea and vomiting. The FDA issued a 'black box' warning on December 5, 2001 regarding the risk of fatal cardiac arrhythmias associated with droperidol. See section on butyrophenones on pages 135–136.

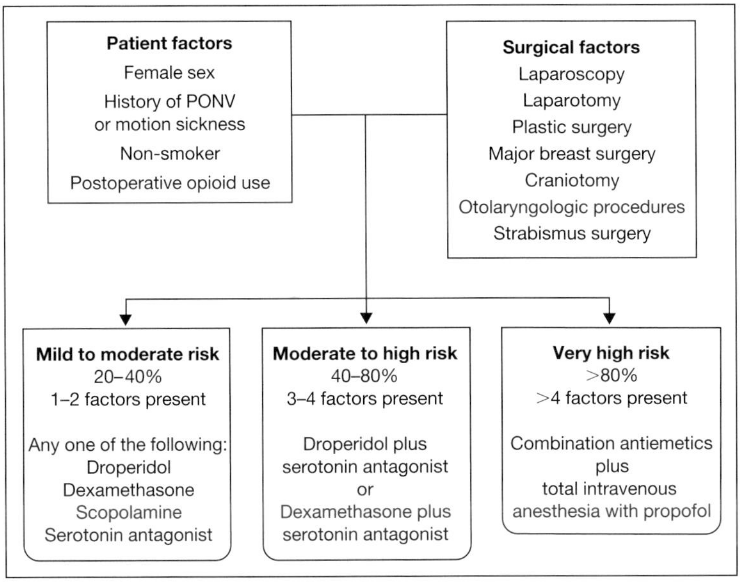

Fig. 3. PONV flow diagram by Gan [59]. Printed with permission. PONV indicates postoperative nausea and vomiting. Percentages denote risk of developing PONV. Consideration should be given to avoid patient and surgical risk factors associated with PONV and other strategies (lower box) to further reduce the incidence. 5-HT_3 antagonists may be preferred antiemetics in operative settings where nursing labor costs are directly related to the length of postanesthesia care unit stay.

predictive scoring system [60] and algorithms [59, 69], the clinical practitioner can choose whether or not to use an antiemetic for prophylaxis and/or treatment, and if so, what antiemetic to use. Antiemetic choices may include droperidol, dexamethasone, scopolamine, a 5-HT_3 receptor antagonist or a combination of these. For patients at low risk, no antiemetic prophylaxis was recommended unless these patients are at risk of medical sequelae from PONV. These patients can be rescued in the PACU with a 5-HT_3 receptor antagonist as needed [62].

As the causes of PONV are complex and multifactorial, routine antiemetic monotherapy for prophylaxis has not been 100% effective for all patients and all types of anesthesia and surgeries. A combination of antiemetics from different drug classes that block different emetic receptors or a multimodal management approach may be necessary to improve antiemetic efficacy and/or treat the difficult PONV patient. In the PONV algorithms, the more costly 5-HT_3 receptor antagonists were generally reserved for rescue therapy, except for pediatric and adult patients who are at moderate to extremely high risk (>60%), when a

$5\text{-}HT_3$ antagonist can be included in the prophylactic combination therapy approach (fig. 2, 3) [59, 62, 69].

Antiemetic Drug Classes

The classes of commonly used antiemetic medications for PONV include anticholinergics, antihistamines, phenothiazines, butyrophenones, antidopaminergics, $5\text{-}HT_3$ receptor antagonists, sedative/anxiolytics and steroids [6]. Medications that may be effective as *prophylactic* antiemetics for nausea and vomiting may be ineffective for the *treatment* of vomiting. An example is droperidol, which is more effective for nausea, while the $5\text{-}HT_3$ antagonists are more effective for vomiting. Antiemetic medications that are used for prophylaxis and treatment in adults and children are listed in table 4.

Anticholinergics

Anticholinergic medications inhibit cholinergic and muscarinic receptors in the pons and cerebral cortex [13]. Atropine and scopolamine are tertiary amines that cross the blood-brain barrier and are effective against motion sickness and PONV [26, 58, 70]. Both scopolamine and atropine appear to be more effective against motion-induced *vomiting* than motion-induced *nausea*. Concurrent premedication with atropine or scopolamine administered with opioids decreases the risk of PONV compared to using opioid premedication alone without anticholinergics. When used as premedication with morphine, scopolamine has more antiemetic efficacy compared to atropine [71]. Scopolamine blocks impulses from the vestibular center to higher areas in the CNS, reticular activating formation and vomiting center. Scopolamine is believed to be effective by altering the CNS imbalance of norepinephrine and acetylcholine that occurs in patients with motion sickness [70, 72]. Glycopyrrolate is a quaternary amine that does not cross the blood-brain barrier and as such does not appear to have antiemetic or antimotion sickness effects [71].

Prophylactic transdermal scopolamine (hyoscine) is more effective for prevention of motion sickness than PONV [70, 71]. To be effective for PONV, scopolamine 1.5 mg transdermal must be placed the previous night or at least 4 h prior to the end of surgery due to its delayed onset of effect [72, 73]. Prophylactic transdermal scopolamine patches have been shown to be effective in preventing PONV due to opioids such as epidural morphine [74, 75]. However, as the emetogenic properties of opioids such as morphine have a longer duration of action than the antiemetic properties of scopolamine, delayed nausea and vomiting may occur when scopolamine's antiemetic effect wears off [74, 75]. Side effects of anticholinergic medications may include sedation,

Table 3. Commonly used antiemetic medications and their side effects

Anticholinergics	
Atropine	Dry mouth
Scopolamine	Dysphoria
Phenothiazines	
Promethazine	Sedation
Prochlorperazine	Hypotension
Chlorpromazine	Dry mouth
Antihistamines	
Diphenhydramine	Sedation
Promethazine	Dry mouth
Cyclizine	
Hydroxyzine	
Butyrophenones	
Droperidol	Sedation, hypotension, dysphoria Extrapyramidal symptoms, ECG effects
Benzamides	
Metoclopramide	Extrapyramidal symptoms
Steroids	
Dexamethasone	Delayed wound healing; postoperative infection (at high doses). These side effects have not been reported at lower, single doses used for PONV
5-HT_3 antagonists	
Ondansetron	Headaches/dizziness
Granisetron	
Tropisetron	
Dolasetron	

dry mouth, blurred vision, mydriasis, urinary retention, hallucinations, CNS excitation, memory loss, confusion and disorientation, especially in the elderly [73, 75] (table 3). Scopolamine is medically contraindicated in patients with cardiac disease and glaucoma, enlarged prostate and intestinal obstruction.

Phenothiazines

Phenothiazines (chlorpromazine, promethazine, prochlorperazine and thiethylperazine) are used as major tranquilizers, sedatives or antiemetics. These medications block dopamine D_2 receptors in the CTZ, have no effect on gastric emptying, and are more effective for PONV than motion sickness [76, 77]. Phenothiazines have a common tricyclic nucleus with an attached chemical group at the No. 10 position that determines antiemetic efficacy [77].

Table 4. Antiemetics used for PONV prophylaxis and treatment in pediatric and adult patients

Pediatrics	Adults
PONV prophylaxis	
Dimenhydrinate	Transdermal scopolamine
Perphenazine	Intramuscular ephedrine
Dexamethasone	Metoclopramide
Ondansetron	Dimenhydrinate
Dolasetron	Promethazine
Droperidol	Prochlorperazine
	Droperidol
	Dexamethasone
	Ondansetron
	Granisetron
	Tropisetron
	Dolasetron
PONV treatment	
Droperidol	Droperidol
Ondansetron	Promethazine
Dolasetron	Metoclopramide
	Intramuscular ephedrine
	Ondansetron
	Dolasetron
	Tropisetron
	Granisetron

Depending on the attached side chain, their chemical structure is either aliphatic (chlorpromazine, promethazine) or heterocyclic (prochlorperazine, perphenazine, thiethylperazine). Heterocyclic phenothiazines have a piperazine ring at the No. 10 position of the tricyclic nucleus. Compared to the heterocyclic phenothiazines, aliphatic phenothiazines are more effective for sedation and less effective as antiemetics. The heterocyclic phenothiazines are more effective antiemetics, but have a greater incidence of extrapyramidal side effects, which include acute dystonia, akathesia, tardive dyskinesia and pseudoparkinsonism [77–81]. Treatment of the extrapyramidal side effects is to discontinue the heterocyclic phenothiazine, administer diphenhydramine, and switch to an aliphatic phenothiazine or a different antiemetic class. The extrapyramidal side effects are less common when heterocyclic phenothiazines are administered in combination with opiates [81].

Promethazine has a long duration of action, causes more sedation, and is more effective for the prevention of motion sickness than for nausea and/or vomiting. Promethazine is considered to be one of the most effective phenothiazines for motion sickness. Its long duration of action makes it preferable to scopolamine [78]. Chlorpromazine is effective for PONV, but not motion sickness and has side effects of sedation and hypotension [80].

Prochlorperazine and perphenazine have similar antiemetic effectiveness; however, perphenazine causes more sedation. Similarly, prochlorperazine and promethazine have similar antiemetic effectiveness, but promethazine causes more sedation. Perphenazine has been shown to be effective for opioid-induced nausea and vomiting [81]. Because of their sedation side effects, the phenothiazines have limitations when used as antiemetics for outpatient surgery.

The neuroleptic malignant syndrome has been reported with the phenothiazines, as well as droperidol and metoclopramide. Patients with neuroleptic malignant syndrome have hyperpyrexia, muscle rigidity, acidosis, autonomic instability, agitation, altered mental status, and anticholinergic side effects that include tachycardia, drowsiness, dry mouth and urinary retention [82].

Butyrophenones

The butyrophenones that have been used for PONV include droperidol and haloperidol. Haloperidol and droperidol have similar PONV effectiveness to the phenothiazines. These antiemetics block dopaminergic D_2 receptors at the CTZ and area postrema. Droperidol and haloperidol also are α-blockers. Side effects may include sedation anxiety, restlessness, hypotension and extrapyramidal syndrome [83]. Droperidol causes a dose-dependent prolongation of the QT interval [84].

A recent United States Food and Drug Administration (FDA) 'black box' warning was issued in December 2001 advising physicians of the risk of fatal cardiac arrhythmias occurring with even low doses of droperidol [85]. Physicians were advised to consider alternative medications for the therapy of nausea and vomiting in patients who may be at high risk for developing cardiac arrhythmias.

McCormick [86] reported that the FDA had examined its database for evidence of cardiovascular events with droperidol around the world. Approximately 100 unique reports of cardiovascular dysrhythmias with approximately 20 unique reports of QT/QTc prolongation and/or torsades de pointes were found. The FDA concluded that this indicated a greater cardiovascular risk than was previously assumed. The FDA cautioned that even low droperidol doses (0.625 mg) should be used only when other first-line antiemetics were ineffective. The results of the FDA review conflicted with the results of PONV comparison studies conducted by Fortney et al. [87] and Tang et al. [88] whose research concluded that droperidol was as safe and effective as ondansetron.

To determine if patients have a prolonged QTc interval, the FDA [85] recommended that prior to receiving droperidol, all patients should have a 12-lead

ECG, with ECG monitoring to continue for 3 h after droperidol is administered. Because of these strong recommendations, the international use of droperidol has decreased. Further research is necessary to determine droperidol's effect on the ECG and its role as an antiemetic. Alternatives to droperidol include diphenhydramine, hydroxyzine, scopolamine, chlorpromazine, promethazine, prochlorperazine, the 5-HT_3 receptor antagonists, and dexamethasone, depending on each clinician's preference. A listing of drugs that may cause a prolonged QT interval can be found in a regularly updated website, www.torsades.org [89].

Chang and Rappaport [86a] reported that, 'although the FDA study was prematurely terminated because of significant neuropsychiatric adverse effects, including dysphoria and anxiety, there were several findings of note.' They report that 'impressive QTc prolongations (approximately 80 ms from baseline) were found in individuals following the 2.5-mg and the 5-mg doses, even though only 7 and 3 subjects, respectively, received these doses. Compared to placebo, the 0.625-mg dose did not appear to have a significant effect on QTc; however, this cannot be considered a definitive finding as only 5 individuals were studied at this dose.' Chang and Rappaport state that, 'additional investigation will be required to further define the relationship between QTc prolongation, potential for dysrhythmia and various doses of droperidol. The FDA is now exploring options to obtain data that satisfy regulatory standards for the demonstration of safety and efficacy at doses lower than 2.5 mg.' Chang and Rappaport urge practitioners to participate in the post-marketing safety assessment process by reporting all potential drug-related adverse events. The web site www.fda.gov/medwatch contains information on reporting adverse events [86a].

Droperidol had been shown to have similar antiemetic effectiveness although with a slower onset of action than haloperidol and phenothiazines for prevention and treatment of PONV [83]. Droperidol 5 mg IM has been shown to be equivalent in antiemetic effectiveness to haloperidol 2 mg IM [90]. Even though it has a shorter plasma half-life than haloperidol, droperidol has longer antiemetic effectiveness (up to 24 h). However, haloperidol's onset of action at the dopaminergic D_2 receptors in the area postrema and CTZ is reportedly more rapid than droperidol's [91]. Both haloperidol and droperidol may cause extrapyramidal side effects which include sedation, anxiety, hypotension and restlessness, especially in young adults and elderly patients [91–94].

Benzamides

The benzamides (metoclopramide, domperidone, benzquinamide) block dopamine D_2 receptors without antihistamine properties [95–97]. Metoclopramide is a procainamide derivative, benzamide prokinetic drug that blocks central dopamine D_2 receptors at the CTZ and area postrema and peripheral D_2 receptors in the GI tract. When used in low doses (10 mg), as for PONV, metoclopramide has few side effects. High doses can cause extrapyramidal symptoms [97, 98].

Lower doses of metoclopramide (10 mg) are used for PONV compared to CINV [83]. The antiemetic efficacy of metoclopramide has been controversial due to different dosing, timing and types of surgery and anesthesia techniques studied. Antiemetic effectiveness has been reported for the control of PONV in the immediate postoperative period when metoclopramide's prokinetic gastric effects increase lower esophageal sphincter tone and gastric motility and counteract the delayed gastric emptying effects of opioids [95, 98]. Because of its short duration of action (1–2 h), low doses of metoclopramide such as 10 mg does not appear to be as effective for PONV prevention when administered prior to the start of anesthesia. While some studies have shown PONV efficacy, a meta-analysis by Henzi et al. [99] has shown that metoclopramide at the doses used for PONV is ineffective as an antiemetic. However, a study by Quaynor and Raeder [99a] determined that metoclopramide 20 mg IV given at the end of laparoscopic cholecystectomy resulted in a similar incidence of PONV compared to ondansetron 8 mg IV. This topic is discussed elsewhere in this book.

Antihistamines

Antihistamines (diphenhydramine, dimenhydrinate, hydroxyzine, cyclizine) are effective for the therapy of vertigo, motion sickness and control of emesis following middle ear surgery [79, 100, 101]. Antihistamines block acetylcholine in the vestibular system and histamine H_1 receptors in the nucleus of the solitary tract [14]. They are the drugs of choice for the control of emesis following middle ear surgery [6].

Antihistamines have antisialogogue and sedative effects making them useful for premedication when combined with opioids and/or hypnotic agents. The dose of opioid and hypnotics should be decreased when used concurrently with antihistamines so as to not delay recovery. Cyclizine has similar effectiveness to promethazine in preventing and treating both the PONV and motion sickness caused by opioids. However, excess sedation from cyclizine can be a side effect, prolonging anesthesia and PACU recovery [100]. The main side effects of antihistamines are sedation, blurred vision, dry mouth and urinary retention [101].

Hydroxyzine has anticholinergic, antihistamine and bronchodilatory effects that are useful for the treatment of motion sickness, vertigo and PONV. Hydroxyzine has antisialogogue and sedation side effects, which make it a good premedication when combined with opioids to supplement their analgesic effect [102].

Benzodiazepines

In adults and children, benzodiazepine premedication (midazolam, lorazepam) appears to have an antiemetic effect [103–105]. Benzodiazepines help decrease patients' anxiety associated with surgery and anesthesia, thereby decreasing nausea and vomiting. Benzodiazepines are believed to achieve this by a decreased α-adrenergic effect, decreasing plasma catecholamines and thereby anxiety [106].

Steroids

While the antiemetic action of steroids is unknown, proposed mechanisms include prostaglandin antagonism, tryptophan depletion, decrease in serotonin brain levels, endorphin release, psychological effects and anti-inflammatory, membrane-stabilizing effects. Chronic treatment with large doses of steroids has been implicated in postoperative infection and delayed wound healing. However, a single small steroid dose does not appear to have these side effects. Two reported common adverse events of dexamethasone following IV dosing, have been cutaneous flushing and perineal itching, which were thought to be due to phosphate in the solution [107].

The plasma half-life of dexamethasone is approximately 4–4.5 h. It is also estimated that 4–5 h are necessary for dexamethasone to be an effective antiemetic for PONV [108]. While the PONV effective dose of dexamethasone has been 8–10 mg IV [108], doses as small as 2.5–5 mg IV have been shown to have similar PONV efficacy when administered prior to the induction of anesthesia [109, 110].

Timing of dexamethasone administration has been shown to be important in regard to PONV antiemetic effectiveness. Asboe et al. [111] determined that betamethasone 12 mg IM when given prior to the start of general anesthesia for ambulatory foot or hemorrhoid surgery produced less PONV and postoperative pain in the first 24 h following surgery. Aouad et al. [112] conducted a comparison study between dexamethasone 0.5 mg/kg IV and placebo at the start of tonsillectomy surgery. Fewer patients who received dexamethasone had emesis in the PACU and on the floor compared to the placebo group. Patients who received dexamethasone also had a faster time to first oral intake and a shorter duration of IV hydration on the floor.

Dexamethasone 1 mg/kg IV was determined by Pappas et al. [113] to significantly decrease the incidence of PONV in children age 2–12 years undergoing tonsillectomy when administered after a mask inhalation induction and before the start of surgery. Wang et al. [114] determined the optimal time of dexamethasone administration by comparing the onset of early versus late PONV. They compared dexamethasone 10 mg IV versus placebo when administered before anesthesia induction versus the end of surgery. When administered before induction, dexamethasone was effective in controlling PONV at 0–2 h in the PACU and at 2–24 h on the floor. When administered at the end of surgery, dexamethasone was effective at 2–24 h on the floor but not at 0–2 h in the PACU.

5-HT$_3$ Receptor Antagonists

Worldwide, the commonly used 5-HT$_3$ receptor antagonists are ondansetron, tropisetron, granisetron and dolasetron. Three new 5-HT$_3$ receptor antagonists currently under investigation are ramositron, azosetron and palamosetron.

The 5-HT$_3$ receptor antagonists have a similar chemical structure compared to serotonin. Serotonin's chemical structure has a six-ring carbon- and five-ring nitrogen-based nucleus. Tropisetron, granisetron, dolasetron and ondansetron all share a similar basic nucleus chemical structure with a different attached side chain (see figure 1 in chapter 3). This chemical nucleus may be hypothesized to be the binding site of the 5-HT$_3$ receptor antagonist and the serotonin receptor.

Because the 5-HT$_3$ receptor antagonists did not have the side effects of the commonly used antiemetics and did not affect laboratory tests or cause drug interactions with other medications, their discovery was considered to be a major advance for the treatment of nausea and vomiting. Headache and dizziness were the most commonly reported side effects of the 5-HT$_3$ receptor antagonists at the doses commonly used for PONV, but were believed to be mild in nature and easily treated with minor analgesics.

In evaluating antiemetics PONV effectiveness, it is important to determine the percent change in efficacy of the study medication compared to placebo, as in nearly all cases, patients have a placebo response. The baseline PONV placebo response rate is often the only indirect indicator of underlying baseline PONV risk. A higher placebo response indicates a high degree of PONV risk in the population studied. Conversely, a low placebo response indicates a low degree of PONV risk. With the introduction and use of the 5-HT$_3$ receptor antagonists, many randomized, controlled trials have determined an improvement in PONV efficacy of only 20–30% above the placebo response when single-agent, monotherapy is used for prophylaxis of PONV.

Ondansetron

Ondansetron was the first 5-HT$_3$ receptor antagonist to be evaluated and approved for PONV. Ondansetron has a peak plasma concentration of 60–90 and 20–30 min after PO and IV administration, respectively. In normal volunteers, its elimination half-life was 4 h. Metabolism is via CYP2D6, 2E1, 1A1, 1A2, 3A4 P_{450} hepatic enzymes with 60% excreted in urine and 25% in feces [115].

The ondansetron 8-mg oral dose was determined by Kenny et al. [116] to be the lowest optimal effective dose for prevention of PONV in female inpatients having gynecological surgery. For PONV prophylaxis, ondansetron 8 or 12 mg was given orally 1–2 h prior to surgery and improved PONV efficacy by 19–23% above the placebo response. McKenzie et al. [117] reported the effectiveness of IV ondansetron for the prevention of PONV following outpatient gynecologic laparoscopy. Prophylactic ondansetron 4 and 8 mg IV improved PONV efficacy by 16–30%. The optimal ondansetron dose was determined to be 4 mg IV given at the start of anesthesia. Scuderi et al. [118] conducted an IV treatment study and determined that all ondansetron IV doses (1, 4, and 8 mg) significantly reduced PONV compared to placebo for the 24-hour period following antiemetic treatment in the PACU. Ondansetron 4 mg IV has been used as the optimal dose for treatment of PONV. However, the minimally effective treatment dose with a 5-HT_3 antagonist appears to be less than the PONV prevention dose. A meta-analysis of ondansetron doses used for treatment of PONV determined that a lower dose of 1 mg IV was effective [119].

In a male-only study by Kovac et al. [120], ondansetron 4 mg IV administered prior to the induction of outpatient anesthesia was determined to be an effective dose for PONV prevention. In children older than 2 years, 0.1 mg/kg orally was effective for prevention [121] and 0.1 mg/kg (<40 kg) and 4 mg (≥40 kg) IV for treatment [122]. Ondansetron 0.1 mg/kg (up to a maximum 4.0 mg in a 40-kg patient) was determined to be the optimal pediatric dose for PONV. Recommended dosing for ondansetron is shown in table 5.

Initially the PONV prevention studies [117, 120] with IV ondansetron were administered prior to the start of anesthesia. Sun et al. [123] and Tang et al. [124] investigated ondansetron's PONV efficacy when administered at the end of surgery. Both studies determined that ondansetron 4 mg IV was significantly more effective when administered at the end of surgery rather than prior to anesthesia induction.

Ondansetron has been evaluated for the IV treatment of PONV secondary to postoperative opioid administration following regional anesthesia. Ondansetron 4 mg IV was determined by Rung et al. [125] to be effective for the treatment of opioid-induced PONV.

Granisetron

Granisetron has a peak plasma concentration following oral and IV administration of 60–90 and 30 min, respectively, with an elimination half-life of 6.3 h. Granisetron is metabolized by the CYP3A P_{450} hepatic enzyme subfamily (CYP3A3/4, CYP3A5, CYP3A7) and excreted 49% and 36% in urine and feces, respectively [126]. Granisetron IV has been shown to be effective for the prevention [127–131, 133–135] and treatment [132] of PONV. Mikawa et al. [127] reported that granisetron administered prophylactically IV was effective in female patients undergoing gynecological surgery. At the start of anesthesia, patients received either IV granisetron 2, 5, 10, 20 μg/kg or placebo. Granisetron was found to significantly decrease the incidence of PONV at doses ≥5 μg/kg IV. The 5 μg/kg granisetron dose (which would be 0.35 mg for a 70-kg patient) was determined to be the optimal dose for prevention of PONV.

Table 5. Recommended dosing of antiemetic agents [135a]. Reprinted with permission

Class	Drug	Route	Initial average dose	Frequency/timing	Adverse effects
Anticholinergics	Scopolamine	IM, IV	Adult: 0.2–0.65 mg	q6–8 h	Sedation, dry mouth, restlessness, central cholinergic syndrome
		TD patch	Adult: 1.5 mg	q72 h (apply 4 h before exposure)	
Phenothiazines	Chlorpromazine	IM, IV	Adult: 25–50 mg	q4–6 h	Sedation, EPS, hypotension, restlessness, anticholinergic syndrome
			Child: 0.5–1.0 mg/kg/dose	q6–8 h	
			Max.: 5–12 y (22.7–45.5 kg): 75 mg/day		
			Max.: <5 y (22.7 kg): 40 mg/day		
		PO	Adult: 10–25 mg	q4–6 h	
			Child: 0.5–1.0 mg/kg/dose	q4–6 h	
	Promethazine	IM, IV, PO	Adult: 12.5–25 mg	q4–8 h	Sedation, EPS, hypotension, restlessness, anticholinergic syndrome
			Child: (<12 y) 0.25–0.5 mg/kg	q6–8 h	
	Perphenazine	IM	Adult: 2.5–5 mg	q6 h	Sedation, EPS, hypotension, restlessness
		IV	Adult: 1 mg	q1–2 min (max. 5 mg)	
		PO	Adult: 2–4 mg	q4–6 h	
	Prochlorperazine	IV	Adult: 2.5–10 mg (max. 40 mg/day)		Sedation, EPS, hypotension, restlessness
		IM, PO	Adult: 5–10 mg	q3–4 h	
		IM	Child: 0.1–0.15 mg/kg/dose	q4–6 h	
		PO	Child: (<10 kg): 0.5 mg/kg/24 h in 3–4 divided doses		
Antihistamines	Cyclizine	IM, IV, PO	Adult: 25–50 mg	q4–6 h	Sedation, dry mouth, restlessness
	Hydroxyzine	PO	Adult: 25–50 mg	q6 h	Sedation, dry mouth, restlessness
		IM	Adult: 25–100 mg	At start of anesthesia	Do not give IV or SC (significant anticholinergic effects)
	Diphenhydramine	IM, IV	Adult: 10–50 mg (max. 300 mg/day)	q2–4 h	Sedation, dry mouth, restlessness
		PO	Adult: 25–50 mg	q6–8 h	
Butyrophenones	Droperidol	IM, IV	Adult: 0.625–2.5 mg (prevention)	At start of anesthesia	Sedation, hypotension, EPS, restlessness, neurolyptic malignant syndrome
			Adult: 0.625–1.25 mg (treatment)		
	Haloperidol	IV	Adult: 7 μg/kg (prevention)	At start of anesthesia	
		IM	Adult 0.5–4 mg (prevention)	15 min before anesthesia	
			Adult: 1.0 mg (treatment)		

Table 5 (continued)

Class	Drug	Route	Initial average dose	Frequency/timing	Adverse effects
Benzamides	Metoclopramide	IV, IM	Adult: 10–20 mg (prevention) Adult 10–20 mg (treatment)	At end of surgery	Sedation, restlessness, EPS
	Domperidone	IV, IM	Adult: 4–10 mg (treatment)		Sedation, restlessness, EPS
	Benzquinamide	IM	Adult: 25–50 mg (0.5–0.75 mg/kg)	15 min before end of anesthesia	Do not give IV (tachycardia, hypertension, cardiac arrhythmias)
		PO	Adult: 100 mg	q6–8 h	
Corticosteroids	Betamethasone	IM	Adult: 12 mg (prevention)	At start of anesthesia	Adrenal suppression, wound healing
	Dexamethasone	IV	Adult: 8 mg (prevention)	At start of anesthesia	
5-HT_3 receptor antagonists	Ondansetron	PO	Adult: 8–16 mg	1–2 h before anesthesia	Headache, dizziness
		IV	Adult: 4 mg (prevention)	At start of anesthesia	
		IV	Adult: 4 mg (treatment) Child: 0.1 mg/kg (max. 4 mg) [prevention and treatment]		
	Granisetron	IV	Adult: 1 mg (prevention)	At start or end of anesthesia	Headache, dizziness
		IV	Adult: 1 mg (treatment)		
	Tropisetron	IV	Adult: 5 mg (prevention)	At start of anesthesia	Headache, dizziness
		IV	Adult: 2 mg (treatment)		
	Dolasetron	PO	Adult: 100 mg (prevention)	1–2 h before anesthesia	Headache, dizziness
		IV	Adult: 12.5 mg (prevention)	15–30 min before end of anesthesia	
		IV	Adult: 12.5 mg (treatment)		
		PO	Child: 1.2 mg/kg (max. 100 mg) [prevention]	1–2 h before anesthesia	
		IV	Child: 0.35 mg/kg (max. 12.5 mg) [prevention and treatment]	15–30 min before end of anesthesia (prevention)	

5-HT = Serotonin (5-hydroxytryptamine); EPS = extrapyramidal symptoms; IM = intramuscular; IV = intravenous; max. = maximum dosage; PO = orally; q*x*h = every *x* hours; SC = subcutaneous; TD = transdermal.

Wilson et al. [128] conducted a randomized, double-blind, dose-ranging study to determine the optimal dose and safety of granisetron for PONV prophylaxis on patients having an open cholecystectomy, open gynecological or vaginal hysterectomy procedures. These patients received either IV granisetron 0.1, 1.0, 3.0 mg or placebo. Antiemetic prophylaxis with a single IV dose of 1.0 or 3.0 mg resulted in a significant reduction in the numbers of patients who experienced nausea and vomiting compared to placebo. Granisetron was believed to be safe and well tolerated. The optimal granisetron dose for PONV prevention was determined to be 1.0 mg IV (table 5).

Fujii et al. [129–131] conducted three studies on the prevention of PONV following major gynecologic surgery comparing the effectiveness of granisetron, droperidol or metoclopramide administered immediately prior to anesthesia in female patients with a history of prior PONV [129], motion sickness [130], or during menstruation [131]. Two studies compared the prophylactic efficacy of IV granisetron 2.5 mg, droperidol 1.25 mg or metoclopramide 10 mg in female patients with a history of postoperative emesis [129] and motion sickness [130]. A third study by Fujii et al. [131] compared the prophylactic antiemetic efficacy of IV droperidol 25 μg/kg, metoclopramide 0.2 mg/kg or granisetron 40 μg/kg in women during menstruation. In all three studies, granisetron was determined to be more effective than droperidol or metoclopramide for the prevention of PONV.

Taylor et al. [132] conducted a dose-ranging IV treatment study comparing granisetron versus placebo. All granisetron doses were found to be effective. Patients who received granisetron doses of 0.1, 1.0 or 3.0 mg experienced no vomiting versus placebo (38, 46, 49 vs. 20%, respectively) in the first 24 h following drug administration. The 0.1-mg granisetron dose was determined to be the lowest effective dose for treatment of PONV. There was a linear and statistically significant correlation between the control of vomiting and the granisetron dose. Granisetron was determined to be well tolerated. The most common adverse experiences were headache, pain, anemia and constipation. However, the incidence of adverse experience was not different between the granisetron and placebo groups. Other studies conducted by Fujii et al. [133, 134] in children determined that granisetron 40 μg/kg IV was the effective dose for POV prevention. Cieslak et al. [135] also conducted a POV prevention study in pediatric patients and determined that granisetron was effective in controlling vomiting. Recommended dosing of granisetron is shown in table 5 [135a].

Tropisetron

Tropisetron is an indole compound with a chemical structure, efficacy, and side effect profile similar to the other 5-HT_3 receptor antagonists. Tropisetron is metabolized by hepatic CYP2D6 P_{450} enzyme. Due to polymorphism of this enzyme, some patients are thought to metabolize tropisetron more rapidly (ultrametabolizers) than other patients [135b]. Metabolic excretion of tropisetron is approximately 80% in the urine and 15% in the feces.

Tropisetron has an elimination half-life of 8–12 h [136] and has been studied for prevention [137–139] and treatment [140] of PONV in adults. Tropisetron has been found effective for prevention of PONV after breast [137] and gynecologic surgery [138] when a 5-mg IV dose was administered prior to the start of anesthesia [137, 138]. Zomers et al. [139] determined that tropisetron 5 mg was effective for prevention of PONV following gynecological surgery. Alon et al. [140] determined that tropisetron 2 mg IV was the optimal effective dose for the treatment of PONV following a variety of abdominal and non-abdominal surgeries (table 5).

Dolasetron

Dolasetron is a pseudopelletirine chemical compound that is converted by the plasma enzyme carbonyl reductase to the active form which is hydrodolasetron. This very rapid enzyme reaction results in a dolasetron half-life of 9 min, making dolasetron undetectable in the serum 2–4 h after IV administration. Peak serum concentrations of hydrodolasetron are found 30 and 60 min after IV and oral administration, respectively. Hydrodolasetron is metabolized by hepatic CYP2D6 and CYP3A P_{450} enzymes with a plasma half-life of approximately 7.1 (6.9–7.3) and 7.9 (7.2–8.1) h for the oral and IV formulations, respectively. Hydrodolasetron is responsible for most (87%) of the antiemetic effect of dolasetron. Metabolic excretion of dolasetron is 67% in the urine and 33% in the feces [141, 142].

Warriner et al. [143] compared oral dolasetron 25, 50, 100 and 200 mg administered 1–2 h prior to anesthesia with placebo in 730 adult, female inpatients. Oral dolasetron 100 mg administered 1–2 h prior to surgery had a statistical improvement above the placebo response. A similar oral dolasetron prevention study was conducted by Diemunsch et al. [144]. With the results of these two studies, the recommended prophylactic oral dose of dolasetron was determined to be 100 mg administered 1–2 h prior to the start of anesthesia.

The recommended timing of IV dolasetron for PONV prophylaxis is 15–30 min before the end of surgery. Graczyk et al. [145] conducted a PONV prevention study on the effect of IV dolasetron 12.5, 25 or 50 mg administered at the end of surgery in 635 female outpatients undergoing laparoscopic gynecologic surgery. The dolasetron doses were found to improve PONV efficacy above placebo by 19–20%. Dolasetron 12.5 mg administered 15–30 min IV before the end of surgery was determined to be the optimal dose.

Kovac et al. [146] reported the results of 1,030 adults (722 females, 308 males) in an outpatient, dose-ranging (12.5, 25, 50, 100 mg) dolasetron IV PONV treatment study. Dolasetron 12.5 mg IV was determined to be the optimal dose. With dolasetron 12.5 mg IV, there was an improvement of 28% above the placebo response for early emesis (0–2 h), and 24% for late emesis (2–24 h). Diemunsch et al. [147] evaluated 337 adult male and female patients in a dolasetron PONV treatment study. Patients were treated with IV dolasetron or placebo if nausea lasted more than 10 min or they had one emetic episode within 2 h in the PACU. All dolasetron groups were significantly superior to placebo. The optimal dolasetron dose for treatment of established PONV was determined to be 12.5 mg IV [141].

The recommended oral dolasetron dose for PONV prevention in pediatric patients 2–16 years old is 1.2 mg/kg up to a maximum dose of 100 mg and given 1–2 h before the start of surgery. The recommended IV dolasetron dose in pediatric patients is 0.35 mg/kg, up to a maximum dose of 12.5 mg administered 15 min before the end of anesthesia for PONV prevention, or as soon as nausea or vomiting presents for PONV treatment [141, 142, 148]. Recommended dosing of dolasetron is shown in table 5.

Non-Traditional Antiemetic Therapy

Ephedrine

Intramuscular (IM) ephedrine appears to be an effective alternative antiemetic for PONV, especially when the PONV may be related to fluid dehydration and orthostatic hypotension that may occur with position changes in the PACU. Rothenberg et al. [149] compared ephedrine 0.5 mg/kg IM with droperidol 0.04 mg/kg IM or saline IM. Ephedrine was determined to have similar efficacy to droperidol and to have significantly more effectiveness than placebo, without blood pressure or sedation side effects. Another study by Naguib et al. [150] compared the effect of ephedrine 0.5 mg/kg IM compared to propofol 0.25 mg/kg IV for the prevention of PONV following laparoscopic surgery. Both propofol IV and ephedrine IM were determined to have better antiemetic effectiveness without hemodynamic changes compared to placebo.

Propofol

Patients who receive propofol appear to have less PONV [151–154]. Subhypnotic IV doses of thiopentone 1.0 mg/kg IV versus propofol 0.5 mg/kg IV was compared by Myles et al. [151] for antiemetic effectiveness at the end of outpatient middle ear surgery. Propofol 0.5 mg/kg IV provided PONV prophylaxis against retching and vomiting for the first 6 h. While the antiemetic effect of propofol is unknown, a plasma propofol concentration of 343 ng/ml achieved with a 10-mg IV bolus followed by an infusion of 10 μg/kg/min was determined by Gan et al. [153] to be necessary to obtain a 50% reduction in postoperative nausea. Intraoperative IV propofol has been determined by Gan et al. [154] to be as effective as ondansetron 4 mg IV in preventing PONV during the first 6 postoperative hours.

PONV Comparison Studies

Studies have compared the antiemetic efficacy of the more traditional, older antiemetics to the newer 5-HT_3 receptor antagonists. A comparison PONV prevention study by Sniadach and Alberts [155] compared droperidol 20 μg/kg IV versus ondansetron 4 mg IV administered prior to anesthesia for outpatient gynecologic laparoscopy. They found similar antiemetic effectiveness between droperidol and ondansetron, with no difference in sedation. Fortney et al. [87] found similar conclusions comparing ondansetron 4 mg IV with IV droperidol 0.625 and 1.25 mg. Both droperidol doses had similar antiemetic effectiveness as ondansetron 4 mg, and all antiemetics were significantly better than placebo. The best antiemetic effectiveness was obtained with droperidol 1.25 mg IV, with no increase in sedation or other side effects. In women undergoing inpatient minor gynecologic surgery, Grond et al. [156] compared ondansetron 8 mg IV with droperidol 2.5 mg IV for PONV prophylaxis. More patients who received droperidol 2.5 mg IV had no emesis compared with the ondansetron 8 mg group. Desilva et al. [157] compared IV ondansetron 4 mg, droperidol 1.25 mg, perphenazine 5 mg and metaclopramide 10 mg for PONV prevention after major gynecological surgery. Metaclopramide was found to be ineffective. While droperidol and perphenazine effectively prevented nausea, droperidol, perphenazine and ondansetron prevented emesis. Because of the lack of side effects, Desilva et al. [157] considered perphenazine to be the best choice of the four antiemetics evaluated for prophylaxis following total abdominal hysterectomy. A study conducted by Danner et al. [158] between dolasetron and droperidol determined that dolasetron had similar but not superior antiemetic efficacy compared to droperidol.

Korttila et al. [159] conducted an IV PONV prevention study comparing dolasetron 25 mg, dolasetron 50 mg, and ondansetron 4 mg with placebo. All study doses were administered prior to anesthesia induction. The dolasetron 50 mg and ondansetron 4 mg doses were determined to have similar antiemetic effectiveness and were significantly more effective than dolasetron 25 mg or placebo. The Korttila et al. [159] protocol design differed from other dolasetron IV PONV prevention studies such as that of Gracyzk et al. [145] in which dolasetron 12.5 mg was administered 15–30 min prior to the end of surgery.

The timing of the dolasetron dose in the Korttila et al. [159] study was designed to conform with the FDA approved pre-anesthesia induction dosing schedule of ondansetron at the time the study was conducted.

Naguib et al. [160] compared ondansetron 4 mg, granisetron 3 mg, tropisetron 5 mg, metoclopramide 10 mg and placebo in which all study doses were administered IV at the start of anesthesia. Ondansetron, granisetron and tropisetron were found to have similar antiemetic effectiveness, and all were similarly more effective than metoclopramide and placebo.

Zarata et al. [161] compared PONV effectiveness and cost of IV ondansetron 4 and 8 mg, and dolasetron 12.5 and 25 mg, in which all doses were administered 30 min before the end of ENT surgery. These researchers concluded that, after taking into consideration the factors of dose, cost and operation of the ambulatory surgery center, dolasetron 12.5 mg IV had similar PONV efficacy to the other study doses, but was more cost-effective than dolasetron 25 mg and ondansetron 4 or 8 mg IV.

Walker [162] completed a PONV retrospective review of the medical charts of 59 adult patients who had a total abdominal hysterectomy or laparoscopic cholecystectomy and received either IV dolasetron 12.5 mg or ondansetron 4 mg. Walker concluded that there was no significant difference in PONV efficacy between of IV dolasetron 12.5 mg and IV ondansetron 4 mg for the prevention of PONV.

Robertson et al. [163] conducted a comparative PONV treatment study in 92 patients between dolasetron 12.5 mg IV and ondansetron 4 mg IV following outpatient surgery. On the basis of greater patient satisfaction and a lower requirement for rescue antiemetic medications, these researchers concluded that dolasetron 12.5 mg IV had better efficacy than ondansetron 4 mg IV following treatment for PONV in the PACU.

Combination Antiemetic Therapy

The 5-HT_3 receptor antagonists have improved the therapy of PONV. However, with only a 20–30% improvement in efficacy above the placebo response, they have not been the complete solution for PONV when used as monotherapy. The numerous emetic receptors and neurochemicals in the CNS suggest that a combination and/or multimodal antiemetic approach would help improve efficacy, especially in the moderate to extremely high risk or difficult-to-treat PONV patient. The use of antiemetic combinations in preventing PONV has become popular, as overall, the combination of antiemetic medications acting at different emetogenic receptors has significantly improved effectiveness compared to monotherapy acting at a single receptor.

Combining the older antiemetics such as antihistamines, phenothiazines, anticholinergics or butyrophenones had a disadvantage because of the additive side effects such as hypotension, sedation, dry mouth and extrapyramidal symptoms. Numerous studies [164–168] have determined the effectiveness of the 5-HT_3 receptor antagonists when used in combination with other antiemetics without these side effects.

McKenzie et al. [164–166] completed three combination antiemetic studies and determined that the prevention of PONV was significantly more effective when ondansetron was combined with dexamethasone compared to ondansetron without dexamethasone. The combination of ondansetron combined with droperidol was found to be more effective than with either antiemetic alone. Similarly, Fujii et al. [167–169] combined granisetron with droperidol or dexamethasone and determined that antiemetic effectiveness of the combination was improved over using each antiemetic alone. Eberhart et al. [170] conducting a meta-analysis of 26 randomized, controlled studies in 2,561 patients and determined that dexamethasone increased the efficacy of the partner antiemetic drug.

Multimodal PONV Management

Often, even combination antiemetic therapy may not be effective for the extremely high risk or difficult-to-treat PONV patient. Following the principles of pain management, combination antiemetic therapy and IV hydration, the anesthetic management for the difficult PONV patient at high risk for PONV has evolved into a multimodal PONV management technique. Simple techniques, such as administering ≥80% oxygen to patients who are having abdominal GI surgery [171], and adequate IV hydration (20 ml/kg) have been found to be effective methods to lower the incidence of PONV and are an important part of multimodal PONV management. An important finding by Suntheralingham et al. [51] was that, in outpatient surgery of less than 2 h duration, patients who received a crystalloid infusion of 20 ml/kg IV had a lower incidence of nausea at 30 and 60 min post-PACU discharge, compared to patients receiving the lower IV infusion rate of 2 ml/kg.

For the difficult PONV patient, a recommended multimodal approach to lower the baseline PONV risk is to avoid N_2O, avoid reversal of muscle relaxants, use propofol for anesthesia induction and maintenance, limit opioids, use non-steroidal anti-inflammatory drugs, administer oxygen at $FiO_2 \geq 80\%$ and use combination (double or triple) antiemetics [62]. For patients in whom an initial dose of antiemetic for the prevention of PONV is ineffective, a repeat dose of the same antiemetic should not be administered; instead, a change to an antiemetic of a different class is recommended. Kovac et al. [172] compared the repeat PACU administration of ondansetron 4 mg IV in whom preoperative prophylactic ondansetron 4 mg IV had been ineffective. They determined that the repeat ondansetron IV dose did not provide additional control of PONV compared to placebo.

Scuderi et al. [173] compared the effect of multimodal PONV management to monotherapy and to no therapy at all in laparoscopic cholecystectomy patients. Group 1 received multimodal therapy of total IV propofol anesthesia and remifentanil with no nitrous oxide or neuromuscular blockade. Intravenous fluid hydration was administered using 25 ml/kg of crystalloid infusion, as well as triple prophylactic antiemetic therapy of IV ondansetron 1 mg, droperidol 0.625 mg and dexamethasone 10 mg. The surgeons performed local anesthesia infiltration at the incision site, and ketorolac 30 mg IV was administered at the end of surgery. Group 2 received only ondansetron 4 mg IV for PONV prophylaxis. Group 3 received no PONV prophylaxis. The multimodal management group (group 1) had no vomiting and only 1 patient had nausea. Groups 2 and 3 had a significantly higher incidence of nausea and vomiting. In addition, patients in the multimodal group were discharged from the PACU earlier than the other groups.

Adverse Side Effects Profile

Depending on the total dose administered and the frequency, the older, more traditional antiemetics have adverse side effects. The butyrophenones (droperidol) and phenothiazines (promethazine) may cause sedation, hypotension and/or extrapyramidal symptoms. The anticholinergics (scopolamine) and antihistamines (diphenhydramine) may cause dry mouth, drowsiness, sedation, and/or restlessness. The substituted benzamides (metoclopramide) may cause extrapyramidal symptoms. The 5-HT_3 receptor antagonists as a class have been found to be safe at the usual doses used for PONV, with no dose-related sedation or extrapyramidal reactions and no effect on vital signs. The most common side effects (in $\leq$2% of patients) of the 5-HT_3 antagonists have been relatively minimal and include headache and dizziness [6, 174] (table 3).

ECG Effects of the 5-HT_3 Receptor Antagonists

Adverse pro-arrhythmic effects caused by the 5-HT_3 receptor antagonists are not easy to determine in cancer patients receiving chemotherapy or patients undergoing surgery. ECG changes of acute, asymptomatic, reversible, dose-dependent prolongation of the PR, QRS and QTc intervals have been reported with dolasetron and the other 5-HT_3 antagonists. The 5-HT_3 antagonists as a class block sodium and/or potassium channels [175]. Benedict et al. [176] reported the ECG parameters in normal volunteers of IV dolasetron mesylate compared to IV ondansetron and found a statistically significant increase in QTc intervals with both 5-HT_3 receptor antagonists. These ECG effects appear to be dose-related. Dolasetron was found to predominantly alter QRS duration, indicative of ventricular depolarization, while ondansetron predominantly caused prolongation of the JT interval, indicative of ventricular repolarization. At the lower doses commonly used for PONV compared to CINV, and compared to placebo, these reported ECG effects were believed by clinical practitioners to be asymptomatic, minor, transient and not clinically significant.

Kuryshev et al. [175] evaluated the effect of ondansetron, granisetron and dolasetron on human sodium and potassium channel inhibition using an in vitro electrophysiological model. Drugs that block potassium channels may cause a prolonged QT interval. Drugs that block sodium channels may cause a widening of the QRS interval. Kuryshev et al. concluded that all the 5-HT_3 receptor antagonists tested blocked human cardiac sodium channels. They hypothesized that this could be clinically relevant when depolarized/ischemic tissue or high heart rates are present. This appears to confirm that the ECG changes of the 5-HT_3 receptor antagonists are a dose-dependent, class-related effect whose relevancy depends on medical comorbidities, patient population, dose administered, physical condition of patient, concurrent medications and hepatic CYP2D6 enzyme metabolism [175].

The 5-HT_3 receptor antagonists do not have drug interactions with the commonly used anesthetics and do not prolong anesthesia or delay PACU discharge. They have little or no affinity for other peripheral or central receptors, including α, β, benzodiazepine GABA, dopamine D_2, histamine or other 5-HT receptors.

NK_1-Receptor Antagonists

Initially, a new class of antiemetics, the neurokinin (NK_1) receptor antagonists, or neurokinins, was expected to replace the 5-HT_3 antagonists. Because substance P is the most likely endogenous ligand for the NK_1 receptor, the development of non-peptide NK_1 receptor antagonists increased interest in these compounds as antiemetics [177]. The NK_1 antagonists were believed to act at multiple sites of action in the CNS and in the periphery and have broad antiemetic activity with a common NK_1 receptor-mediated link. Several initial studies had determined effectiveness of the NK_1 antagonists in chemotherapy [178] and PONV [179].

PONV Management Summary

Various factors relate to the etiology and incidence of PONV. These factors are part of the patient, anesthesia, surgery and PACU management. Different types of surgical procedures and anesthetics cause different degrees of PONV risk. Common causes of PONV after PACU discharge are the initiation of oral opioids and patient movement. No antiemetic is 100% effective for all surgeries and patient populations. There may be a need to use different types or combinations of antiemetics in different types of patients and surgical procedures. In patients with a high risk for PONV, a combination or multimodal antiemetic approach should be used considering efficacy, side effects and cost.

Routine antiemetic prophylaxis does not work in every patient and is not needed for every patient. The decision of which prophylactic antiemetic to use can be determined based on the analysis of the expected PONV frequency and determining the PONV risk. When costs were analyzed in comparative PONV antiemetic studies, no difference in efficacy or cost savings were determined when using the 5-HT_3 receptor antagonists alone versus droperidol, suggesting that lower cost antiemetics should be the first choice for PONV management. Further research is needed to determine the overall effects of new antiemetic medications and lower emetogenic anesthesia techniques on issues of cost, patient satisfaction, quality of life and outcome.

Overall, the 5-HT_3 receptor antagonists as a class are safe and well tolerated. The 5-HT_3 receptor antagonists as a class have similar antiemetic efficacy and safety. Adverse events, when they occur, are usually mild, self-limiting, transient and rarely require discontinuation of the drug. Headache is the most common side effect (although <2%). Headache is frequently reported as mild to moderate and easily treated with mild analgesics. Hemodynamic changes are uncommon. The 5-HT_3 antagonists have no effect on vital signs (heart rate, blood pressure, respiratory rate). ECG changes such as prolonged QT_c interval have been observed with all the 5-HT_3 antagonists as a class, but have been judged to be dose-related and clinically insignificant at the doses commonly used for PONV.

For low baseline PONV risk patients, prophylaxis does not always give the best efficacy. For patients with a low baseline PONV risk, it is recommended to not use PONV prophylaxis but to treat in PACU if needed, as antiemetics used for treatment of PONV are more cost-effective than if used for prevention. In order to lower the baseline PONV risk, for initial PONV management during the pre-anesthesia, induction and intraoperative periods, one should consider regional anesthesia, use anxiolytics such as midazolam, limit opioids and eliminate the use of nitrous oxide. Use hypnotic medications such as propofol that allow a slow, smooth recovery. Avoid or limit medications with high PONV potential

Table 6. PONV management summary

Different surgeries and anesthetics have different baseline PONV risk potentials
Individual patients' PONV risk can be unpredictable
Common PONV causes after PACU discharge are oral opioids and/or patient movement
No antiemetic medication or technique is 100% effective in all patients
Use antiemetics of a different class/receptor site if first antiemetic is ineffective
5-HT_3 receptor antagonists are important additions to therapy for PONV – they have similar effectiveness and safety but differences in cost
Use combination multimodal antiemetic therapy in difficult PONV patients
Remember simple things: hypoxia, dehydration, orthostatic hypotension, motion, anxiety, pain, swallowing of blood, etc. that can cause PONV
Review the weight of patient. Has an adequate dose of antiemetic been administered?

such as opioids, and use prophylactic antiemetics as indicated, based on a PONV scoring system and estimated baseline PONV risk. Use the older prophylactic antiemetic medications first and 5-HT_3 antagonists second for moderate and extremely high-risk adult and pediatric patients based on a PONV risk score. Give combination antiemetics at end of operation (except dexamethasone) rather than at induction (dexamethasone). Administer oxygen at $FiO_2 \geq 80\%$, adequate IV hydration of 20–25 ml/kg, avoid hypotension, maintaining blood pressure to decrease the chance of orthostatic hypotension.

For PONV management in the PACU, ensure pain control with the use of pain medications such as opioids and/or non-steroidal anti-inflammatory agents. Treat the simple things first. Ensure adequate oxygenation ($\geq 80\%$ FiO_2), IV hydration, and avoid orthostatic hypotension. Avoid tight-fitting oxygen masks, encouraging patients to breathe slowly and avoid hyperventilation. Minimize patient movement, if possible, and avoid using unnecessary oropharyngeal suctioning and oral airways, as these devices/techniques may stimulate the gag reflex. Avoid the use of muscle relaxants and/or reversal of neuromuscular block if possible. If needed, use of smaller doses of neostigmine ($<$2.5 mg) is recommended. Administer antiemetic medications as needed depending on the degree of the patient's PONV risk. The minimally effective 5-HT_3 antagonist treatment dose for PONV appears to be less than the PONV prevention dose.

If PONV persists, one should consider additional antiemetic treatment options. As most PONV studies for FDA new drug applications were performed on patients who weighed between 40 and 80 kg, a higher antiemetic dose may be required if the patient weighs more than 80 kg. Consider switching to a different antiemetic class that acts at a different receptor site if the first antiemetic was not effective. Evaluate the IV fluid status and consider an IV fluid challenge to avoid orthostatic blood pressure changes. Propofol 10–20 mg IV or ephedrine 25–50 mg IM can be administered in the difficult PONV patient to minimize or prevent further nausea and/or vomiting. Ensure adequate pain relief and minimize the anxiety level of the patient. Use non-steroidal anti-inflammatory drugs such as COX-2 inhibitors or benzodiazepines such as midazolam if needed. It is important to determine the type of surgery and whether blood has been swallowed by the patient as blood in the stomach is a strong emetogenic stimulus. If so, gastric suctioning is recommended (table 6).

References

1 Kapur PA: The big 'little problem'. Anesth Analg 1991;73:243–245.
2 Macario A, Weinger M, Carney S, Kim A: Which clinical anesthesia outcomes are important to avoid? Anesth Analg 1999;89:652–658.
3 Koivuranta M, Läärä E, Snare L, Alahuhta S: A survey of postoperative nausea and vomiting. Anaesthesia 1997;52:443–449.
4 Gold BS, Kitz DS, Lecky JH, et al: Unanticipated admission to the hospital following ambulatory surgery. JAMA 1989;262:3002–3010.
5 Carroll NV, Miederhoff P, Cox FM, et al: Postoperative nausea and vomiting after discharge from outpatient surgery centers. Anesth Analg 1995;80:903–909.
6 Watcha MF, White PF: Postoperative nausea and vomiting: Its etiology, treatment and prevention. Anesthesiology 1992;77:162–184.
7 Borison HL, Wang SC: Physiology and pharmacology of vomiting. Pharm Rev 1953;5:192–230.
8 Wang SC, Borison HL: The vomiting center: A critical experimental analysis. Arch Neurol Psychiatry 1950;63:928–941.
9 Borison HL, McCarthy LE: Neuropharmacology of chemotherapy-induced emesis. Drugs 1983:25(suppl 1):8–17.
10 Borison HL: Area postrema: Chemoreceptor circumventricular organ of the medulla oblongata. Prog Neurobiol 1989;32:351–90.
11 Stefanini E, Clement-Cormier Y: Detection of receptors in the area postrema. Eur J Pharmacol 1981;74:257–260.
12 Atweh SF, Kuhar MJ: Autoradiographic localization of opiate receptors in the rat brain. II. The brain stem. Brain Res 1977;129:1–12.
13 Wamsley JK, Lewis MS, Young WS, et al: Autoradiographic localization of muscarinic cholinergic receptors in rat brainstem. J Neurosci 1981;1:176–191.
14 Palacios JM, Wamsley JK, Kuhar MJ: The distribution of histamine H_1-receptors in the rat brain: An autoradiographic study. Neuroscience 1981;6:15–17.
15 Andrews PLR, Davis CJ, Binham S, et al: The abdominal visceral innervation and the emetic reflex: Pathways, pharmacology and plasticity. Can J Physiol Pharmacol 1990;668:325–345.
16 Peroutke SJ, Snyder SH: Antiemetics: Neurotransmitter receptor binding predicts therapeutic action. Lancet 1982;i:658–659.
17 Tramèr MR: A rational approach to the control of postoperative nausea and vomiting: Evidence from systemic reviews. I. Efficacy and harm of antiemetic intervention and methodological issues. Acta Anaesthesiol Scand 2001;45:4–13.
18 Tramèr MR: A rational approach to the control of postoperative nausea and vomiting: Evidence from systematic reviews. II. Recommendations for prevention and treatment and research agenda. Acta Anaesthesiol Scand 2001;45:14–19.
19 McCarthy BG, Peroutka SJ: Differentiation of the muscarinic cholinergic receptor subtypes in human cortex and pons: Implications for anti-motion sickness therapy. Aviat Space Environ Med 1988;49:63–66.

20 Philip BK: Etiologies of postoperative nausea and vomiting. Pharm Ther 1997;22(suppl):18–25.

21 Jenkins JC, Lahay D: Central mechanisms of vomiting related to catecholamine response: Anaesthetic implication. Can Anaesth Soc J 1971;18:434–441.

22 Haigh CG, Kaplan LA, Durham JA: Nausea and vomiting after gynecological surgery: A meta-analysis of factors affecting their incidence. Br J Anaesth 1993;71:512–522.

23 Palazzo MGA, Strunin L: Anaesthesia and emesis. I. etiology. Can Anaesth Soc J 1984;31: 178–187.

24 Bellville J: Postanesthetic nausea and vomiting. Anesthesiology 1961;22:773–780.

25 Bellville JW, Bross IDJ, Howland WS: Postoperative nausea and vomiting. IV. Factors related to postoperative nausea and vomiting. Anesthesiology 1960;21:186–193.

26 Clarke RSJ: Nausea and vomiting. Br J Anaesth 1984;56:19–27.

27 Jones RM: Desflurane and sevoflurane: Inhalation anesthetics for this decade? Br J Anaesth 1990;65:527–536.

28 Ghouri AF, Bodner M, White PF: Recovery profile after desflurane-nitrous oxide versus isoflurane-nitrous oxide in outpatients. Anesthesiology 1991;74:419–424.

29 Tramèr M, Moore A, McQuay H: Omitting nitrous oxide in general anaesthesia: Meta-analysis of intraoperative awareness and postoperative emesis in randomized controlled trials. Br J Anaesth 1996;76:186–193.

30 Pandit UA, Malviya S, Lewis IH: Vomiting after outpatient tonsillectomy and adenoidectomy in children: The role of nitrous oxide. Anesth Analg 1995;80:230–233.

31 Melnick BM, Johnson LS: Effect of eliminating nitrous oxide in outpatient anesthesia. Anesthesiology 1987;67:982–984.

32 Felts JA, Poler SM, Spitznagel EL: Nitrous oxide, nausea and vomiting after outpatient gynecologic surgery. J Clin Anesth 1990;2:168–171.

33 Eger EI: Anesthesia uptake and action. Baltimore, Williams & Wilkins, 1981, pp 171–177.

34 Watcha MF, Simeon RM, White PF, et al: Effect of propofol on the incidence of postoperative nausea and vomiting after strabismus surgery in pediatric outpatients. Anesthesiology 1991;75: 204–209.

35 Korttila K, Ostman P, Faure E, et al: Randomized comparison of recovery after propofol-nitrous oxide versus thiopentone-isoflurane-nitrous oxide anaesthesia in patients undergoing ambulatory surgery. Acta Anaesthesiol Scand 1990;34:400–403.

36 Doze VA, Westphal LM, White PF: Comparison of propofol with methohexital for outpatient anesthesia. Anesth Analg 1986;65:1189–1195.

37 Tramèr M, Moore A, McQuay H: Propofol anaesthesia and postoperative nausea and vomiting: Quantitative systematic review of randomized controlled studies. Br J Anaesth 1997;8978:247–255.

38 Thompson GE, Renington JM, Millman BS, et al: Experience with outpatient anesthesia. Anesth Analg 1973;52:881–897.

39 White PF, Dwonsky WA, Horai Y, Treron AJ: Comparison of continuous infusion fentanyl or ketamine versus thiopental: Determining the mean effective serum concentrations for outpatient surgery. Anesthesiology 1983;59:54–59.

40 Kestin IG, Dorje P: Anesthesia for evacuation of retained products of conception: Comparison between alfentanil plus etomidate and fentanyl plus thiopentone. Br J Anaesth 1987;59:364–368.

41 Horrigan RW, Moyers JR, Johnson BA, et al: Etomidate versus thiopental with and without fentanyl: A comparative study of awakening in man. Anesthesiology 1980;52:362–364.

42 Fragen RJ, Caldwell N: Comparison of a new formulation of etomidate with pentothal – Side effects and awakening times. Anesthesiology 1979;50:242–244.

43 King MJ, Milazkievicz R, Carli F, et al: Influence of neostigmine on postoperative vomiting. Br J Anaesth 1988;61:403–406.

44 Child CS: Prevention of neostigmine-induced colonic activity: A comparison of atropine and glycopyrronium. Anaesthesia 1984;39:1083–1085.

45 Tramèr M, Fuchs-Buder T: Omitting reversal of neuromuscular blockade: Effect on postoperative nausea and vomiting and risk of residual paralysis. A systematic review. Br J Anaesth 1999;82: 379–386.

46 Bonica JJ, Crepps W, Monk B, et al: Postoperative nausea and retching and vomiting. Anesthesiolgoy 1958;19:532–540.

47 Crocker JS, Vandam LD: Concerning nausea and vomiting during spinal anesthesia. Anesthesiology 1959;20:587–590.
48 Green NM: Physiology of spinal anesthesia, ed 3. Baltimore, Williams & Wilkins, 1981, pp 258–260.
49 Anderson R, Krogh K: Pain as a major cause of postoperative nausea. Can Anaesth Soc J 1976;23:366–369.
50 Yogendran S, Asokumar B, Cheng DC, Chung F: A prospective randomized double-blinded study of the effect of intravenous fluid therapy on adverse outcomes in outpatient surgery. Anesth Analg 1995;80:682–686.
51 Suntheralingham Y, Buvanendran A, Cheng DCH, et al: A prospective randomized double-blinded study of the effect of intravenous fluid therapy on adverse outcomes on outpatient surgery. Anesth Analg 1995;80:682–686.
52 Purkis IE: Factors that influence postoperative vomiting. Can Anaesth Soc J 1974;11:335–353.
53 Vandenberg AA, Lambourne A, Yazji NS, Laghani NA: Vomiting after ophthalmic surgery: Effects of intraoperative antiemetics and postoperative oral fluid restriction. Anaesthesia 1987; 42:270–276.
54 Dent SJ, Ramachandra V, Stephen CR: Postoperative vomiting: Incidence, analysis and therapeutic measures in 3,000 patients. Anesthesiology 1955;16:564–572.
55 Conroe JH, Dripps RD: Reactions to morphine in ambulatory and bed patients. Surg Gynecol Obstet 1948;87:221–224.
56 Rowley MP, Brown TCK: Postoperative vomiting in children. Anaesth Intensive Care 1982; 10:309–313.
57 Lerman J: Surgical and patient factors involved in postoperative nausea and vomiting. Br J Anaesth 1992;69(suppl 1):24–32.
58 Dundee JW, Moore J, Nicholl RM: Studies of drugs given before anaesthesia. II. A method for the assessment of their influence on the course of anaesthesia. Br J Anaesth 1962;34: 523–526.
59 Gan TJ: Postoperative nausea and vomiting – Can it be eliminated? JAMA 2002;287:1233–1236.
59a Koivuranta M, Läärä E, Snare L, et al: A survey of postoperative nausea and vomiting. Anaesthesia 1997;52:443–449.
60 Apfel CC, Läärä E, Koivuranta M, Greim CA, Roewer N: A simplified risk score for predicting postoperative nausea and vomiting. Anesthesiology 1999;91:693–700.
61 Sinclair DR, Chung F, Mezei G: Can postoperative nausea and vomiting be predicted? Anesthesiology 1999;91:109–118.
62 Gan TJ, Myers T, Apfel C, et al: Consensus guidelines for the management of postoperative nausea and vomiting. Anesth Analg 2003 (in press).
63 Derrico C, Voepellewis TD, Siewert M, Malviya S: Prolonged recovery stay and unplanned admission of the pediatric surgery outpatient – An observational study. J Clin Anesth 1998;10:482–487.
64 Smessaert A, Schehr CA, Artusio JF Jr: Nausea and vomiting in the immediate postanesthesia period. JAMA 1959;170:2072–2076.
65 Honkavaara P: Effect of transdermal hyoscine on nausea and vomiting during and after middle-ear surgery under local anesthesia. Br J Anaesth 1996;76:749–750.
66 Vance JP, Neill RS, Norris W: The incidence and aetiology of postoperative nausea and vomiting in a plastic surgical unit. Br J Plast Surg 1973;26:336–339.
67 Thompson DP, Ashley FL: Face-lift complications: A study of 922 cases performed in a 6-year period. Plast Reconstr Surg 1978;61:40–49.
68 Stein JM: Factors affecting nausea and vomiting in the plastic surgery patient. Plast Reconstr Surg 1982;70:505–511.
69 Watcha MF: The cost-effective management of postoperative nausea and vomiting. Anesthesiology 2000;92:931–933.
70 Golding JF, Scott JR: Comparison of the effects of a selective muscarinic receptor antagonist and hyoscine (scopolamine) on motion sickness, skin conductance and heart rate. Br J Clin Pharmacol 1997;43:633–637.
71 Dundee JW, Kirwan MK, Clarke RSJ: Anaesthesia and premedication as factors in postoperative vomiting. Acta Anaesthesiol Scand 1965;9:223–231.

72 Tigerstedt I, Salmela L, Aromaa U: Double-blind comparison of transdermal scopolamine, droperidol and placebo against postoperative nausea and vomiting. Acta Anaesthesiol Scand 1988; 32:454–457.
73 Bailey PL, Streisand JB, Pace NL, et al: Transdermal scopolamine reduces nausea and vomiting after outpatient laparoscopy. Anesthesiology 1999;72:977–980.
74 Loper KA, Ready LB, Dorman GH: Prophylactic transdermal scopolamine patches reduce nausea in postoperative patients receiving epidural morphine. Anesth Analg 1989;68:144–146.
75 Kotelko DM, Rottman RL, Wright WC, et al: Transdermal scopolamine decreases nausea and vomiting following cesarean section in patients receiving epidural morphine. Anesthesiology 1989;71:675–678.
76 Wood C: Antimotion sickness and antiemetic drugs. Drugs 1979;17:471–479.
77 Dundee JW, Moore J, Love WJ, et al: Studies of drugs given before anaesthesia. VI. The phenothiazine derivatives. Br J Anaesth 1965;37:332–352.
78 Dillon GP: Clinical evaluation of promethazine for prevention of postoperative vomiting. Am Pract Digest Treatment 1958;8:1571–1575.
79 Dundee JW, Assaf FAE, Loan WB, et al: A comparison of the efficacy of cyclizine and perphenazine in reducing the emetic effects of morphine and pethidine. Br J Clin Pharmacol 1975;2:81–85.
80 Howat DDC: Anti-emetic drugs in anaesthesia. Anaesthesia 1960;15:289–297.
81 Splinter WM, Roberts DJ: Perphenazine decreases vomiting by children after tonsillectomy. Can J Anaesth 1997;44:1308–1310.
82 Caroff SN: The neuroleptic malignant syndrome. J Clin Psychiatry 1980;41:679–681.
83 Loeser EA, Bennett G, Stanley TH, et al: Comparison of droperidol, haloperidol and prochlorperazine as postoperative antiemetics. Can Anaesth Soc J 1979;26:125–127.
84 Lischke V, et al: Droperidol causes a dose-dependent prolongation of the QT interval. Anesth Analg 1994;79:983–986.
85 FDA Strengthens Warnings for Droperidol. http://www.fda.gov/bbs/topics/ANSWERS/2001/ANSO1123.html (accessed Jan 17, 2003)
86 McCormick CG. FDA Alert: Current FDA report on droperidol status and basis for black box warning. Am Soc Anesthesiol Newsl 2002;66:19–20.
86a Chang N, Rappaport B: FDA alert: Update on droperidol and the FDA. Am Soc Anesthesiol Newsl 2002;66:25.
87 Fortney JT, Gan TJ, Craczyk S, et al: A comparison of the efficacy, safety and patient satisfaction of ondansetron versus droperidol as emetic for elective outpatient surgical procedures. S3A-409 and S3A-0410 Study Groups. Anesth Analg 1998;86:731–738.
88 Tang J, Watcha MF, White PF: A comparison of costs and efficacy of ondansetron and droperidol as prophylactic antiemetic therapy for elective outpatient gynecologic procedures. Anesth Analg 1996;83:304–313.
89 Woosley RL: Drugs that prolong QTc and/or induce torsades de pointes (online). Available from URL: http://www.torsades.org (accessed March 10, 2003).
89a http://www.fda.gov/medwatch: Information on reporting adverse events (accessed March 10, 2003).
90 Ross WT, Franz JA: Prevention of post-operative nausea and vomiting by haloperidol or droperidol (abstract). Anesth Analg 1990;70:S335.
91 Barton MD, Libonati M, Cohen PJ: The use of haloperidol for treatment of postoperative nausea and vomiting: A double-blind, placebo-controlled trial. Anesthesiology 1975;42:508–512.
92 Lehmann KA, Van Peer A, Ikonomakis M, et al: Pharmacokinetics of droperidol in surgical patients under different conditions of anesthesia. Br J Anaesth 1988;61:297–301.
93 Rita L, Goodarzi M, Seleny F: Effect of low-dose droperidol on postoperative vomiting in children. Can Anaesth Soc J 1981;28:259–262.
94 Wetchler BV, Collins IS, Jacob L: Antiemetic effects of droperidol on the ambulatory surgery patient. Anesthesiol Rev 1982;9:23–26.
95 Harrington RA, Hamilton CW, Brogden RM, et al: Metoclopramide: An updated review of its pharmacological properties and clinical use. Drugs 1983;25:451–494.
96 Madej TH, Simpson KH: Comparison of the use of domperidone, droperidol and metoclopramide in the prevention of nausea and vomiting following major gynaecological surgery. Br J Anaesth 1986;58:884–887.

97 Kauste A, Tuominen M, Heikkinen H, et al: Droperidol, alizapride and metoclopramide in the prevention and treatment of postoperative emetic sequelae. Eur J Anaesth 1986;3:1–9.
98 Assaf RA, Clarke RS, Dundee JW, et al: Studies of drugs given before anesthesia. XXIV. Metoclopramide with morphine and pethidine. Br J Anaesth 1974;46:514–519.
99 Henzi I, Walder B, Tramèr MR: Metoclopramide in the prevention of postoperative nausea and vomiting – A quantitative systematic review of randomized placebo-controlled studies. Br J Anaesth 1999;83:761–771.
99a Quaynor H, Raeder JC: Incidence and severity of postoperative nausea and vomiting are similar after metoclopramide 20 mg and ondansetron 8 mg given by the end of laparoscopic cholecystectomies. Acta Anaesth Scand 2002;46:109–113.
100 Dundee JW, Assaf RAE, Loan WB, et al: A comparison of the efficacy of cyclizine and perphenazine in reducing the antiemetic effects of morphine and pethidine. Br J Clin Pharmacol 1975;2:81–85.
101 Bellville JW, Howland WS, Bross IDJ. Postoperative nausea and vomiting. III. Evaluation of the antiemetid drugs fluphenazine (prolixin) and promethazine (phenergan) and comparison with triflupromazine (vesprin) and cyclizine (marezine). JAMA 1960;172:1488–1493.
102 McKenzie R, Wadhwa RK, Lim Uy NT, et al: Antiemetic effectiveness of intramuscular hydroxyzine compared with intramuscular droperidol. Anesth Analg 1981;60:783–788.
103 DiFlorio T: The use of midazolam for persistent postoperative nausea and vomiting. Anesth Intensive Care 1992;20:383–386.
104 Splinter WM, MacNeill HB, Menard EA: Midazolam reduces vomiting after tonsillectomy in children. Can J Anaesth 1995;42:201–203.
105 Khalil SN, Berry JM, Howard G, et al: The antiemetic effect of lorazepam after outpatient strabismus surgery in children. Anesthesiology 1992;77:915–919.
106 Giacalone VF: Antianxiety/sedative drugs: The benzodiazepines. Clin Podiatr Med Surg 1992; 9:465–479.
107 Lopez-Olaondo L, Carrascosa F, Pueyo FJ: Advances in antiemetic pharmacology. Review Course Lectures. European Society of Anaesthesiologists 8th Annual Meeting, Vienna, April 2000, pp 251–258.
108 Henzi I, Walder B, Tramèr MR: Dexamethasone for the prevention of postoperative nausea and vomiting: A qualitative systematic review. Anesth Analg 2000;90:186–194.
109 Liu K, Hsu CC, Chia YY: The effective dose of dexamethasone for antiemesis after major gynecological surgery. Anesth Analg 1999;89:1316–1318.
110 Wang JJ, Ho ST, Lee SC, et al: The use of dexamethasone for preventing postoperative nausea and vomiting in females undergoing thyroidectomy: A dose-ranging study. Anesth Analg 2000; 91:1404–1407.
111 Asboe V, Raeder JC, Groegaard B: Betamethasone reduces postoperative pain and nausea after ambulatory surgery. Anesth Analg 1998;87:319–323.
112 Aouad MT, Siddik SS, Rizk LB, et al: The effect of dexamethasone on postoperative vomiting after tonsillectomy. Anesth Analg 2001;92:636–640.
113 Pappas AL, Sukhani R, Hotaling AJ, et al: The effect of perioperative dexamethasone on the immediate and delayed postoperative morbidity in children undergoing adenotonsillectomy. Anesth Analg 1998;87:57–61.
114 Wang JJ, Ho ST, Tzeng JI, Tang CS: The effect of timing of dexamethasone administration on its efficacy as a prophylactic antiemetic for postoperative nausea and vomiting. Anesth Analg 2000; 91:136–139.
115 Zofran® (ondansetron hydrochloride – package insert). Research Triangle Park, GlaxoSmithKline, 2001.
116 Kenny GNC, Oates JDL, Lesser J, et al: Efficacy of orally administered ondansetron in the prevention of postoperative nausea and vomiting: A dose-ranging study. Br J Anaesth 1992;68: 466–470.
117 McKenzie R, Kovac A, O'Connor T, et al: Comparison of ondansetron versus placebo to prevent postoperative nausea and vomiting in women undergoing ambulatory gynecologic surgery. Anesthesiology 1993;78:21–28.
118 Scuderi P, Wetchler B, Sung YF, et al: Treatment of postoperative nausea and vomiting after outpatient surgery with the 5-HT_3-receptor antagonist ondansetron. Anesthesiology 1993;78:15–20.

119 Tramèr M, Moore RA, Reynolds DJM, McQuay HG: A quantitative systematic review of ondansetron in treatment of established postoperative nausea and vomiting. BMJ 1997;314: 1088–1092.
120 Kovac A, Pearman M, Khalil S, et al: Ondansetron prevents postoperative emesis in male outpatients. J Clin Anesth 1996;8:644–651.
121 Rose JB, Brenn BR, Corddry DH, et al: Preoperative oral ondansetron for pediatric tonsillectomy. Anesth Analg 1996;83:558–562.
122 Khalil S, Rodarte A, Weldon BC, et al: Intravenous ondansetron in established postoperative emesis in children. Anesthesiology 1996;85:204–206.
123 Sun R, Klein KW, White PF: The effect of timing of ondansetron administration in outpatients undergoing otolaryngologic surgery. Anesth Analg 1997;84:331–336.
124 Tang J, Wang B, White PF, et al: The effect of timing of ondansetron administration on its efficacy, cost-effectiveness and cost-benefit as a prophylactic antiemetic in the ambulatory setting. Anesth Analg 1998;86:274–282.
125 Rung GW, Claybon L, Hord A, et al: Intravenous ondansetron for postsurgical opioid-induced nausea and vomiting. Anesth Analg 1997;84:832–838.
126 Kytril® injection (granisetron hydrochloride – package insert). Nutley, Roche Laboratories, Inc, 2000.
127 Mikawa K, Takao Y, Nishina K, et al: Optimal dose of granisetron for prophylaxis against postoperative emesis after gynecological surgery. Anesth Analg 1997;85:652–656.
128 Wilson AJ, Diemunsch P, Lindeque BG, et al: Single-dose intravenous granisetron in the prevention of postoperative nausea and vomiting. Br J Anaesth 1996;76:515–518.
129 Fujii Y, Saitoh Y, Tanaka H, et al: Prevention of PONV with granisetron, droperidol or metoclopramide in patients with postoperative emesis. Can J Anaesth 1998;45:153–156.
130 Fujii Y, Toyooka H, Tanaka H: Prevention of PONV with granisetron, droperidol and metoclopramide in female patients with history of motion sickness. Can J Anaesth 1997;44:820–824.
131 Fujii Y, Toyooka H, Tanaka H. Prevention of postoperative nausea and vomiting in female patients during menstruation: Comparison of droperidol, metoclopramide and granisetron. Br J Anaesth 1998;80:248–249.
132 Taylor AM, Rosen M, Diemunsch PA, et al: A double-blind, parallel-group, placebo-controlled, dose-ranging, multicenter study of intravenous granisetron in the treatment of postoperative nausea and vomiting in patients undergoing surgery with general anesthesia. J Clin Anesth 1997;9: 658–663.
133 Fujii Y, Tanaka H: Preoperative oral granisetron for the prevention of vomiting following paediatric surgery. Paediatr Anaesth 2002;12:267–271.
134 Fujii Y, Tanaka H: Granisetron reduces post-operative vomiting in children: A dose-ranging study. Eur J Anaesthesiol 1999;16:62–65.
135 Cieslak GD, Watcha MF, Phillips MB, et al: The dose-response relationship of granisetron for the prophylaxis of pediatric postoperative emesis. Anesthesiology 1996;85:1076–1085.
135a Kovac A: Prevention and treatment of postoperative nausea and vomiting. Drugs 2000;59: 213–243.
135b Kaiser R, Sezen O, Papies A, et al: Patient-tailored antiemetic treatment with 5-hydroxytryptamine 3 receptor antagonists according to cytochrome P-450 2D6 genotype. J Clin Oncol 2002;20: 2805–2811.
136 Simpson K, Spencer CM, McClellan KJ: Tropisetron: An update of its use in the prevention of chemotherapy-induced nausea and vomiting. Drugs 2000;59:1297–1315.
137 Chan MTV, Chui PT, Ho WS, et al: Single-dose tropisetron for preventing postoperative nausea and vomiting after breast surgery. Anesth Analg 1998;87:931–935.
138 Alon E, Kocian R, Nett PC, et al: Tropisetron for the prevention of postoperative nausea and vomiting in women undergoing gynecologic surgery. Anesth Analg 1996;82:338–341.
139 Zomers PJ, Langenberg CJ, de Grujin KM: Tropisetron for postoperative nausea and vomiting after gynaecological surgery. Br J Anaesth 1993;71:677–680.
140 Alon E, Buchser E, Herrera E, et al: Tropisetron for treating established postoperative nausea and vomiting: A randomized, double-blind, placebo-controlled study. Anesth Analg 1998;86: 617–623.

141 Anzemet® injection (dolasetron mesylate – package insert). Kansas City, Aventis Pharmaceuticals, Inc, 2002.
142 Balfour JA, Goa KL: Dolasetron: A review of its pharmacology and efficacy in the management of nausea and vomiting induced by chemotherapy, radiotherapy or surgery. Drugs 1997;54:273–298.
143 Warriner CB, Knox D, Belo S, et al: Prophylactic oral dolaetron mesylate reduces postoperative nausea and vomiting after abdominal hysterectomy. Can J Anaesth 1997;44:1167–1173.
144 Diemunsch P, Korttila K, Leeser J, et al: Oral dolasetron mesylate for prevention of postoperative nausea and vomiting: A multicenter, double-blind, placebo-controlled study. The Oral Dolasetron PONV Prevention Study Group. J Clin Anesth 1998;10:145–152.
145 Gracyzk SG, McKenzie R, Kaller S, et al: Intravenous dolasetron for the prevention of postoperative nausea and vomiting after outpatient laparoscopic gynecologic surgery. Anesth Analg 1997;84:325–330.
146 Kovac AL, Scuderi P, Boerner TF, et al. Treatment of postoperative nausea and vomiting with single intravenous doses of dolasetron mesylate: A multicenter trial. Anesth Analg 1997;84: 546–552.
147 Diemunsch P, Leeser J, Feiss P, et al: Intravenous dolasetron mesylate ameliorates postoperative nausea and vomiting. Can J Anaesth 1997;44:173–181.
148 Lerman J, Sims C, Sikich N, et al: Pharmacokinetics of the active metabolite (MDL 74,156) of dolasetron mesylate after oral or intravenous administration to anesthetized children. Clin Pharmacol Ther 1996;60:485–492.
149 Rothenberg DM, Parnass SM, Litwack K, et al: Efficacy of ephedrine in the prevention of postoperative nausea and vomiting Anesth Analg 1991;72:58–61.
150 Naguib K, Osman HA, Al-Khayat HL, et al: Prevention of postoperative nausea and vomiting following laparoscopic surgery: ephedrine vs. propofol. Middle East J Anaesthesiol 1998;14: 219–230.
151 Myles PS, Hendrata M, Bennett AM, et al: Postoperative nausea and vomiting. Propofol or thiopentone: Does choice of induction agent affect outcome? Anaesth Intensive Care 1996;24: 355–359.
152 Hamunen K, Vaalamo MO, Maunuksela EL: Does propofol reduce vomiting after strabismus surgery in children? Acta Anaesthesiol Scand 1997;41:973–977.
153 Gan TJ, Glass PSA, Howell ST, et al: Determination of plasma concentrations of propofol associated with 50% reduction of postoperative nausea. Anesthesiology 1997;87:779–784.
154 Gan TJ, Ginsberg B, Grant AP, et al: Double-blind, randomized comparison of ondansetron and intraoperative propofol to prevent postoperative nausea and vomiting. Anesthesiology 1996;85: 1036–1042.
155 Sniadach MS, Alberts MS: A comparison of the prophylactic antiemetic effect of ondansetron and droperidol on patients undergoing gynecologic laparoscopy. Anesth Analg 1979;85:797–800.
156 Grond S, Lynch J, Diefenbach C, et al: Comparison of ondansetron and droperidol in the prevention of nausea and vomiting after inpatient minor gynecologic surgery. Anesth Analg 1995;81: 603–607.
157 Desilva PH, Darvish AH, McDonald SM, et al: The efficacy of prophylactic ondansetron, droperidol, perphenazine and metoclopramide in the prevention of nausea and vomiting after major gynecologic surgery. Anesth Analg 1995;81:139–143.
158 Danner K, Becker HG, Best B, Madler C: Prophylaxis of nausea and vomiting after thyroid surgery: Comparison of oral and intravenous dolasetron with intravenous droperidol and placebo. Anaesth Intensive Med 2001;36:425–430.
159 Korttila K, Clergue F, Leeser J, et al: Intravenous dolasetron and ondansetron in prevention of postoperative nausea and vomiting: A multicenter, double-blind, placebo-controlled study. Acta Anaesthesiol Scand 1997;42:914–922.
160 Naguib M, el-Bakry AK, Khoshim MH, et al: Prophylactic antiemetic therapy with ondansetron, tropisetron, granisetron and metoclopramide in patients undergoing laparoscopic cholecystectomy: A randomized, double-blind comparison with placebo. Can J Anaesth 1996;43:226–231.
161 Zarata E, Watcha M, White PF, et al: Comparative cost-effectiveness of dolasetron and ondansetron for prophylaxis of postoperative nausea and vomiting after ambulatory surgery (abstract). Anesthesiology 1999;91:A3.

162 Walker JB: Efficacy of single-dose intravenous dolasetron versus ondansetron in the prevention of postoperative nausea and vomiting. Clin Ther 2001;23:932–938.
163 Robertson CR, McLeskey CH, Meyer T, et al: IV dolasetron vs. ondansetron for the treatment of PONV in ambulatory surgery patients (abstract). Anesthesiology 1999;91:A4.
164 McKenzie R, Tantisira B, Karambelkar DJ, et al: Comparison of ondansetron with ondansetron plus dexamethasone in the prevention of postoperative nausea and vomiting. Anesth Analg 1994; 79:961–964.
165 McKenzie R, Riley TJ, Tantisira B, et al: Effect of propofol for induction and ondansetron with or without dexamethasone for the prevention of nausea and vomiting after major gynecologic surgery. J Clin Anesth 1997;9:15–20.
166 McKenzie R, Uy NTL, Riley TJ, Hamilton DL: Droperidol/ondansetron combination controls nausea and vomiting after tubal banding. Anesth Analg 1996;83:1218–1222.
167 Fujii Y, Toyooka H, Tanaka H: Prevention of postoperative nausea and vomiting with a combination of granisetron and droperidol. Anesth Analg 1998;86:613–616.
168 Fujii Y, Tanaka H, Toyooka H: Granisetron-dexamethasone combination reduces postoperative nausea and vomiting. Can J Anaesth 1995;42:387–390.
169 Fujii Y, Tanaka H, Toyooka H: The effects of dexamethasone on antiemetics in female patients undergoing gynecologic surgery. Anesth Analg 1997;85:913–917.
170 Eberhart LH, Morin AM, Georgieff M: Dexamethasone for prophylaxis of postoperative nausea and vomiting. A meta-analysis of randomized controlled studies. Anaesthetist 2000;49:713–720.
171 Greif RE, Laciny S, Rapf B, et al: Supplemental oxygen reduces the incidence of postoperative nausea and vomiting. Anesthesiology 1999;91:1246–1252.
172 Kovac A, O'Connor T, Pearman M, et al: Efficacy of repeat intravenous dosing of ondansetron in controlling postoperative nausea and vomiting: A randomized, double-blind, placebo-controlled multicenter trial. J Clin Anesth 1999;11:453–459.
173 Scuderi P, James R, Harris L, et al: Multimodal management prevents early postoperative vomiting after outpatient laparoscopy. Anesth Analg 2000;91:1408–1414.
174 Sung YF: Risks and benefits of drugs used in the management of postoperative nausea and vomiting. Drug Saf 1996;14:181–197.
175 Kuryshev YA, Brown AM, Wang L, et al: Interactions of the 5-hydroxytryptamine-3 antagonist class of antiemetic drugs with human cardiac ion channels. J Pharmacol Ther 2000;295:614–620.
176 Benedict CR, Arbogast R, Martin L, et al: Single-blind study of the effects of intravenous dolasetron mesylate versus ondansetron on electrocardiographic parameters in normal volunteers. J Cardiovasc Pharmacol 1996;28:53–59.
177 Diemunsch P, Grelot L: Potential of substance P antagonists as antiemetics. Drugs 2000;60: 533–546.
178 Navari RM, Reinhardt RR, Gralla RJ, et al: Reduction of cisplatin-induced emesis by a selective neurokinin-1-receptor antagonist. N Engl J Med 1999;340:190–195.
179 Diemunsch P, Schoeffler P, Bryssine B, et al: Antiemetic activity of the NK_1 receptor antagonist GR205171 in the treatment of established postoperative nausea and vomiting after major gynecological surgery. Br J Anaesth 1999;82:274–276.

Anthony L. Kovac, MD
Department of Anesthesiology, University of Kansas Medical Center
3901 Rainbow Blvd, Kansas City, KS 66160-7415 (USA)
E-Mail akovac@kumc.edu

Donnerer J (ed): Antiemetic Therapy.
Basel, Karger, 2003, pp 161–168

Metoclopramide for the Control of Postoperative Nausea and Vomiting

Iris Henzi, Martin R. Tramèr

Division d'Anesthésiologie, Département APSIC,
Hôpitaux Universitaires Genève, Suisse

History of Metoclopramide

Metoclopramide (methoxychloroprocainamide) has been used as an antiemetic for almost 40 years. The molecule was first described by Justin-Besançon and Laville in 1964, and the first clinical trials on its efficacy were published by Tourneu et al. in 1964 and by Boisson and Albott in 1966 [1]. Initially, metoclopramide was used as a treatment of nausea and vomiting in association with migraine and severe headache. In this setting, the combination of metoclopramide with an analgesic proved to be very efficacious with a short delay of action. Later, metoclopramide was used for the control of sickness due to radiation therapy and chemotherapy, and for the prevention and treatment of postoperative nausea and vomiting (PONV). Today, metoclopramide is probably one of the most popular antiemetic drugs in anesthetic practice. It is sold as Primperan (France, Switzerland), Paspertin (Germany, Switzerland), Maxolon (UK), and Reglan (USA).

Pharmacokinetics

After oral administration, the peak plasma concentration of metoclopramide is reached after about 1 h [2]. After rectal administration, the peak plasma concentration is delayed (1–3 h) due to an incomplete absorption [3]. The average bioavailability of oral metoclopramide is about 50% with an important interindividual variability. This variability is probably due to individual differences in the hepatic elimination (first-pass metabolism). Metoclopramide passes the blood-brain barrier. It is almost entirely (80%) eliminated by the kidneys. The elimination half-time is 4–5 h after oral administration, and is 2–4 h after intravenous or intramuscluar administration [4]. Metoclopramide is well tolerated when given intravenously, intramuscularly, orally, or rectally.

Pharmacodynamics

Metoclopramide is part of the benzamide family, and is chemically derived from the local anesthetic procaine. Indeed, metoclopramide has shown a local anesthetic effect in both experimental [5] and clinical studies [6]. The antiemetic property of metoclopramide is mainly due to its interaction with dopaminergic (D_2) and serotoninergic (5-HT_3 and 5-HT_4) receptors. Metoclopramide also has a gastrointestinal prokinetic effect through cholinergic stimulation. This effect consists of an increased tension in the lower esophageal sphincter and at the gastric fundus, an increase in gastric and small intestinal motility, and a relaxation of the pylorus and duodenum during contraction of the stomach [7]. The gastrokinetic effect is mediated by an antagonism at the D_2 and 5-HT_3 receptors and by activation of the 5-HT_4 receptor [8, 9].

5-HT_3 Receptor

The role of the 5-HT_3 receptor in the control of the PONV is poorly understood. The presence of the 5-HT_3 receptor has been proven indirectly by the antiemetic effect of ondansetron, an antagonist of the 5-HT_3 receptor [10]. The 5-HT_3 receptor is localized in the central nervous system (CNS), on vagal abdominal sensory endings (the main site for antiemetic action of 5-HT_3 receptor antagonists), on sympathetic neurons, and in enterochromaffin cells in the mucosa of the upper gastrointestinal tract which are responsible for inducing nausea and vomiting. Enterochromaffin cells are rich in serotonin, and can mainly be found in the intestinal mucosa; less serotonin can be found in the plexus myentericus [11]. Cytostatic agents (e.g., cisplatin) or irradiation can induce a liberation of serotonin and sensitize the 5-HT receptors. Antagonists of the 5-HT_3 receptor, like metoclopramide, counteract these effects. The affinity of metoclopramide for the 5-HT_3 receptors is weak and dose-dependent, however, the optimal dose of metoclopramide to recruit 5-HT_3 receptors in humans is unknown.

5-HT_4 Receptor

The pharmacological profile of these receptors was found to be similar to that of 5-HT receptors, located in the CNS or peripherally. Neural and non-neural 5-HT_4 receptors have been demonstrated in the gastrointestinal tract. It is interesting to point out that drugs like metoclopramide or cisapride, besides acting as agonists at the 5-HT_4 receptor level, also possess antagonistic properties [12]. Theoretically, a combination of 5-HT_4 receptor agonist with A5-HT_3 antagonist seems to produce three major benefits [13]: (1) there is improved relief of chemotherapy-induced nausea and vomiting by inhibition of 5-HT secretion from enterochromaffin cells and blockade of intestinal vagal afferent activation; (2) due to the prokinetic effect mediated by 5-HT, there is an improvement of the motility of the upper gastrointestinal tract, and thus a re-installation of normal peristalsis, and (3) no constipation will result which represents a frequent adverse side effect of pure 5-HT_3 receptor antagonism.

D_2 Receptor

The main binding site of metoclopramide is the dopamine receptor, localized in the CNS and in nonspecific cholinergic neurons. Coupling of metoclopramide on the receptor leads to an antagonism [14]. It results in an antiemetic effect and a blockage of inhibitory vagal efferences of the gastrointestinal tract. Although there are no specific dopaminergic neurons in the gastrointestinal tract, two dopamine agonists, apomorphine and levodopa, have shown to inhibit gastrointestinal motility and to diminish gastric expulsion [15]. This effect, however, is not considered to be of clinical relevance.

The dopaminergic receptors of the chemoreceptor trigger zone can be activated by opioids, cytostatic drugs, bacteria toxins, radiation, and metabolic disorders (uremia, hypoxemia). These receptors play an important role in the transmission of an emetogenic stimulation to the vomiting center, and represent a point of action for many antiemetic drugs. With metoclopramide, alizapride, droperidol, or domperidone, for instance, the dopaminergic effect of many emetogenic stimuli can be blocked. The inhibitory effect is due to an acetylcholine secretion of postganglionic nerves that can be observed with all D_2 agonists [16]. There is evidence that metoclopramide sensitizes gastrointestinal smooth muscles to the effects of acetylcholine, which explains the observation that metoclopramide requires a background cholinergic activity to be effective.

Other Effects

Metoclopramide stimulates the secretion of prolactin through a mechanism that is not well understood [17]. Metoclopramide also inhibits the vestibular nucleus, resulting in an antivertigo effect [18].

Metoclopramide for the Control of PONV

Postoperative Nausea and Vomiting

In contrast to sickness related to radiotherapy or chemotherapy, there is no animal model to study PONV. Thus, for the PONV setting, data on the efficacy of antiemetic drugs have to be derived from clinical trials. PONV is often underestimated as a medical problem because it is self-limiting (it usually stops spontaneously after 24 h), it never becomes chronic, and it almost never kills. However, 10% of the population undergoes surgery every year [19], and about 30% of them will suffer from PONV [20]. This is 200,000 people in the UK alone every year. There is evidence that surgical patients prefer postoperative pain [21] to PONV, and would be willing to pay considerable amounts of money for an effective antiemetic [22]. About 1% of patients undergoing ambulatory surgery are admitted overnight because of uncontrolled PONV [20]. Thus, there is a need for antiemetic interventions that are efficacious, safe and cheap.

Methods

The Endpoints

Nausea is defined as a subjective and uncomfortable sensation that is sometimes associated with a hyperactivity of the autonomous vagal system with subsequent pallor, profuse transpiration, hypersalivation, and occasionally arterial hypotension and bradycardia. Nausea is often followed by the need to vomit. Vomiting is the violent rejection of the contents of the stomach through the mouth. Nausea and vomiting can often be observed independently, and thus can be studied independently. It is important to note that nausea is not merely a mild bout of vomiting.

The Systematic Review

Systematic reviews aim to assess the best possible scientific evidence about the effects of healthcare interventions. The basic methodology can be divided into a systematic (i.e., unbiased) search for reports of randomized, controlled trials; the methodological scoring of retrieved reports using predefined validity criteria; extraction of data, and the analysis of data from independent trials using biostatistical methods (i.e., meta-analysis). The systematic search is a crucial step in this process; it includes the search in electronic databases (Medline, Embase, Cochrane Controlled Trials Register, etc.), hand-searching of journals, reviewing bibliographies of retrieved reports, and contact with authors and manufacturers. A valid estimation of antiemetic efficacy has to include information about the comparison (e.g., metoclopramide compared with placebo), the tested dose and route of administration (e.g., 10 mg i.v.), the endpoint (e.g., prevention of postoperative nausea), and the length of the observation period (e.g., antinausea efficacy in the immediate postoperative period). Two observation periods have been arbitrarily defined for the PONV setting, a 'short' period (efficacy up to 6 h after surgery) and a 'long' period (up to 48 h after surgery) [23]. As an estimate of efficacy, the number-needed-to-treat (NNT) may be calculated which indicates how many patients have to receive an intervention (e.g., metoclopramide 10 mg) for one to profit compared with doing nothing, or with another antiemetic. In the PONV setting, an NNT of 5 or less to prevent (or to treat) PONV compared with placebo may be regarded as a clinically relevant degree of efficacy.

The systematic review is a powerful tool to further our understanding on the efficacy of interventions and their likelihood of harm when there are lots of data from numerous smaller trials, and when there are unresolved questions. Systematic reviews have become valuable sources for rational decision-making and patient care. The antiemetic efficacy of metoclopramide in the PONV setting has been evaluated in several systematic reviews [24–28] – these are briefly discussed below.

Prevention of PONV with Metoclopramide – Evidence from Active Controlled Trials

Three systematic reviews have investigated the relative efficacy of metoclopramide compared with other antiemetic drugs based on data from active controlled trials (i.e., A vs. B design without a placebo group) [26–28]. They all came to the conclusion that metoclopramide was less efficacious than the modern 5-HT_3 receptor antagonists (setrons). These analyses, however, were unable to provide information on dose responsiveness, on optimal dose, and on adverse drug reactions. This lack of information is related to the inherent weakness of many active controlled trials [29]. The idea of active controlled trials is that an experimental drug 'A' (here metoclopramide) was directly compared with a gold standard drug 'B', and that placebos that may be perceived unethical may be avoided. Unfortunately, there is no gold standard in the PONV setting. Thus, the choice of the comparator substance will always be arbitrary. Also, since there is no placebo group in such trials, the baseline risk (or the underlying risk) remains unknown. In a randomized placebo-controlled trial, the incidence of nausea and vomiting in patients receiving a placebo may be regarded as an indicator of the true underlying risk of PONV in the study population. If the control (placebo) event rate was high, we would assume that the investigated cohort represented a high-risk setting. If this event rate was low, it most likely represented a low-risk setting. This stratification remains obscured in active controlled trials. For rational decision-making in the PONV setting, efficacy data from placebo-controlled trials are needed.

Prevention of PONV with Metoclopramide – Evidence from Placebo-Controlled Trials

The prophylactic antiemetic efficacy of metoclopramide and its likelihood to harm have been investigated in a systematic review of randomized placebo-controlled trials [24]. In 66 studies, 3,260 patients received 18 different regimens of metoclopramide, and 3,006 controls received placebo or no treatment. 6,000 adults and children have been investigated in over 60 relevant studies. In adults, the best-documented regimen was 10 mg i.v. With this regimen, NNTs to prevent nausea or vomiting up to 6 h after surgery were about 9, and up to 48 h were about 10. Other doses of metoclopramide (5, 15, 20 and 30 mg) were studied in single small trials only, however they did not show any superiority of metoclopramide compared with placebo for the prevention of PONV.

In children, the best-documented regimen was 0.25 mg/kg i.v. (which corresponds to about 18 mg in an adult with a body weight of 70 kg). The antivomiting efficacy of metoclopramide in the immediate postoperative period was slightly better than in adults; the NNT to prevent early vomiting was about 6. No sensible conclusion could be drawn on the long-term effects since five trials only investigated late efficacy in children. Also, no data were available on metoclopramide's antinausea efficacy, as in pediatric studies, nausea is usually not investigated.

There was no increased risk of adverse reactions that may be attributed to interaction of metoclopramide with the dopamine receptor (e.g., extrapyramidal symptoms, or sedation and drowsiness), neither in adults nor in children.

These data do provide strong evidence that metoclopramide, in the doses described in these trials, has no clinically relevant antiemetic effect for the prevention of PONV. The most likely explanation for his result (absence of efficacy and absence of harm) is that the doses were too low. In chemotherapy, metoclopramide doses about 50 times higher are used. A large randomized dose-finding study is needed to establish dose responsiveness and to define the optimal dose of metoclopramide for the prevention of PONV. In the mean time, metoclopramide cannot be recommended as a worthwhile prophylaxis of PONV.

Treatment of Established PONV

One systematic review investigated the efficacy of all available antiemetic interventions for the treatment of established PONV symptoms [25]. There were four main results of this systematic review. First, compared with the plethora of prevention trials in the PONV setting (there are over one thousand studies in the world's literature), only 18 valid placebo-controlled trials on the treatment of PONV could be retrieved. Second, the well-documented 5-HT_3 receptor antagonists were efficacious to some extent in preventing further vomiting in a vomiting patient after surgery; they showed less efficacy in preventing further nausea in a nauseated patient. Third, over wide ranges of doses there was weak evidence only of dose responsiveness with all the 5-HT_3 receptor antagonists tested. And finally, for metoclopramide and for other classic antiemetics that have been widely used for decades, there was a lack of evidence on their therapeutic efficacy in the postoperative period. Only one valid placebo-controlled trial (in 185 patients) could be retrieved on the efficacy of metoclopramide in the treatment of established PONV [30]. Thus, as for prevention, a large randomized dose-finding study is needed to establish dose responsiveness and to define the optimal dose of metoclopramide for the treatment of established PONV symptoms. In the mean time, metoclopramide cannot be recommended as a worthwhile treatment of PONV.

Conclusions

Metoclopramide is an old drug and has been used for many years in anesthetic practice in an attempt to prevent and to treat PONV. Metoclopramide possesses several favorable antiemetic properties: antagonism of the D_2 and 5-HT_3 receptors, agonism of the 5-HT_4 receptor, and a prokinetic gastrointestinal effect. Thus, in theory, metoclopramide should be the perfect antiemetic. However, looking at all valid and relevant randomized controlled studies reveals that there is no prophylactic efficacy with the most frequently used dose of metoclopramide (10 mg i.v.), and that there is a lack of evidence of any efficacy for the treatment of established PONV symptoms. Unless large studies show with confidence that metoclopramide is of any relevant benefit for the control of PONV, its use in daily anesthetic practice cannot be recommended.

References

1 Sanger GJ, King FD: From metoclopramide to selective gut motility stimulants and 5-HT_3 receptor antagonists. Drug Des Deliv 1988;3:273–295.
2 Ross-Lee LM, Eadie MJ, Hooper WD, Bochner F: Single-dose pharmacokinetics of metoclopramide. Eur J Clin Pharmacol 1981;20:465–471.
3 Block W, Pingoud A, Khan M, Kjellerup P: The pharmacokinetics, bioequivalence and bioavailability of different formulations of metoclopramide in man. Azneimittelforschung 1981;31: 1041–1045.
4 Graffner C, Lagerstroem PO, Lundberg P, Roenn O: Pharmacokinetics of metoclopramide intravenously and orally determined by liquid chromatography. Br J Clin Pharmacol 1979;8:469–474.
5 Wei-Wu P, Mok MS, Da-Peng Chang, Min-Ho Huang: Local anesthetic effect of tramadol, metoclopramide and lidocaine following intradermal injection. Reg Anesth Pain Med 1998;23:580–583.
6 Picard PR, Tramèr MR: Prevention of pain on injection with propofol: Quantitative systematic review. Anesth Analg 2000;90:936–939.
7 Schulze-Delrieu K: Metoclopramide. Drug therapy. N Engl J Med 1981;305:28–32.
8 Costall B, Naylor RJ: Neuropharmacology of emesis in relation to clinical response. Br J Cancer Suppl 1992;19:2–8.
9 Clarke DE, Craig DA, Fozard JR: The 5-HT_4 receptor: Naughty, but nice. Trends Pharmacol Sci 1989;10:385–386.
10 Raftery S, Sherry E: Total intravenous anaesthesia with propofol and alfentanil protects against postoperative nausea and vomiting. Can J Anaesth 1992;39:37–40.

11 Furness JB, Casta M: Identification of gastrointestinal neurotransmitters; in Bertaccini EG (ed): Mediators and Drugs in Gastrointestinal Motility. Handbook of Experimental Pharmacology. Berlin, Springer, 1982, vol 59/I, pp 383–462.
12 Tonini M, Rizzi CA, Manzo L, Onori L: Novel enteric 5-HT_4 receptors and gastrointestinal prokinetic action. Pharmacol Res 1991;24:5–14.
13 Tonini M: 5-HT_4 receptor involvement in emesis; in Reynolds DJM, Andrews PLR, Davis CJ (eds): Serotonin and the Scientific Basis of the Anti-Emetic Therapy. Oxford, Oxford Clinical Communications, 1995, pp 192–199.
14 Pinder RM, Brogden RN, Sawyer PR, Speight TM, Avery GS: Metoclopramide: A review of its pharmacological properties and clinical use. Drugs 1976;12:81–131.
15 Berkowitz DM, McCallum RW: Interaction of levodopa and metoclopramide on gastric emptying. Clin Pharmacol Ther 1980;27:414–420.
16 Kusunoki M, Taniyama K, Tanaka C: Dopamine regulation of [^{3}H]acetylcholine release from guinea-pig stomach. J Pharmacol Exp Ther 1985;234:713–719.
17 Fang VS, Zimo DA, Byyny R: Pituitary response to metoclopramide in the rat. J Endocrinol 1977; 74:155–156.
18 Gonzalez CG, Palomero JMS, Finamore PH: Estudio clinico de la asociacion dimenhidrinato-metoclopramida-piridoxina en el campo otorrinolaringologico. Ann Otol Rhinol Laryngol Iberoam 1977;4:135–140.
19 Clergue F, Auroy Y, Pequignot F, Jougla E, Lienhart A, Laxenaire MC: French survey of anesthesia in 1996. Anesthesiology 1999;91:1509–1520.
20 Tramèr MR: A rational approach to the control of postoperative nausea and vomiting: Evidence from systematic reviews. I. Efficacy and harm of antiemetic interventions and methodological issues. Acta Anaesthesiol Scand 2001;45:4–13.
21 Van Wijk MGF, Smalhout B: A postoperative analysis of the patient's view of anaesthesia in a Netherlands' teaching hospital. Anaesthesia 1990;45:679–682.
22 Gan T: How much are patients willing to pay to avoid postoperative nausea and vomiting? Anesth Analg 2001;92:393–400.
23 Tramèr M, Moore A, McQuay H: Prevention of vomiting after paediatric strabismus surgery: A systematic review using the numbers-needed-to-treat method. Br J Anaesth 1995;75:556–561.
24 Henzi I, Walder B, Tramèr MR: Metoclopramide in the prevention of postoperative nausea and vomiting – A quantitative systematic review of randomised placebo-controlled trials. Br J Anaesth 1999;83:761–771.
25 Kazemi-Kjellberg F, Henzi I, Tramèr MR: Treatment of established postoperative nausea and vomiting: A quantitative systematic review. BMC Anesthesiol 2001;1:2.
26 Tramèr MR, Reynolds DJM, Moore RA, McQuay HJ: When placebo-controlled trials are essential and equivalence trials are inadequate. BMJ 1998;317:775–780.
27 Domino KB, Anderson EA, Polissar NL, Posner KL: Comparative efficacy and safety of ondansetron, droperidol and metoclopramide for preventing postoperative nausea and vomiting: A meta-analysis. Anesth Analg 1999;88:1370–1379.
28 Loewen PS, Marra CA, Zed PJ: 5-HT_3 receptor antagonists vs. traditional agents for the prophylaxis of postoperative nausea and vomiting. Can J Anaesth 2000;47:1008–1018.
29 Ellenberg SS, Temple R: Placebo-controlled trials and active-control trials in the evaluation of new treatments. 1. Ethical and scientific issues. Ann Intern Med 2000;133:455–463.
30 Korttila K, Kauste A, Auvinen J: Comparison of domperidone, droperidol and metoclopramide in the prevention and treatment of nausea and vomiting after balanced general anesthesia. Anesth Analg 1979;58:396–400.

Iris Henzi, MD
Division d'Anesthésiologie, Département APSIC
Hôpitaux Universitaires, CH–1211 Genève 14 (Switzerland)
Tel. +41 22 3827415, Fax +41 22 3827511, E-Mail iris.henzi@hcuge.ch

Donnerer J (ed): Antiemetic Therapy.
Basel, Karger, 2003, pp 169–178

Prevention of Delayed Nausea and Emesis Induced by Chemotherapy

Fausto Roila

Medical Oncology Division, Policlinico Hospital, Perugia, Italy

Introduction

Delayed emesis has been arbitrarily defined as emesis that begins or persists more than 24 h after chemotherapy. Until recently, little attention had been addressed to the delayed emesis phenomenon. This is because primarily it is a less severe event than acute emesis; delayed emesis occurs when the patients are at home and away from direct observation of the oncologists; an animal model for the study of this condition was not available until recently [1, 2]. The inevitable consequence of this has been that only a few, and often not well-conducted studies, have been published on this topic.

The pathophysiology of delayed emesis is unknown. Though not proven, various mechanisms have been postulated:

(1) *Disruption of the blood-brain barrier:* Antineoplastic agents, especially cisplatin, can disrupt the blood-brain barrier, determining a mild and reversible cerebral edema. The increased intracranial pressure may potentiate other emetic inputs. This has been demonstrated in the dog after cisplatin administration via the carotid artery [3]. The documented activity of corticosteroids in the treatment of cerebral edema and delayed emesis gives some support to this hypothesis.

(2) *Disruption of gastrointestinal motility and/or permeability:* Chemotherapeutic agents, in particular cisplatin, can cause temporary disturbances of gastrointestinal tract function, such as hypomotility and gastroparesis, that are capable of inducing protracted nausea and vomiting [4, 5].

(3) *Role of endogenous or exogenous adrenal hormones:* It has been shown that urinary cortisol excretion is inversely related and noradrenaline excretion is directly related to the intensity of chemotherapy-induced delayed

nausea [6, 7]. Furthermore, it has been suggested that corticosteroids, used for the prevention of acute emesis, after their abrupt discontinuation, can bring about adrenal failure which may be responsible for the occurrence of delayed emesis [8].

(4) *Accumulation of emetogenic metabolites from chemotherapeutic agents:* It has been postulated that delayed emesis may be the result of an accumulation of metabolites of chemotherapy agents (those of cisplatin have been identified in the body fluid and tissues over 24 h after its administration) or of the hypomagnesemia induced by cisplatin.

It is likely that delayed emesis is a multifactorial phenomenon with the relative contribution of each of the above-mentioned factors or others not yet determined.

Incidence, Pattern and Prognostic Factors of Delayed Emesis

The incidence and characteristics of delayed emesis differ among patients receiving highly (i.e., cisplatin) or moderately (i.e., carboplatin and cyclophosphamide) emetogenic chemotherapy.

Cisplatin induces a biphasic pattern of emesis. Generally, vomiting begins with a short latency period of 2–3 h and peaks around 6–8 h following cisplatin administration. This acute phase lasts about 10–12 h before subsiding. It is followed by a separate phase occurring about 18–24 h after chemotherapy that is the delayed emesis phase. The incidence of delayed emesis after cisplatin chemotherapy varied from 40 to 90% of patients in different studies. The incidence and intensity of symptoms peaked during the 48- to 72-hour period following its administration, then decreased during the subsequent days [9, 10]. In any case, the symptoms experienced during the delayed phase are less severe than during the acute phase.

Differently from cisplatin, the emetic symptoms in patients submitted to moderately emetogenic chemotherapy follow a monophasic pattern. The onset of emesis after carboplatin and cyclophosphamide occurs with a latency period of 6–12 h, longer than that observed with cisplatin. Symptoms are most intense in the first 24 h, but nausea and vomiting can persist over a 24- to 36-hour period [11].

Data on the incidence of delayed emesis in patients treated with moderately emetogenic chemotherapy are scanty. In a large study by the Italian Group for Antiemetic Research, evaluating patients submitted to cyclophosphamide, doxorubicin, epirubicin and carboplatin, on days 2–5 when patients were monitored without receiving any antiemetic prophylaxis, the incidence of moderate-severe nausea and vomiting was approximately 20 and 25%, respectively [12].

Differences in incidence of delayed emesis are commonly observed among studies and can be explained by some patient/treatment characteristics which represent important prognostic factors. Only a few studies have evaluated the prognostic factors conditioning delayed emesis. The most important prognostic factor is obtaining complete protection from nausea and vomiting during the first 24 h [10, 13]. Other important prognostic factors are the administered dose of cisplatin and sex: in fact, delayed emesis is significantly more frequent in patients receiving higher cisplatin doses ($>90\,mg/m^2$) and in females [14].

Prophylaxis of Delayed Emesis

The results of comparative blind studies specifically planned to evaluate different antiemetic treatments in the prevention of delayed emesis will be presented. Studies that have as primary objective the evaluation of different antiemetic drugs in the prevention of acute emesis, and in which the same drugs were continued in the following days, will not be reported. This is because in such studies the superiority of one drug with respect to another in the prophylaxis of delayed emesis could mean either that the drug is superior or that the superiority of a drug is due to better results obtained with this drug in the first 24 h that persist in the following days and, therefore, to a dependence effect. To distinguish these two results, a multifactorial analysis comparing the results obtained in the prevention of delayed emesis balancing those obtained in the prophylaxis of acute emesis should be carried out. Unfortunately, this analysis was not performed in such studies.

In evaluating antiemetic efficacy against delayed emesis, considering the different incidence and characteristics of the phenomenon, it is necessary to plan studies in which patients submitted to cisplatin chemotherapy are clearly separated from those submitted to moderately emetogenic chemotherapy. Instead, two recently published studies enrolled both types of patients [15, 16]. In these studies from day 2 to day 5, all patients received dexamethasone (4 or 10 mg orally) and were randomized to granisetron (1 or 2 mg orally) or metoclopramide (10 or 20 mg three times a day). Complete protection from delayed emesis was similar with both regimens (68 vs. 55% and 81 vs. 84%, respectively, with granisetron and metoclopramide).

Cisplatin

Comparative studies evaluating the efficacy of antiemetics different from 5-HT_3 receptor antagonists in the prevention of delayed emesis are summarized in table 1 [14, 17–20]. In Roila's study [14], orally administered metoclopramide

Table 1. Cisplatin-induced delayed emesis: Comparative studies without 5-HT_3 antagonists

Study	Patients, n	Cisplatin dose mg/m^2	Antiemetics	CP %	Results: vomiting	Results: nausea	Ref.
SB	120	≥50	MTC DEX PL	69.0 65.4 56.7	MTC = DEX = PL	MTC and DEX > PL	14
DB	60	≥60	ACTH PL	67.0 43.0	ACTH > PL	ACTH = PL	17
DB	152	60–120	ACTH 1 mg ACTH 2 mg + 1mg after 72 h PL	62.0 71.4 35.3	ACTH 2 mg ≥ ACTH 1 mg > PL	ACTH 2 mg ≥ ACTH 1 mg > PL	18
DB	91	120	MTC + DEX DEX PL	52.0 35.0 11.0	MTC + DEX > DEX > PL	MTC + DEX and DEX > PL	19
SB	63	60–120	DEX ALZ + DEX MTC + DEX	44.0 30.0 70.0	MTC + DEX > ALZ +DEX and DEX	MTC + DEX = ALZ + DEX = DEX	20

SB = Single-blind; DB = double-blind; PL = placebo; ALZ = alizapride; MTC = metoclopramide; DEX = dexamethasone; CP = complete protection from delayed vomiting.

(20 mg × 4/day) and dexamethasone (1 mg × 4/day) were compared with placebo in 120 patients. Complete protection from nausea, but not from vomiting, was significantly increased by both dexamethasone and metoclopramide with respect to placebo. In Passalacqua's two studies [17, 18], ACTH (1 or 2 mg i.m.) induced significant superior complete protection from vomiting, but not from nausea, with respect to placebo.

From these data it appears clear that the efficacy showed by metoclopramide, dexamethasone or ACTH, when used alone, although superior to placebo in the prevention of delayed nausea or vomiting, is often of limited clinical significance.

In Kris' study [19], a combination of orally administered metoclopramide (0.5 mg/kg × 4/day on days 2–5) plus dexamethasone (8 mg twice/day on days 2 and 3 after cisplatin and 4 mg twice/day on days 4 and 5) was shown more efficacious than dexamethasone alone and placebo in 90 patients submitted to 120 mg/m^2 of cisplatin. Complete protection from delayed vomiting was obtained in 52, 35 and 11% of patients, respectively.

Table 2. Cisplatin-induced delayed emesis: Efficacy of 5-HT_3 antagonists

Study	Patients, n	Cisplatin dose mg/m^2	Antiemetics	CP %	Results: vomiting	Results: nausea	Ref.
DB	48	≥100	OND PL	40.0 33.0	OND ≥ PL	OND = PL	22
DB	538	≥70	OND PL	36.0 26.0	OND ≥ PL	OND ≥ PL	23
DB	434	≥50	DEX + PL DEX + GRAN	35.0 38.0	GRAN + DEX = DEX	GRAN + DEX = DEX	24
DB	619	≥69	DEX + PL DEX + GRAN	58.4 57.2	GRAN + DEX = DEX	GRAN + DEX = DEX	25

DB = Double-blind; CP = complete protection from delayed vomiting; OND = ondansetron; GRAN = granisetron; DEX = dexamethasone; PL = placebo.

These results have been confirmed by Moreno's study [20] which compared metoclopramide plus dexamethasone (at the same doses of Kris' study, but dexamethasone was administered intramuscularly instead of orally) to alizapride plus dexamethasone or dexamethasone alone. In both these studies the superiority of the metoclopramide plus dexamethasone combination with respect to dexamethasone alone was shown regarding complete protection from vomiting, but not nausea.

In any case, this combination should be considered the standard preventive treatment for cisplatin-induced delayed emesis.

Nonetheless, as shown in two large studies in 249 and in 522 patients followed for three consecutive cycles of cisplatin chemotherapy, prevention of delayed vomiting is far from being optimal, as about 40–60% of patients had delayed nausea and/or vomiting despite treatment with metoclopramide plus dexamethasone [13, 21].

The role of the 5-HT_3 receptor antagonists in the prevention of cisplatin-induced delayed emesis has now been clarified. In fact, the results of the published studies evaluating 5-HT_3 receptor antagonists were controversial until recently.

The efficacy of the 5-HT_3 receptor antagonists with respect to placebo is reported in table 2. In Gandara's study [22], ondansetron showed an antiemetic efficacy not significantly different from placebo even if complete protection from vomiting was slightly superior.

In Navari's study [23], carried out in 538 patients, ondansetron 8 mg orally twice reduced significantly the mean number of emetic episodes during

Table 3. Cisplatin-induced delayed emesis: Efficacy of 5-HT_3 antagonists plus dexamethasone

Study	Patients, n	Cisplatin dose mg/m^2	Antiemetics	CP %	Results: vomiting	Results: nausea	Ref.
DB	527	≥50	GRAN + PL GRAN + DEX	58.0 78.9	GRAN + DEX > GRAN	GRAN + DEX > GRAN	26
DB	236	≥50	OND + PL OND + DEX	50.0 63.0	OND + DEX ≥ OND	OND + DEX ≥ OND	27
DB	322	≥50	MTC + DEX OND + DEX	60.0 62.0	MTC + DEX = OND + DEX	MTC + DEX = OND + DEX	28

DB = Double-blind; CP = complete protection from delayed vomiting; OND = ondansetron; GRAN = granisetron; DEX = dexamethasone; MTC = metoclopramide; PL = placebo.

days 2–3 after cisplatin with respect to placebo, but complete protection from delayed vomiting and nausea was only slightly superior to placebo. The analysis of these studies suggests that 5-HT_3 receptor antagonist activity in the prevention of delayed emesis is probably not as good as it is in the prevention of acute emesis and that their efficacy, when used alone, is, at best, only moderate.

Furthermore, in two other studies [24, 25] the addition of a 5-HT_3 antagonist to dexamethasone did not increase complete protection from delayed vomiting and nausea with respect to dexamethasone alone. On the other hand, as shown in table 3, the addition of dexamethasone to a 5-HT_3 antagonist increased the complete protection from delayed nausea and vomiting with respect to a 5-HT_3 antagonist alone [26, 27].

Finally, in a double-blind randomized study, oral ondansetron (8 mg every 12 h on days 2–4) combined with dexamethasone showed antiemetic activity similar to that of standard metoclopramide plus dexamethasone in the prevention of cisplatin-induced delayed emesis, and these two regimens should be considered the antiemetic prophylaxis of choice for delayed emesis [28].

Considering the higher cost, metoclopramide remains the standard treatment, but, according to the results of this study, ondansetron is to be preferred in patients who do not tolerate metoclopramide or who have emesis in the first 24 h.

Moderately Emetogenic Chemotherapy

Only a few double-blind studies have been published on the prevention of delayed emesis due to moderately emetogenic chemotherapy (table 4).

Table 4. Delayed emesis induced by moderately emetogenic chemotherapy: Comparative studies with 5-HT_3 antagonists

Study	Patients, n	Antiemetics	CP %	Results		Ref.
				vomiting	nausea	
DB	189	OND PL	60.0 42.0	OND > PL	OND > PL	29
DB	139	GRAN PL	67.1* 49.3*	GRAN > PL		30
DB	618**	DEX + OND** DEX PL	91.8 87.4 76.8	DEX + OND and DEX > PL	DEX + OND and DEX > PL	33
	87***	DEX + OND*** DEX	40.9 23.3	DEX + OND = DEX	DEX + OND = DEX	

DB = Double-blind; CP = complete protection from delayed vomiting; *no vomiting and no nausea; **patients without and ***with acute vomiting and/or moderate-severe nausea; PL = placebo; GRAN = granisetron; OND = ondansetron; DEX = dexamethasone.

Kaizer's [29] and Guillem's [30] studies, carried out in 189 and 139 patients, showed the superiority of ondansetron and granisetron with respect to placebo (complete protection from vomiting in 60 vs. 42% and in 67.1 vs. 49.3% of patients).

Koo's study [31] in 98 patients showed the better antiemetic activity of dexamethasone with respect to no therapy (complete protection from vomiting in 57 and 33% of patients, respectively), while in Pater's [32] study the addition of a 5-HT_3 antagonist (ondansetron or dolasetron) to dexamethasone did not increase complete protection from delayed emesis with respect to dexamethasone alone. Unfortunately, these were both open studies.

Finally, the Italian Group for Antiemetic Research [33] carried out a double-blind study in which patients, 24 h after chemotherapy, were divided into two groups: patients who did not have either acute vomiting or moderate-to-severe nausea (the low-risk group) and patients who had one or both (the high-risk group). Patients in the low-risk group were then randomly assigned to receive from day 2 to day 5 after chemotherapy: oral placebo, 4 mg of dexamethasone given orally twice daily, or 8 mg of ondansetron in combination with 4 mg of dexamethasone, given orally twice daily. Patients in the high-risk group were randomly assigned to receive oral dexamethasone alone or in combination with ondansetron at the same doses as those used in the low-risk group.

Among the 618 patients in the low-risk group, complete protection from both delayed vomiting and moderate-to-severe nausea was significantly superior in those who received ondansetron plus dexamethasone (91.8%) and those who received dexamethasone (87.4%) than in those who received placebo (76.8%). Significantly more patients receiving ondansetron plus dexamethasone reported constipation.

Therefore, for low-risk group patients dexamethasone alone seems preferable because it is similarly efficacious, better tolerated and less costly with respect to its combination with ondansetron.

In the 87 patients of the high-risk group, complete protection achieved with ondansetron plus dexamethasone (40.9%) was superior, but not statistically significant, with respect to those achieved with dexamethasone alone (23.3%). Therefore, more studies are needed in this subgroup of patients to identify the optimal antiemetic prophylaxis.

Conclusions

In the last 10 years, despite the achievement of important results in the prevention of chemotherapy-induced nausea and vomiting, delayed emesis remains a challenge for antiemetic research, as the results obtained with the most efficacious regimens available are still unsatisfactory, particularly in cisplatin-treated patients.

In the prevention of cisplatin-induced delayed emesis with the two most efficacious treatments (a combination of oral dexamethasone with metoclopramide or ondansetron), about 40–60% of patients continue to have delayed nausea and vomiting.

In the prevention of delayed emesis induced by moderately emetogenic chemotherapy, an antiemetic prophylaxis with dexamethasone should be recommended for all patients even if only one fourth of those having acute vomiting or moderate-severe nausea achieve complete protection from delayed emesis.

In the coming years, better control of delayed emesis may be possible with the development of new and more efficacious antiemetic drugs for delayed emesis. A possible neurotransmitter of delayed emesis has recently been identified: substance P, a neuropeptide found within the central and peripheral nervous system. When substance P is released as a result of emetogenic stimuli, it binds to a specific NK_1 receptor, and mediates nausea and vomiting. In the ferret, selective antagonists of NK_1 receptors have been shown to block chemotherapy-induced emesis. These antagonists are still being evaluated as antiemetics for the prophylaxis of chemotherapy-induced acute and delayed emesis and the results of phase III comparative studies are awaited with interest.

References

1 Milano S, Blower P, Romain D, Grélot L: The piglet as a suitable animal model for studying the delayed phase of cisplatin-induced emesis. J Pharmacol Exp Ther 1995;274:951–961.

2 Rudd JA, Naylor RJ: Effects of 5-HT_3 receptor antagonists on models of acute and delayed emesis induced by cisplatin in the ferret. Neuropharmacology 1994;33:1607–1608.

3 Neuwelt EA, Glasberg M, Frankel E: Neurotoxicity of chemotherapeutic agents after blood-barrier modification: Neuropathological studies. Ann Neurol 1983;14:316–324.

4 Allan SG, Smyth JF: Small intestinal mucosal toxicity of cisplatinum. Comparison of toxicity with platinum analogues and dexamethasone. Br J Cancer 1986;53:355–360.

5 Cunningham D, Morgan RJ, Mills PR: Functional and structural changes of the human proximal small intestine after cytotoxic therapy. J Clin Pathol 1985;38:265–270.

6 Fredrikson M, Hursti T, Furst CJ, Steineck G, Borjesson S, Wikblom M, Peterson C: Nausea in cancer chemotherapy is inversely related to urinary cortisol excretion. Br J Cancer 1992;65: 779–780.

7 Fredrikson M, Hursti TJ, Steineck G, Furst CJ, Borjesson S, Peterson C: Delayed chemotherapy-induced nausea is augmented by high levels of endogenous noradrenaline. Br J Cancer 1994;70: 642–645.

8 Alberola V, Garcia J, Lluch A, Cervantes A, Carbonell F, Pascual A, Gomez J, Garcia-Conde J: Relation between adrenal failure and delayed emesis in patients receiving dexamethasone to prevent gastrointestinal toxicity of high-dose cisplatin. Cancer Chemother Pharmacol 1986; suppl 1: A2.

9 Gralla RJ, Itri LM, Pisko SE, Squillante AE, Kelsen DP, Braun DW, Bordin LA, Braun TJ, Young CW: Antiemetic efficacy of high-dose metoclopramide: Randomized trials with placebo and prochlorperazine in patients with chemotherapy-induced nausea and vomiting. N Engl J Med 1981;305:905–909.

10 Kris MG, Gralla RJ, Clark RA, Tyson LB, O'Connell JP, Wertheim MS, Kelsen DP: Incidence, course and severity of delayed nausea and vomiting following the administration of high-dose cisplatin. J Clin Oncol 1985;3:1379–1384.

11 Martin M: The severity and pattern of emesis following different cytotoxic agents. Oncology 1996;53(suppl 1):26–31.

12 The Italian Group for Antiemetic Research: Delayed emesis induced by moderately emetogenic chemotherapy: Do we need to treat all patients? Ann Oncol 1997;8:561–567.

13 Italian Group for Antiemetic Research: Cisplatin-induced delayed emesis: Pattern and prognostic factors during three subsequent cycles. Ann Oncol 1994;5:585–589.

14 Roila F, Boschetti E, Tonato M, Basurto C, Bracarda S, Picciafuoco M, Patoia L, Santi E, Penza O, Ballatori E, Del Favero A: Predictive factors of delayed emesis in cisplatin-treated patients and efficacy and tolerability of metoclopramide or dexamethasone. Am J Clin Oncol 1991; 14:238–242.

15 Aapro MS, Sessa C, Thurlimann B, De Pree C, Bernhard J, Maibach R: SAKK90/95: A randomized double-blind trial to compare the clinical efficacy of granisetron to metoclopramide both combined to dexamethasone in the prophylaxis of chemotherapy-induced delayed emesis. Proc ASCO 2000;19:600A.

16 Jara C, Hernandez M, Alonso C, Fernandez A, Gomez-Aldaravi JL, Mayordomo JI: Dexamethasone with oral granisetron or metoclopramide in preventing chemotherapy-induced delayed emesis: A randomised, double-blind trial. Proc ASCO 1999;18:592A.

17 Passalacqua R, Cocconi G, Bella M, Monici L, Michiara M, Bandini N, Bacchi M: Double-blind, randomized trial for the control of delayed emesis in patients receiving cisplatin: Comparison of placebo vs. adrenocorticotropic hormone. Ann Oncol 1992;3:481–485.

18 Passalacqua R, Cocconi G, Caminiti C, Silingardi V, Bella MA, Bichisao E, Michiara M, Malavasi V, Donati D, Di Costanzo F, Rocca A, Di Sarra S, Scaglione F, Fraschini F: Double-blind, multicenter, randomized trial to compare the effect of two doses of adrenocorticotropic hormone versus placebo in controlling delayed emesis after high-dose cisplatin in adult patients with cancer. J Clin Oncol 1997;15:2467–2473.

19 Kris MG, Gralla RJ, Tyson LB, Clark RA, Cirrincione C, Groshen S: Controlling delayed emesis: Double-blind, randomized trial comparing placebo, dexamethasone alone, and metoclopramide plus dexamethasone in patients receiving cisplatin. J Clin Oncol 1989;7:108–114.
20 Moreno I, Rosell R, Abad A, Barnadas A, Carles J, Ribelles N, Solano V, Font A: Comparison of three protracted antiemetic regimens for the control of delayed emesis in cisplatin-treated patients. Eur J Cancer 1992;28A:1344–1347.
21 Italian Group for Antiemetic Research: Prevention of cisplatin-induced delayed emesis: Still unsatisfactory. Support Care Cancer 1999;8:229–232.
22 Gandara DR: Progress in the control of acute and delayed emesis induced by cisplatin. Eur J Cancer 1991;27(Suppl 1):9–11.
23 Navari RM, Madajewicz S, Anderson N, Tchekmedyian NS, Whaley W, Garewal H, Beck TM, Chang AY, Greenberg B, Caldwell KC, Huffman DH, Gould JR, Carron G, Ossi M, Anderson EM: Oral ondansetron for the control of cisplatin-induced delayed emesis: A large, multicenter, double-blind, randomized comparative trial of ondansetron versus placebo. J Clin Oncol 1995;13:2408–2416.
24 Latreille J, Pater J, Johnston D, Laberge F, Stewart D, Rusthoven J, Hoskins P, Findlay B, McMurtie E, Yelle L, Williams C, Walde D, Ernst S, Dhaliwal H, Warr D, Shepherd F, Mee D, Nishimura L, Osoba D, Zee B for the National Cancer Institute of Canada Clinical Trials Group: Use of dexamethasone and granisetron in the control of delayed emesis for patients who receive highly emetogenic chemotherapy. J Clin Oncol 1998;16:1174–1178.
25 Goedhals L, Heron JF, Kleisbauer JP, Pagani O, Sessa C: Control of delayed nausea and vomiting with granisetron plus dexamethasone or dexamethasone alone in patients receiving highly emetogenic chemotherapy: A double-blind, placebo-controlled, comparative study. Ann Oncol 1998;9:661–666.
26 The Italian Multicenter Study Group: A double-blind randomized study comparing intramuscular granisetron with intramuscular granisetron plus dexamethasone in the prevention of delayed emesis induced by cisplatin. Anticancer Drugs 1999;10:465–470.
27 Gridelli G, Ianniello GP, Ambrosini G, Mustacchi G, Pedicini T, Farris A, Jacobelli S, Rossi G, Boni C, D'Aprile M, De Lena M, Di Carlo A, Bonsignori M, Silingardi V, Catalano G, Mosconi M, Olivieri A, Bianco AR: Ondansetron versus ondansetron plus dexamethasone in the prophylaxis of delayed emesis over three courses of cisplatin chemotherapy: Results of a double-blind randomized study. Proc ASCO 1996;15:545.
28 The Italian Group for Antiemetic Research: Ondansetron versus metoclopramide, both combined with dexamethasone, in the prevention of cisplatin-induced delayed emesis. J Clin Oncol 1997; 15:124–130.
29 Kaizer L, Warr D, Hoskins P, Latreille J, Lofters W, Yau J, Palmer M, Zee B, Levy M, Pater J: Effect of schedule and maintenance on the antiemetic efficacy of ondansetron combined with dexamethasone in acute and delayed nausea and emesis in patients receiving moderately emetogenic chemotherapy: A phase III trial of the National Cancer Institute of Canada Clinical Trials Group. J Clin Oncol 1994;12:1050–1057.
30 Guillem V, Carrato A, Rifà J, Lopez-Lopez R, Barneto I, Gomez-Bernal A, Soriano V, Luque A, Aranda E: High efficacy of oral granisetron in the total control of cyclophosphamide-induced prolonged emesis. Proc ASCO 1998;17:46A.
31 Koo WH, Ang PT: Role of maintenance oral dexamethasone in prophylaxis of delayed emesis caused by moderately emetogenic chemotherapy. Ann Oncol 1996;7:71–74.
32 Pater JL, Lofters WS, Zee B, Dempsey E, Walde D, Moquin J-P, Wilson K, Hoskins P, Guevin RM, Verma S, Navari R, Krook JE, Hainsworth J, Palmer M, Chin C: The role of the 5-HT_3 antagonists ondansetron and dolasetron in the control of delayed onset nausea and vomiting in patients receiving moderately emetogenic chemotherapy. Ann Oncol 1997;8:181–185.
33 The Italian Group for Antiemetic Research: Dexamethasone alone or in combination with ondansetron for the prevention of delayed nausea and vomiting induced by chemotherapy. N Engl J Med 2000;342:1554–1559.

Fausto Roila, MD, Medical Oncology Division
Policlinico Hospital, Via Brunamonti, I–06122 Perugia (Italy)
Tel. +39 75 5783968, Fax +39 75 5720990, E-Mail roila.fausto@libero.it

Donnerer J (ed): Antiemetic Therapy.
Basel, Karger, 2003, pp 179–191

Prophylaxis of Radiation-Induced Emesis

Ernesto Maranzano

Radiation Oncology Center, Policlinico Hospital, Terni, Italy

Introduction

Nausea and vomiting are distressing side effects overall when they last days or weeks. Radiation-induced emesis (RIE) is often considered to be less frequent and less severe than nausea/vomiting encountered in patients receiving chemotherapy. However, this issue has only been addressed in a few studies. It is possible that sometimes in clinical practice radiation oncologists underestimate the problem and do not ask their patients about nausea and vomiting [1]. There are at least two important reasons for paying attention to RIE: (1) a radiotherapy course may last 4–7 weeks and, if untreated, sickness produces adverse effects, such as dehydration, electrolyte imbalance and/or malnutrition, which are liable for a worsening of the patient's quality of life, and (2) nausea and/or vomiting may cause an interruption in the treatment with possible unfavorable effects on tumor control when radiotherapy is delivered with curative intent [2, 3].

Acute emesis is seen more frequently with radiotherapy. The latent period ranges from 0.5 to 4 h and is shorter when higher radiotherapy doses are administered. Prolonged emesis lasting 2–3 days is reported by up to 40% of patients. Anticipatory emesis induced by radiotherapy is extremely rare. Generally, the highest incidence of RIE is registered in the trials in which total body irradiation (TBI), upper half-body irradiation (HBI), upper or whole abdomen irradiation and radiosurgery to the area postrema were administered. Instead, the emetogenic potential of radiotherapy is considered moderate in radiotherapy of the thorax, pelvis and lower HBI, and low in radiotherapy of head and neck, extremities, brain and skin [4].

The purpose of this paper is to discuss the pathophysiology of RIE, the risk factors of RIE, the strategies to reduce RIE and the guidelines suggested by

MASCC (Multinational Association of Supportive Care in Cancer) and ASCO (American Society of Clinical Oncology) for the antiemetic prescription.

Pathophysiology of RIE

The exact mechanism of RIE remains unclear. Possible mechanisms are: (1) activation of the chemoreceptor trigger zone (CTZ) either directly or indirectly; (2) peripheral stimulation of the gastrointestinal (GI) mucosa and GI neurotransmitter receptors that activate the vomiting center; (3) vestibular mechanisms; (4) cortical mechanisms (i.e., direct cerebral activation due to radiotherapy to the brain or radiosurgery, or psychogenic activation), and (5) alterations of taste and smell [5]. It was suggested that the critical organs responsible for RIE were in the upper abdomen and the underlying mechanism might be related to a toxin released by degradation of tumor protein [6–8]. Hypothetically there can be two different pathophysiological mechanisms working together in the RIE: (1) passive cell damage mechanism in terms of release of transmitters that induce emesis, and (2) active functional defense mechanism through release of mediators by functioning cells [9].

Some of the neurotransmitters located in the area postrema of the brain or in visceral tissues that may be excited and lead to emesis include dopamine, histamine, substance P, norepinephrine, neurotensin, prostaglandins, gastrin and serotonin. When released, these substances stimulate afferent visceral fibers, an action that then initiates sensory signals to the CTZ [5]. The enterochromaffin cells of the mucosa have a high serotonin (5-hydroxytryptamine, 5-HT_3) content. Damage of the enterochromaffin cells of the GI tract by toxins and/or irradiation leads to release of serotonin, which may initiate the emetogenic response. It has been suggested that serotonin may mediate emesis via mechanisms involving the 5-HT_3 receptors, vagus and greater splanchnic nerve, and the CTZ [9]. The correlation of RIE and increased levels of 5-hydroxyindoleacetic acid, a metabolite of serotonin, after TBI, HBI and upper abdominal irradiation, strongly suggests that the mechanism of RIE is related to the release of serotonin. This mechanism is probably involved when radiotherapy is applied to the abdomen, whereas radiosurgery of the area postrema or brain irradiation most likely induces vomiting/nausea from a direct injury to the CTZ [5].

Factors Influencing RIE and Observational Trials

The frequency, severity and onset of RIE can be patient-related and therapy-related [9]. Age, gender, tolerance of previous therapy, anxiety and alcohol intake are risk factors for emesis. The risk of RIE is high in female patients, those younger than 50 years, patients who have a previous history of poorly controlled emesis and/or who are anxious, whereas it is low in those with high alcohol consumption [2, 9]. Among therapy-related factors, the site of radiotherapy is important and the incidence of RIE is high when the radiation field encompasses the upper abdomen. Emesis occurs more frequently when patients receive treatment to larger fields (e.g., TBI or HBI) and in doses higher than 5 Gy [9]. Other factors influencing RIE are reported (total dose, dose rate, fractionation, patient positioning, radiation technique, energy, beam quality, general health status of the patient) but seem to be less important than those already discussed [9]. Worthy of note is to consider that the data regarding incidence of RIE and factors influencing it come from small randomized clinical trials evaluating the efficacy of various antiemetic drugs in preventing RIE, and therefore cannot be considered as representative of the general population undergoing radiotherapy for cancer [1].

The incidence of RIE has been evaluated in only two observational trials [1, 10]. Feyer et al. [10] coordinated the first one which was carried out in patients submitted to fractionated radiotherapy 'between thorax and pelvis'. Only 15% of patients received antiemetic prophylaxis. The incidence of nausea and vomiting, recorded in 297 of 1,387 patients who entered the study, was 38 and 36%, respectively. These values refer to 269 of 297 evaluable patients who did not receive an antiemetic prophylaxis. Of the remaining 28 cases treated with an antiemetic prophylaxis, 61% experienced nausea and 57% vomiting. This high incidence of emesis in the group treated with antiemetics can be explained by a higher individual risk profile (most frequent abdominal irradiation, larger irradiated volume) of these patients [10]. Considering that this report is available only as an abstract, it is impossible to understand the actual significance of these results.

The other observational trial on incidence of RIE was carried out by the Italian Group for Antiemetic Research in Radiotherapy (IGARR) which analyzed 934 consecutive patients submitted to all types of radiotherapy (all irradiated sites, fractionation schedules, dose per fraction, field size) [1]. The IGARR study evidenced that the overall cumulative incidence of vomiting and nausea occurred in about 40% of patients undergoing radiotherapy. The median start time of vomiting and/or moderate-severe nausea was 8 days (range 1–47), and the median duration was 3 days for vomiting and 4 days for nausea. Among patients who had vomiting, the median number of emetic episodes per patient and per day was 8 (range 1–246) and 3 (range 1–60), respectively. The incidence of RIE was analyzed according to patient and radiotherapy-related characteristics to identify the more important risk factors. At multivariate analysis, the irradiated site and radiation field size (>400 cm^2) were the significant radiotherapy-related risk factors, whereas previous chemotherapy was the only patient-related factor. Many characteristics, such as gender, kinetosis, alcohol intake, setting, dose per fraction and fractionation schedule, were also examined, but they did not influence RIE. Considering the irradiated site, not only the patients submitted to abdominal radiotherapy were at major risk of vomiting and nausea (71%), but also those receiving treatment to the thorax, brain, head and neck, and pelvis (49, 40, 40, and 39%, respectively). Unfortunately, RIE was not evaluable either in patients submitted to TBI or HBI due to the small number of patients who received these therapies. According to the results of this trial, it is possible to divide the emetogenic potential of radiotherapy on the basis of irradiated site, field size and previous chemotherapy. However, the irradiated site remains the most important prognostic factor used in clinical practice for defining the risk profile of patients. The IGARR study evidenced this relationship between irradiated site and emetogenic risk: (a) upper abdomen irradiation is the 'most emetogenic' regimen (probably together with TBI and HBI), (b) the emetogenic potential is 'moderate' in thorax, pelvis, brain, and head and neck radiotherapy, and (c) 'low' in radiotherapy of extremities and skin [1]. This epidemiological trial on RIE monitored also the prescription of antiemetics in clinical practice and evidenced the attitude of radiotherapists in prescribing antiemetic drugs only in a few (14%) patients, mostly as a rescue, and that 5-HT_3 antagonists, rather than other antiemetics, are generally used [1].

Strategies to Reduce RIE

The primary prevention of RIE is suggested by Feyer et al. [9] using 3-D treatment planning, multileaf collimators and dose-volume histograms to reduce the volume of normal tissues encompassed in the irradiated fields. Although we can expect a lower incidence of nausea/vomiting if innovative radiotherapy techniques are used, it should be confirmed by clinical controlled trials.

The secondary prevention implies the assessment of emetogenic risk and the prescription of antiemetic therapy either as prophylaxis or as rescue. Randomized clinical trials on antiemetics in radiotherapy are briefly reported.

Three randomized reports on RIE in patients treated with fractionated radiotherapy to the abdomen and thorax were published before the introduction of 5-HT_3 antagonists. In the first study, 39 patients were randomized to receive oral metoclopramide or nabilone. In the second, 89 patients were treated with oral metoclopramide, prochlorperazine or placebo, and in the third, 11 patients received tetrahydrocannabinol or prochlorperazine [11–13].

Table 1. Randomized clinical trials with 5-HT_3 antagonists in patients submitted to upper abdomen irradiation

Group (first author)	Patients, n	Radiotherapy regimen	Antiemetic randomization	Percent of complete response	Results
Priestman, 1990 [18]	121	8–10 Gy single fraction	OND 8 mg × 3/day p.o. for 5 days MTC 10 mg × 3/day p.o. for 5 days	68 39	OND better than MTC
Bey, 1996 [16]	50	At least 6 Gy single fraction	DOL 0.3 mg/kg i.v. DOL 0.6 mg/kg i.v. DOL 1.2 mg/kg i.v. Placebo	100* 93* 83* 54*	DOL better than placebo
Priestman, 1993 [19]	135	1.8 Gy/day for at least 5 fractions	OND 8 mg × 3/day p.o. PCP 10 mg × 3/day p.o.	61 35	OND better than PCP (for vomiting)
Franzen, 1996 [17]	111	At least 1.7 Gy/day for ≥10 fractions	OND 8 mg × 2/day p.o. Placebo	67 45	OND better than placebo
Aass, 1997 [15]	23	2 Gy/day to 30 Gy in 15 fractions	TRO 5 mg/day p.o. MTC 10 mg × 3/day p.o.	91 50	TRO better than MTC
Lanciano, 2001 [20]	260	10–30 fractions (1.8–3 Gy/fraction)	GRAN 2 mg/day Placebo	57.5 42	GRAN better than placebo

*Complete plus major response. OND = Ondansetron; MTC = metoclopramide; DOL = dolasetron; TRO = tropisetron; GRAN = granisetron; PCP = prochlorperazine; administered p.o. (orally) or i.v. (intravenously).

Only one randomized study has been carried out with 43 patients submitted to single-fraction palliative radiotherapy to the thoracic and/or lumbar spine. In this study, chlorpromazine was compared with two different doses of levonantrol [14]. All these studies enrolled a small number of patients (median 46) and showed no difference among the various compounds determining a limited antiemetic efficacy (complete protection of vomiting in about 50% of cases).

In the last decade, the 5-HT_3 antagonists have been used in clinical practice to treat RIE. Tables 1 and 2 show randomized trials with 5-HT_3 antagonist in patients submitted to radiotherapy with single or fractionated regimens.

Table 2. Randomized clinical trials with 5-HT_3 antagonists in patients submitted to TBI and HBI

Group (first author)	Patients, n	Radiotherapy regimen	Antiemetic randomization	Percent of complete response	Results
Tiley, 1992 [24]	20	10.5 Gy TBI-single fraction	OND 8 mg i.v. Placebo	90* 50*	OND better than placebo
Prentice, 1995 [21]	30	7.5 Gy TBI-single fraction	GRAN 3 mg i.v. versus MTC 20 mg i.v. + DEX 6 mg/m^2 i.v. + LOR 2 mg i.v.	53 13	GRAN better than MTC + DEX + LOR
Spitzer, 1994 [22]	20	1.2 Gy × 3/day TBI-11 fractions to a total dose of 13.2 Gy	OND 8 mg × 3/day p.o. Placebo	50 0	OND better than placebo
Sykes, 1997 [23]	66	8–12.5 Gy HBI-single fraction	OND 8 mg × 2 p.o. versus CLP 25 mg × 3 p.o. + DEX 6 mg × 3 p.o.	94 34	OND better than CLP + DEX
Spitzer, 2000 [25]	34	1.2 Gy × 3/day TBI-11 fractions to a total dose of 13.2 Gy	OND 8 mg × 3/day p.o. versus GRAN 2 mg × 1/day p.o.	47 61	No difference

*All patients received intravenous dexamethasone (8 mg) and phenobarbitone (60 mg/m^2). OND = Ondansetron; GRAN = granisetron; MTC = metoclopramide; LOR = lorazepam; CLP = chlorpromazine; DEX = dexamethasone; administered (p.o.) orally or (i.v.) intravenously.

Different compounds and a wide range of doses and schedules have been used. Antiemetics were generally started 1–2 h before radiotherapy and usually continued until the end of irradiation when a fractionated regimen of dose was adopted. The oral route was prevalent (73%). The six published trials regarding patients submitted to upper abdomen irradiation showed that 5-HT_3 antagonists achieved significantly greater protection from RIE than metoclopramide, phenotiazines or placebo (table 1) [15–20]. Also, in patients treated with TBI or HBI, 5-HT_3 antagonists gave a significantly greater protection from RIE than placebo or conventional antiemetics (table 2) [21–25].

Only in one randomized trial on antiemetic prophylaxis in fractionated TBI did the protection from emesis achieved using ondansetron last for the entire treatment period (4 days) [22]. But the other randomized trials on antiemetic prophylaxis in patients undergoing fractionated TBI or radiotherapy to the upper abdomen showed that 5-HT_3 antagonist is less effective as treatment continues. Priestman et al. [18] reported that ondansetron becomes less effective after the first week, and Franzen et al. [17] after the third week of radiotherapy. It has also been shown in chemotherapy studies that the efficacy of 5-HT_3 antagonists diminishes with repeated courses. Headache and/or constipation were the most common adverse events registered with the use of 5-HT_3 antagonists. Sometimes rather than constipation, 5-HT_3 antagonists reduced the frequency of diarrhea, a troublesome side effect due to acute radiation enteric toxicity [9, 17, 26, 27].

In chemotherapy-induced emesis, corticosteroids (above all dexamethasone) are also suggested as single agents for the prevention of delayed emesis, or in combination with a 5-HT_3 antagonist for patients receiving highly emetogenic chemotherapy [28, 29]. Their widespread availability, low cost, and benefit make corticosteroids very interesting antiemetic drugs. To date in radiotherapy no prospective randomized studies have been published evaluating the addition of corticosteroid to the 5-HT_3 antagonist in comparison to the 5-HT_3 antagonist alone. Regarding the use of dexamethasone as a single agent for the prophylaxis of RIE, a double-blind study has recently been published [30]. Patients enrolled received fractionated radiotherapy to the upper abdomen and oral dexamethasone (2 mg × 3/day) or placebo only in the first week of radiotherapy even though the courses lasted up to 6 weeks. Complete protection from RIE was significantly better in the dexamethasone group with acceptable side effects, but with no overall positive effect on global quality of life. Considering that the majority of emetic episodes occurred early in the treatment, it is possible that prophylactic antiemetics may not be necessary for a full course of radiotherapy but only for the first week [30]. More studies evaluating the efficacy of steroids, compared to 5-HT_3 antagonists, or in combination may answer these questions.

The role of antiemetics given on an as-needed basis has not been investigated in randomized trials. Two open pilot studies have evaluated the use of a rescue treatment using a 5-HT_3 antagonist in patients failing to achieve relief with common antiemetics [31, 32]. In the first study, 4 patients who had RIE after prophylaxis with prochlorperazine and metoclopramide received rescue treatment with ondansetron. All patients achieved complete protection from vomiting [31]. In the second study, 34 patients experiencing RIE during fractionated radiotherapy to the abdomen were treated with tropisetron which controlled vomiting in 73% of cases [32]. The potential role of 5-HT_3 antagonists as rescue medication has been suggested in these reports.

Table 3. MASCC and ASCO risk levels according to irradiated site and suggested antiemetic drug prescription

Risk level	MASCC	ASCO	Antiemetic drug prescription
High	Total body irradiation Upper half body irradiation Abdominal bath Total nodal irradiation	Total body irradiation	MASCC and ASCO: prophylaxis with $5\text{-}HT_3$ antagonists ± dexamethasone
Moderate	Upper abdomen Lower thorax region Pelvis Lower half body irradiation	Hemibody irradiation Upper abdomen Abdominal-pelvic Mantle Cranium (radiosurgery) Craniospinal	MASCC: prophylaxis or rescue with $5\text{-}HT_3$ antagonists ± dexamethasone ASCO: prophylaxis with dopamine receptor antagonists or $5\text{-}HT_3$ antagonists
Low	Head and neck Extremities Cranium	Cranium Breast Head and neck Extremities Pelvis Thorax	MASCC and ASCO: rescue with dopamine receptor antagonists or $5\text{-}HT_3$ antagonists

MASCC = Multinational Association of Supportive Care in Cancer; ASCO = American Society of Clinical Oncology.

Consensus Conference Guidelines

Two Consensus Conferences on Antiemetic Therapy were recently organized, the first in Europe under the auspices of MASCC, the other one in the USA held by an ASCO expert panel [28, 33, 34]. Although many ASCO experts were involved in defining the MASCC guidelines, some differences exist between the two guidelines, both in the definition of radiation emetic risk categories and in the antiemetic prophylaxis suggested. These controversies are due to a lack of systematic evaluation of RIE by an adequate number of prospective randomized trials. In table 3 the different classification of emetic potential of radiotherapy according to irradiated site as well the suggested antiemetic drug prescription in the MASCC and ASCO guidelines are shown. The following differences in the emesis risk groups are the most important: (1) the ASCO guidelines classified only TBI at high risk, whereas MASCC ones added to this group abdominal bath, HBI and total nodal irradiation, and (2) moderate risk categories were quite different, too: thorax and pelvis were classified as at low risk by ASCO and at moderate risk by MASCC guidelines.

In table 3, MASCC and ASCO antiemetic prophylaxis are also reported according to emetogenic potential of radiotherapy. Two therapeutic attitudes are suggested: prophylaxis, giving the antiemetic drug(s) before each radiotherapy fraction, or rescue, on an as-needed basis therapy beginning as soon as symptoms (usually nausea) develop. If for high and low risk levels the antiemetics suggested by the two guidelines are similar, for patients at moderate risk level there are clear differences because MASCC suggests prophylaxis or rescue treatment with 5-HT_3 antagonists eventually associated with dexamethasone, whereas ASCO suggests only prophylaxis with dopamine receptor antagonists or 5-HT_3 antagonists without dexamethasone. Several double-blind studies comparing a 5-HT_3 antagonist with a placebo or a dopamine antagonist for the prevention of emesis induced by fractionated irradiation of the upper abdomen have been published. These studies have found that the 5-HT_3 antagonist is better [15–20]. It is strange that in this case the ASCO guidelines suggest using either a 5-HT_3 antagonist or a dopamine antagonist, implying that the two drug classes have the same efficacy. Furthermore, the ASCO guidelines suggest the use of antiemetics on an as-needed basis for head and neck, thorax and pelvis irradiation, classified as low risk level sites, after the demonstration by IGARR observational trial that the incidence of RIE in this case is over to 40%.

In my opinion, considering that MASCC rather than ASCO risk group classifications are more similar to those of the IGARR observational trial, MASCC guidelines could be considered as a starting point for the prescription of antiemetics in clinical practice. The results of other prospective clinical trials, aimed at identifying which patients submitted to radiotherapy require antiemetic prophylaxis or rescue and what the optimal treatment is, are necessary.

Discussion

The IGARR observational trial evidenced that in clinical practice only a minority of patients undergoing radiotherapy received antiemetic treatment, and that rescue treatment was more often used than prophylaxis. This pattern of utilization of antiemetics might have been due to an underevaluation of the clinical relevance of RIE or a 'wait-and-see' attitude which seems to be preferred by radiation oncologists [1]. The introduction of the 5-HT_3 receptor antagonists induced a significant improvement in the control of RIE. The 5-HT_3 receptor antagonists offer better antiemetic prophylaxis than placebo [16, 17, 20, 22, 24] or older antiemetic drugs [15, 18, 19, 21, 23, 25] in patients undergoing radiotherapy with moderate to high emetogenic potential. In all these patient categories, 5-HT_3 antagonists should be considered the antiemetic treatment of choice [2, 3, 5]. However, the recent published guidelines for the use of antiemetics, differ somewhat both in classifying radiation emetogenic risk categories, and regarding the indications for the use of antiemetic drugs [28, 33]. Starting from the most important questions to be solved on RIE, some suggestions are given for clinical practice and for planning future trials:

(1) *Which categories of patients must be considered at greater risk of developing RIE?* Considering that MASCC rather than ASCO group categories are similar to classification of the IGARR observational trial, in my opinion, MASCC guidelines should be considered for the prescription of antiemetics in clinical practice. Although IGARR trial evidenced a high incidence of RIE after upper abdomen irradiation and a moderate incidence after cranium, head and neck, thorax and pelvis irradiation, the future trials on RIE should concern patients submitted to abdomen, pelvis and thorax radiotherapy considering their prevalence in radiation oncology clinical practice.

(2) *Which antiemetics are most effective in the treatment of these patients, which is the optimal dose, and how long must antiemetics be given?* When patients are submitted to high-moderate emetogenic radiotherapy, the 5-HT_3 antagonists should be the drugs of choice given prophylactically 1–2 h before each radiotherapy fraction, at standard dose, and for the whole treatment course.

(3) *The addition of dexamethasone increases the efficacy of 5-HT_3 antagonists?* Although in radiotherapy no prospective randomized studies have been published evaluating the addition of corticosteroid to the 5-HT_3 antagonist in comparison to the 5-HT_3 antagonist alone, in clinical practice, as in the treatment of highly emetogenic chemotherapy, dexamethasone should be added to the 5-HT_3 antagonist for categories of patients at high risk of RIE (i.e., TBI, HBI, and abdominal irradiation). However, other trials should be planned to examine if the addition of dexamethasone to the 5-HT_3 antagonist can give better results in high-moderate risk profile patient categories.

(4) *When is prophylaxis better and when is rescue antiemetic therapy better?* The use of a rescue antiemetic treatment is interesting if we weigh up the better cost-effectiveness ratio with respect to prophylaxis. Certainly rescue therapy must begin as soon as symptoms (usually nausea) develop. Patients submitted to radiotherapy of low emetogenic risk (e.g., breast and extremities) do not require any antiemetic prophylaxis; however, if vomiting or nausea are registered during the radiotherapy course, rescue antiemetic medication (serotonin or

dopamine receptor antagonists) should be administered. The effectiveness of the rescue in patients at high-moderate risk of developing emesis is under discussion and no randomized study regarding this problem was published. The IGARR is presently carrying out a double-blind randomized clinical trial comparing prophylactic ondansetron (8 mg orally twice a day for the entire radiotherapy course) plus dexamethasone (2 mg orally three times a day for the first 5 days) versus the same schedule of ondansetron and dexamethasone given as a rescue treatment in patients undergoing fractionated radiotherapy to the upper abdomen. The main goal of this ongoing trial is to verify if an as-needed based antiemetic therapy can be as effective as the prophylaxis for patients irradiated to the abdomen [30].

Many questions on RIE remain unanswered, and other prospective controlled trials are needed for their solution.

References

1 The Italian Group for Antiemetic Research in Radiotherapy: Radiation-induced emesis: A prospective observational multicenter Italian trial. Int J Radiat Oncol Biol Phys 1999;44:619–625.

2 Roila F, Ciccarese G, Palladino MA, De Angelis V: Prevention of radiotherapy-induced emesis. Tumori 1998;84:274–278.

3 Maranzano E: Radiation-induced emesis: A problem with many open questions. Tumori 2001;87: 213–218.

4 Stewart A: Antiemetics in radiotherapy. Extended abstract book of Consensus Conference on Antiemetic Therapy, Perugia, April 28–29, 1997, pp 98–104.

5 Berger AM, Clark-Snow RA: Adverse effects on treatment: Nausea and vomiting; in De Vita VT Jr, Hellman S, Rosenberg SA (eds): Cancer Principles and Practice of Oncology, ed 6. Philadelphia, Lippincott Williams & Wilkins, 2001, pp 2869–2880.

6 Court-Brown WM: Symptomatic disturbance after single therapeutic dose of x-rays. Br J Med 1953;i:802–805.

7 Danjoux E, Rider WD, Fitzpatrick PJ: The acute radiation syndrome. Clin Radiol 1979;30: 581–584.

8 Scarantino WC, Ornitz RD, Hoffman LG, Anderson RF: Radiation-induced emesis: Effects of ondansetron. Semin Oncol 1992;6:38–43.

9 Feyer CP, Stewart AL, Titlbach OJ: Aetiology and prevention of emesis induced by radiotherapy. Support Care Cancer 1998;6:253–260.

10 Feyer CP, Titlbach OJ, Wilkinson J, Budach V: Gastrointestinal reactions in radiotherapy. Support Care Cancer 1996;4:249.

11 Priestman SG, Priestman TJ, Canney PA: A double-blind randomised cross-over comparison of nabilone and metoclopramide in the control of radiation-induced nausea. Clin Radiol 1987;38: 543–544.

12 Sokol GH, Greenberg HM, McCarthy S, Sledjessky L, Lyman G: Radiation-induced nausea: The comparative efficacy of oral metoclopramide versus prochlorperazine and placebo. A double-blind randomized study. Proc ASCO 1986;5:249.

13 Ungerleider JT, Andrysiak TA, Fairbanks LA, Tesler AS, Parker RG: Tetrahydrocannabinol vs. prochlorperazine. The effects of two antiemetics on patients undergoing radiotherapy. Radiology 1984;150:598–599.

14 Lucraft HH, Palmer MK: Randomized clinical trial of levonantrodol and chlorpromazine in prevention of radiotherapy-induced vomiting. Clin Radiol 1982;33:621–622.

15 Aass N, Hatun DE, Thoresen M, Fossa SD: Prophylactic use of tropisetron or metoclopramide during adjuvant abdominal radiotherapy of seminoma stage I: A randomised, open trial in 23 patients. Radiother Oncol 1997;45:125–128.
16 Bey P, Wilkinson PM, Resbeut M, Bourdin S, Le Floch O, Hahne W, Claverie N: A double-blind, placebo-controlled trial of intravenous dolasetron mesilate in the prevention of radiotherapy-induced nausea and vomiting in cancer patients. Support Care Cancer 1996;4:278–383.
17 Franzen L, Nyman J, Hagberg H, Jacobsson M, Sorbe B, Nyth AL, Lomberg H, Henriksson R: A randomised placebo controlled study with ondansetron in patients undergoing fractionated radiotherapy. Ann Oncol 1996;7:587–592.
18 Priestman TJ, Roberts JT, Lucraft H, Collis CH, Adams M: Results of a randomized, double-blind comparative study of ondansetron and metoclopramide in the prevention of nausea and vomiting following high-dose upper abdominal irradiation. Clin Oncol 1990;2:71–75.
19 Priestman TJ, Roberts JT, Upadhyaya BK: A prospective randomized double-blind trial comparing ondansetron versus prochlorperazine for the prevention of nausea and vomiting in patients undergoing fractionated radiotherapy. Clin Oncol 1993;5:358–363.
20 Lanciano R, Sherman DM, Michalski J, Preston AJ, Yocom K, Friedman C: The efficacy and safety of once-daily kytril (granisetron hydrolchloride) tablets in the prophylaxis of nausea and emesis following fractionated upper abdominal radiotherapy. Cancer Invest 2001;19:763–772.
21 Prentice HG, Cunningham S, Gandhi L, Cunningham J, Collis C, Hamon MD: Granisetron in the prevention of irradiation-induced emesis. Bone Marrow Transplant 1995;15:445–448.
22 Spitzer TR, Bryson JC, Cirenza E, Foelber R, Wallerstadt M, Stout C, Kunka RL, Plagge PB, Dubois A: Randomized double-blind, placebo-controlled evaluation of oral ondansetron in the prevention of nausea and vomiting associated with fractionated total-body irradiation. J Clin Oncol 1994;12:2432–2438.
23 Sykes AJ, Kiltie AE, Stewart AL: Ondansetron versus chlorpromazine and dexamethasone combination for the prevention of nausea and vomiting: A prospective, randomised study to assess efficacy, cost effectiveness and quality of life following single-fraction radiotherapy. Support Care Cancer 1997;5:500–503.
24 Tiley C, Powles R, Catalano J, Treleaven J, Eshelby J, Hewetson M, Tait D, Cunningham D: Results of a double-blind, placebo-controlled study of ondansetron as an antiemetic during total body irradiation in patients undergoing bone marrow transplantation. Leuk Lymphoma 1992;7: 317–321.
25 Spitzer TR, Friedman CJ, Bushnell W, Frankel SR, Raschko J: Double-blind, randomized, parallel-group study on the efficacy and safety of oral granisetron and oral ondansetron in the prophylaxis of nausea and vomiting in patients receiving hyperfractionated total body irradiation. Bone Marrow Transplant 2000;26:203–210.
26 Henriksson R, Lomberg H, Istraelsson G, Zackrisson B, Franzen L: The effect of ondansetron on radiation-induced emesis and diarrhoea. Acta Oncol 1992;31:767–769.
27 Maranzano E, Roila F, De Angelis V, Del Duca M, Di Russo A, Fillini C, Mignogna M, Timurian D, Lupattelli M, Latini P, for the Italian Group for Antiemetic Research in Radiotherapy: Vomiting/nausea and diarrhea in radiotherapy: A prospective observational Italian trial. Radiother Oncol 1998;48(suppl 1):181.
28 Gralla R, Osaba D, Kris MG, Kirkbride P, Hesketh PJ, Chinnery LW, Clark-Snow R, Gill DP, Groshen S, Grunberg S, Koeller JM, Morrow GR, Perez EA, Silber JH, Pfister DG, for the American Society of Clinical Oncology: Recommendations for the use of the antiemetics: Evidence-based, clinical practice guidelines. J Clin Oncol 1999;9:2971–2994.
29 The Italian Group for Antiemetic Research: Ondansetron + dexamethasone versus metoclopramide + dexamethasone + diphenhydramine in prevention of cisplatin-induced emesis. Lancet 1992;34:96–99.
30 Kirkbridge P, Bezjak A, Pater J, Zee B, Palmer MJ, Wong R, Cross P, Gulavita S, Blood P, Sun A, Dundas G, Ganguly PK, Lim J, Chowdhury AD, Kumar SE, Dar AR: Dexamethasone for the prophylaxis of radiation-induced emesis: A National Cancer Institute of Canada Clinical Trials Group phase III study. J Clin Oncol 2000;18:1960–1966.
31 Roberts JT: Ondansetron in control of refractory emesis following radiotherapy. Clin Oncol 1992; 4:67–68.

32 Miralbell R, Coucke P, Behroutz F, Blazek N, Melliger M, Philipp S, Wickenhauser R, Gebhard S, Schwabb T, Rosset A, Hagen G, Douglass P, Bieri S, Allal A, Majno S, Bardina A: Nausea and vomiting in fractionated radiotherapy: A prospective on-demand trial of tropisetron rescue for non-responders to metoclopramide. Eur J Cancer 1995;31A:1461–1464.
33 Antiemetic Subcommittee of the Multinational Association of Supportive Care in Cancer (MASCC): Prevention of chemotherapy- and radiotherapy-induced emesis: Results of the Perugia Consensus Conference. Ann Oncol 1998;9:811–819.
34 Maranzano E, Bellavita R: La terapia dell'emesi in radioterapia oncologica. Tumori 2000;86 (suppl 2):43–44.

Ernesto Maranzano, MD
U.O. di Radioterapia Oncologica
Azienda Ospedaliera 'S. Maria'
I–05100 Terni (Italy)
Tel. +39 744 205697, Fax +39 744 205034, E-Mail ernesto.maranzano@libero.it

Donnerer J (ed): Antiemetic Therapy.
Basel, Karger, 2003, pp 192–203

Pharmacotherapy for Nausea and Vomiting in Early Pregnancy

N. Kemal Kuşcu

Celal Bayar University, School of Medicine, Department of Obstetrics and Gynecology, Manisa, Turkey

Introduction

Hyperemesis gravidarum (HG) may be defined as an advanced stage of nausea and vomiting seen commonly in the first trimester of pregnancy. The symptoms may be so serious that the patient may need hospitalization. While 75% of women complain of nausea and vomiting until the 14th week of pregnancy, fortunately the incidence of hyperemesis is only about 1–20 per 1,000 pregnant women. Several risk factors include female sex of the offspring, gravidity number, high daily intake of primarily saturated fat prior to pregnancy, gestational trophoblastic disease and multiple pregnancy [1–3]. Some of these factors point to a high level of steroids such as estradiol and human chorionic gonadotropin. Recurrence and multiple admissions to hospital may be encountered in some cases. Weight loss and abnormal electrolyte levels are the most common problems, and besides these metabolic and endocrine derangements, severe neurological, gastrointestinal and hepatic complications may occur. This chapter will primarily focus on pharmacological treatment of patients with HG.

General Outlines for Initial Management

The patients diagnosed as having HG require hospitalization and are usually exhausted due to fatigue caused by persistent nausea and vomiting. If she is not in negative balance, she may be followed on an outpatient basis and simple measures such as frequent but small feedings, choosing the most favorite food and avoiding foul smells may suffice. Psychological support from both the spouse and the family is of great help. It will be more difficult to overcome the unpleasant effects of the syndrome if the patient has additional socioeconomic problems. In a study comparing safety, efficacy and cost-effectiveness of treating patients at home versus hospitalization, the authors found out that the success rate was similar with a significant reduced cost when patients were treated at home [4].

If >2+ ketonuria is found on dipstick urinary analysis, and the patient loses weight and seems exhausted, she needs to be hospitalized. The negative balance is not only due to malnutrition, but also to weight loss caused by persistent vomiting. She needs caloric intake as well as psychological support from the medical team. If the baby is unexpected or not desired, management may even become worse. The mother should be assured that this hard time with vomiting episodes is temporary, and the problem will be overcome with both medical and psychological management. The growing fetus should also be accepted as a child, and both the patient and her spouse should accept themselves as mother and father. Psychological support from other family members is an additive to the treatment. The patient may be allowed to change her lifestyle according to her desire with flexible leisure and work hours. She may be told that the severe form of hyperemesis will not lead to adverse perinatal outcome as long as medical treatment is supplied.

The intravenous or rectal route may be selected for initial treatment and then changed to the oral form when the symptoms begin to subside. Other medical problems such as gastroenteritis, cholecystitis, pancreatitis, hepatitis, peptic ulcer, pyelonephritis and fatty liver of pregnancy may underlie the symptoms, therefore the patient with ongoing and/or worsening complaints should be evaluated for the correct diagnosis.

The patient must be weighed daily or every other day to see the changes. Urine dipstick analysis will help monitor the nitrogen balance and glucose load given in solutions. In some patients liver enzymes are elevated, but usually do not increase more than 4-fold of the upper normal limit. Therefore, the levels should be followed in these patients. Ultrasonographic evaluation will help to rule out multiple pregnancy, gestational trophoblastic disease and give psychological support to parents by direct visualization of the fetus.

Pharmacotherapy of Hyperemesis

When simple measures fail and the patient feels that she is 'ill' other than 'pregnant', the healthcare provider needs to begin an antiemetic therapy. The treatment can be divided into four headings: (1) ameliorating food intake; (2) electrolyte balance; (3) antiemetic therapy, and (4) vitamin supplementation.

Ameliorating Food Intake

As the patient is in a negative balance, she must receive either oral or parenteral food. A short course for oral intake may be tried first, but if persistent vomiting exists, peripheral or central venous access should be begun. In addition, presence of ≥2+ ketonuria measured on a dipstick urine analysis may necessitate parenteral support. Besides energy supplementation, electrolyte replacement is crucial for the deficit and acid-base imbalances.

Daily intake of a nonpregnant and pregnant woman must be around 2,200 and 2,500 kcal respectively. Calories supply energy and whenever caloric intake is inadequate, protein, which is vital for fetal growth and development, is metabolized to meet the energy demand. Therefore, the initial step in taking care of the hyperemetic patient should be adequate nutrition. If she does not tolerate oral feeding, fluid therapy with additional vitamins should be considered.

The most favorite food is advised for the hyperemetic woman, especially during the recovery phase. Small but frequent feedings should be ingested. In severe cases, chewing small ice cubes may help tolerate food intake and alleviate nausea. Foul smells and fatty, fried, spicy and undesired foods must be avoided in both the acute and recovery phases. Salty crackers may be well tolerated, and potato chips serve as replacing potassium, folic acid and vitamin C [5]. Meal times can be arranged according to the time of symptoms, such that eating may be preferred when nausea is least severe. Small but frequent fluid intake may be tried between meals. Though iron is not usually supplemented in the first trimester of pregnancy, it should be especially avoided in patients with HG as iron itself may irritate the gastrointestinal system.

Total parenteral nutrition may be necessary in severe cases especially if the symptoms do not resolve within several days of management [6]. Amino acid solutions and 25% dextrose supply protein formation and energy. In addition, electrolytes, a multivitamin solution and a weekly 10% fat solution were administered. Significant nutritional improvement and anabolic state were achieved after treatment. No adverse effect on perinatal outcome such as low birth weight, placental insufficiency and preterm labor, and placental emboli on pathological examination were seen. Thiamine supplementation should be kept in mind in total parenteral nutrition and this type of therapy should be reserved for intractable cases when usual measures fail. A peripherally inserted central catheter was used in 3 women with HG for 28–137 days [7]. The perinatal outcome was satisfactory and this type of venous access was suggested to avoid some risks of subclavian entry with safe administration of long-term parenteral nutrition. Enteral feeding is an alternative approach after the acute symptoms subside with initial therapy [8, 9]. In addition, percutaneous endoscopic gastrostomy was performed in 2 intractable cases with resultant weight gain [10]. The intervention did not cause any complications and the patients tolerated well and

Table 1. Electrolyte concentrations (mEq/l) in each body compartment

	Intracellular	Extracellular	
		intravascular	interstitial
Sodium	10	145	142
Potassium	140	4	4
Calcium	<1	3	3
Magnesium	50	2	2
Chloride	4	105	110
Bicarbonate	10	24	28
Phosphorus	75	2	2

regained their lost weight. This type of nutrition may be reserved for patients in negative balance with promising outcomes. Percutaneous endoscopic gastrostomy was reported to be better than nasogastric feeding as it did not cause sinusitis, epistaxis, negative impact on body image, and gastroesophageal acid reflux.

Electrolyte Balance

The concentration of various electrolytes in different body compartments is seen in table 1. Extracellular fluid, namely the intravascular compartment, supplies energy to the tissues and removes waste products away from them. Therefore, maintenance of a constant volume and pressure is vital, especially in a pregnant woman who not only nourishes herself but also the growing fetus. Daily water intake and loss are approximately 2,500 ml in a normal adult, and the primary route for this loss is urine. In pathological states such as hyperemesis, fluid loss is exacerbated through the gastrointestinal system. Progressive vomiting may lead to hyponatremia with a resultant decrease in urinary sodium output. Severe hyponatremia may cause a shift towards the intracellular compartment and result in lethargy, confusion and seizures. For patients with <10 mEq/l urine sodium concentration, isotonic saline replacement should be the standard therapy (normal daily urinary sodium excretion is 60 mEq/l). The amount of sodium which should be replaced can be calculated according to the following formula:

$$\text{Sodium deficit} = \text{Total body water} \times (130 - \text{present concentration})$$

Total body water is about 50% of body weight in females, but obesity decreases water content. The amount of saline can be calculated by dividing sodium deficit by 154, which is the content of isotonic saline solution. The desired fluid treatment rate is 0.5 mEq/l/h, but this can be raised up to 3-fold in severe cases.

Table 2. Various solutions commonly used for patients with HG

Solution	D g	Na^+ mEq/l	K^+ mEq/l	Cl^- mEq/l	Ca^{2+} mEq/l	Mg^{2+} mEq/l	PO^- mEq/l	Lactate mEq/l	Acetate mEq/l	Gluconate
5% D	5									
20% D	20									
30% D	30									
5% DRL	5	130	4	109	3			28		
Saline										
Isolyte	5	40	35	40			15		20	
Isolyte S		141	5	98		3	1		27	23
Isolyte M		40	35	40			15		20	

D = Dextrose; DRL = dextrose-Ringer lactate.

Increased potassium loss may also be seen due to severe vomiting, and increased sweat formation may contribute to this loss. Urinary potassium excretion may be <20 mEq/l (normal value is 35 mEq/l). Hypokalemia may lead to cardiovascular problems such as dysrhythmia and myocardial dysfunction; neuromuscular problems such as skeletal muscle weakness and tetany, and also hormonal and metabolic derangements. The amount of potassium which should be replaced can be calculated according to the following formula:

Potassium deficit = 50 × (4 − present concentration)
(the coefficient 50 should be replaced with 100 in obese subjects)

Potassium may be added in solutions and administered at a rate of 20–30 mEq/l, but usually it should not exceed 40 mEq/l. Dextrose-containing solutions may lead to hyperglycemia with resultant hyperinsulinemia which enhances membrane-bound Na^+, K^+-ATPase and a shift of potassium towards intracellular compartment. Intravenous replacement rate and maximum daily potassium amount should not exceed 10 mEq/h and 140 mEq/day respectively. Common solutions used for fluid therapy are seen in table 2.

Skin turgor, hydration of mucous membranes and blood pressure point to the degree of hypovolemia. A decrease in blood pressure in normal pregnant women should be kept in mind to avoid false-positive diagnosis in hypotension. Aqueous solutions of low-molecular-weight ions are crystalloid solutions whereas high-molecular-weight substances such as proteins or large glucose polymers are colloid solutions. Colloid solutions mostly remain in the intravascular compartment while crystalloid solutions fill the entire extracellular compartment. In patients with HG, water and caloric loss are mostly associated with electrolyte disturbances and replacement therapy is not only maintained with glucose, but also with isotonic electrolyte solutions. Colloid solutions are not usually indicated in hyperemetic patients unless the patient has severe fluid deficit and hypotension. Dextran 70 and dextran 40 are colloids commonly used to maintain intravascular volume.

One gram of glucose supplies approximately 3.4 kcal. In our daily practice, we administer 30% dextrose in water together with 5% dextrose in water via the same venous access twice daily, and we individualize electrolyte solutions according to the deficits. Though some authors may accept high intravenous dextrose as a precipitating factor for severe neurological complications, we have not seen such a case yet, and the daily calorie requirement needs to be met somehow. Daily sodium, potassium and chloride requirements are roughly 1 mEq/kg. This amount can be added with the calculated loss and given in 24 h.

Antiemetic Therapy

Various antiemetics may be given with vitamin supplementation. Promethazine, prochlorperazine, chlorpromazine, meclizine, droperidol-diphenhydramine and metoclopramide are the most commonly used agents to alleviate nausea and vomiting.

H_1-Receptor Antagonists

Histamine is an important mediator of immediate allergic and inflammatory reactions and functions as a neurotransmitter in certain areas of the brain. Most tissues contain histamine in bound form in granules in mast cells or basophils. The bound form is inactive and released to various stimuli. Histamine interacts with its receptors located on the cellular membrane, and increases intracellular Ca^{2+} through H_1-receptors. The H_1-antagonists, which are used to block the actions of histamine, are lipid-soluble and rapidly absorbed following oral use. They are widely distributed throughout the body including the central nervous system. Duration of action is 4–6 h except meclizine which acts around 12–24 h. H_1-receptor antagonists act by reversible, competitive antagonism at the specific receptor. Some of the actions of these antagonists, including prevention of nausea and vomiting, are not related to the blockade of the receptor. These actions are probably due to having similar structure with the drugs which affect muscarinic cholinoceptor, α-adrenoceptor and serotonin sites. Sedation is a common denominator of H_1-antagonists with different severity depending upon the chemical structure. The subgroups and effects of H_1-antagonists are seen in table 3. Besides sedation, postural hypotension may occur due to adrenoceptor blocking action especially in the phenothiazine group.

In a multianalysis including 24 controlled studies involving more than 200,000 women, no increase in teratogenic risk was observed in the offspring

Table 3. The effects of commonly prescribed anti-histamines

Group	Effects	FDA class	Dose
Ethanolamine			
Dimenhydrinate	Marked sedation, ANV	B_M	50 mg
Diphenhydramine	Marked sedation, ANV	C	25–50 mg
Doxylamine	Marked sedation, ANV	B	1.25–25 mg
Piperazine			
Meclizine	Slight sedation, ANV	B_M	25–50 mg
Phenothiazine			
Promethazine	Marked sedation, ANV	C	10–25 mg

ANV = Anti-nausea and vomiting; FDA = Food and Drug Administration. FDA Classification: B = Either animal reproduction studies have not demonstrated a fetal risk but there are no controlled studies in pregnant women or animal reproduction studies have shown an adverse effect that was not confirmed in controlled studies in women in the first trimester. C = Either studies in animals have revealed adverse effects on the fetus and there are no controlled studies in women or studies in women and animals are not available. Drugs should be only if the potential benefit justifies the potential risk to the fetus.

Subscript M (e.g., B_M): Many drugs have not been given a letter rating by the manufacturers. Subscript M identifies that the rating was given by its own manufacturer in the professional literature.

of patients who received antihistamines in the first trimester [11]. The odds ratio for major malformations was found to be 0.76 (98% CI: 0.60–0.94), and antihistamines were found safe to be prescribed during pregnancy.

Antipsychotic Agents

Chlorpromazine and prochlorperazine are phenothiazine derivative antipsychotic drugs with strong antiemetic effects. They are both included in class C according to the FDA classification. They act by blocking dopamine receptors located on the chemoreceptor trigger zone and the stomach. Another antipsychotic agent, droperidol, is a butyrophenone derivative and is also used for nausea and vomiting. It is a class C_M drug and was used in combination with diphenhydramine in patients with HG [12]. This treatment was safe and more effective than various other antiemetics with fewer re-admissions to the hospital.

Metoclopramide

Metoclopramide, a potent dopamine antagonist, is a class B_M drug. As the drug is effective in stimulating peristalsis of the bowel, it is frequently used to alleviate nausea and promote bowel motion during the postoperative period.

The antiemetic effect is due to centrally acting dopamine antagonism. It also raises lower esophageal sphincter tonus and accelerates gastric emptying and is therefore useful to prevent aspiration in pregnant patients who undergo cesarean section. The most common side effects are somnolence and nervousness. It is frequently used as an antiemetic in pregnant women. In a study involving 301 women, a subcutaneous metoclopramide pump was used on an outpatient basis and was found to be both safe and cost-effective in the treatment of HG [13]. Around 65% of the patients had complete resolution, though 55% of the patients had side effects, most of them were mild and the drug was well tolerated.

Trimethobenzamide

This FDA class C drug acts by inhibiting the chemoreceptor trigger zone, and the duration of action is around 4–6 h. The drug may be given by either oral, parenteral or rectal route. Oral absorption may vary among individuals, therefore the efficacy may be different. Adverse effects such as lethargy, dizziness and diarrhea may be seen with high doses.

Other Agents

We will now discuss some other agents which have been used in clinical trials but not widely used by obstetricians. Diazepam, a sedative-hypnotic benzodiazepine, potentiates GABAergic neurotransmission in both the central nervous system and the spinal cord. This results in a change in chloride ion conductance leading to a decrease in neuronal discharge. The major indication of this class D drug is relief of anxiety and sedation and it has been added to fluid and vitamin therapy in patients with HG [14]. It effectively reduced nausea and no teratogenic effect was observed.

Ondansetron, a class B drug, is a 5-hydroxytryptamine receptor antagonist and used to prevent severe nausea and vomiting during chemotherapy and the postoperative period. Though the drug is usually accepted to be a strong antiemetic, it was not found to be superior to promethazine [15]. Hospital stay, medication doses desired by the patients, decline in the severity of nausea and daily weight gain were similar between the two groups. A patient was reported to receive the drug intermittently in every trimester without any side effects to the fetus [16].

Though adrenocorticotropic hormone had no benefit [17] on HG, universal anti-inflammatory agents, steroids, have been beneficial in refractory cases. Short-acting forms, methylprednisolone and hydrocortisone, were used with high success rates [18, 19]. Oral methylprednisolone was found to be more efficacious than promethazine in reducing the re-admission rate of the patients without any difference in perinatal outcome. Methylprednisolone or promethazine was given to patients in a randomized fashion if nausea and vomiting did not resolve after initial fluid therapy or if it was the second admission of the patient. The patients received oral methylprednisolone 16 mg tid for 3 days, then the dose was tapered by halving of the dose every 3 days. No re-admittance to the hospital was observed in the methylprednisolone group compared with 5 patients who received promethazine. Hydrocortisone led to cessation of vomiting within hours and the regaining of lost weight within days. In this study, the patients were maintained with oral prednisolone therapy up to 45 mg/day. In some patients, oral prednisolone was continued for 10.6 ± 4.7 weeks. Steroids are accepted to affect the chemoreceptor trigger zone and be reserved for intractable nausea and vomiting. Short-term use does not seem to affect adversely birth weight and Apgar scores. In a recent report by Moran and Taylor [20], the authors confirmed weight loss >5% of prepregnant weight to be the best objective clinical indicator of severity, and prednisolone therapy was found to be effective in women with severe HG not only in resolving the symptoms, but also in allowing recovery of muscle mass and muscle strength. Steroid therapy was not associated with decreased birth weight and was considered to be reserved for severe cases. In another study, though steroid therapy improved the symptoms and increased weight gain, the authors concluded that this type of treatment did not lead to complete and rapid remission [21]. In this study, although there was a significant improvement in the sense of well-being and an increased intake of food and weight gain was observed, severity of nausea and amount of vomiting did not decrease significantly. The authors related this result to the limited sample size, premature termination of the study and randomization procedures. The efficacy of the drug has been emphasized, but the authors are contrary to the previous reports where prompt relief was reported.

Ginger was reported to diminish or eliminate the symptoms of HG without any side effects [22], but its mutagenic effects are not known in humans. The degree of nausea and the frequency of vomiting decreased with ginger.

Vitamin Supplementation

Wernicke's encephalopathy and associated thiamine deficiency were reported in pregnant women with HG [23, 24]. The first case had almost total blindness and was confused before diagnosis and responded dramatically to intravenous thiamine and oral multivitamins. In addition, the second case also recovered following thiamine treatment. Thiamine deficiency seems to be the most important factor leading to neurological complications, therefore it should be administered to patients with HG before the advanced stage of the syndrome.

Pyridoxine has been given to resolve the symptoms of HG in various studies [25, 26]. In both studies the severity of nausea was reduced, but a positive effect on vomiting was reported in the study which used a higher dose. A high dose, >75 mg/day, may be harmful. In our daily practice we give pyridoxine orally in a combined form with meclizine. Most of our patients tolerate the drug well and the symptoms subside if not severe.

A recent review by Mazotta and Magee [27] revealed that treatment with doxylamine and pyridoxine, antihistamines or pyridoxine did not have any teratogenic effect on the fetuses whose mothers were exposed to such drugs.

Vitamin K deficiency was reported in a hyperemetic woman who had severe epistaxis [28]. The authors suggested that HG caused inadequate uptake and absorption of vitamin K resulting in coagulopathy and bleeding. In severe cases, vitamin K supplementation may be considered.

Perinatal Outcome

Reduced caloric intake during gestation was reported to stimulate placental growth, optimize fetal growth and well-being later in pregnancy [29]. Placental size was found to be greater in women who were malnourished only in the first trimester [30]. In addition, the offspring of rats underfed in early gestation tended to be larger than those underfed in late pregnancy [31]. Therefore, if severe complications are not seen and the patient responds well to treatment, low birth weight is not expected.

Birth weight, gestational age, preterm delivery, Apgar scores, perinatal mortality and incidence of fetal anomalies did not differ in normal and hyperemetic patients [32]. In another study, no increased risk of growth retardation, congenital anomalies and prematurity was detected [33]. According to these studies, the hyperemetic patient may be assured that she most likely will not face poor perinatal outcome only due to hyperemesis. However, in cases with multiple admissions to the hospital, patients may have a more severe nutritional disturbance, reduced maternal weight gain and birth weight [34].

In summary, vomiting and/or nausea are the most common complaints during early pregnancy, but the severe form, hyperemesis, is quite rare. Most patients with HG require hospitalization and antiemetics, and short-term steroid therapy may be beneficial in intractable cases. Serious complications are rare but medical therapy is mandatory. Vitamin supplementation, especially thiamine and pyridoxine, seems to prevent neurological complications and help treatment. Hyperthyroidism may accompany about 60% of patients which may not require specific therapy. *Helicobacter pylori* infection was reported to occur in these patients and appropriate antibiotics may cure the infection. Enteral feeding is an alternative therapy for patients who do not tolerate oral ingestion.

References

1 Signorello LB, Harlow BL, Wang S, Erick MA: Saturated fat intake and the risk of severe hyperemesis gravidarum. Epidemiology 1998;9:636–640.

2 Askling J, Erlandsson G, Kaijser M, Akne O, Ekborn A: Sickness in pregnancy and sex of child. Lancet 1999;354:2053.

3 Vilming B, Nesheim BI: Hyperemesis gravidarum in a contemporary population in Oslo. Acta Obstet Gynecol Scand 2000;79:640–643.

4 Naef RW 3rd, Chauhan SP, Roach H, Roberts WE, Travis KH, Morrison JC: Treatment for hyperemesis gravidarum in the home: An alternative to hospitalization. J Perinatol 1995;15: 289–292.

5 Erick M: Battling morning (noon and night) sickness: New approaches for treating an age-old problem. J Am Diet Assoc 1994;94:147–148.

6 Levine MG, Esser D: Total parenteral nutrition for the treatment of severe hyperemesis gravidarum: Maternal nutritional effects and fetal outcome. Obstet Gynecol 1988;72:102.

7 Greenspoon JS, Rosen DJD, Ault M: Use of the peripherally inserted central catheter for parenteral nutrition during pregnancy. Obstet Gynecol 1993;81:831–834.

8 Boyce RA: Enteral nutrition in hyperemesis gravidarum: A new development. J Am Diet Assoc 1992;92:733.

9 Hsu JJ, Clark-Glena R, Nelson DK, Kim CH: Nasogastric enteral feeding in the management of hyperemesis gravidarum. Obstet Gynecol 1996;88:343–346.

10 Godil A, Chen YK: Percutaneous endoscopic gastrostomy for nutrition support in pregnancy associated with hyperemesis gravidarum and anorexia nervosa. J Parenter Enteral Nutr 1998;22: 238–241.

11 Seto A, Einarson T, Koren G: Pregnancy outcome following first trimester exposure to antihistamines: Meta-analysis. Am J Perinatol 1997;14:119–124.

12 Nageotte MP, Briggs GG, Towers CV, Asrat T: Droperidol and diphenhydramine in the management of hyperemesis gravidarum. Am J Obstet Gynecol 1996;174:1801–1805.

13 Buttino L, Gambon C: Home subcutaneous metochlopramide therapy for hyperemesis gravidarum. Prim Care Update Ob Gyns 1998;5:189.

14 Ditto A, Morgante G, la Marca A, De Leo V: Evaluation of treatment of hyperemesis gravidarum using parenteral fluid with or without diazepam. A randomized study. Gynecol Obstet Invest 1999;48:232–236

15 Sullivan CA, Johnson CA, Roach H, Martin RW, Stewart DK, Morrison JC: A pilot study of intravenous ondansetron for hyperemesis gravidarum. Am J Obstet Gynecol 1996;174:1565–1568.

16 Tincello DG, Johnstone MJ: Treatment of hyperemesis gravidarum with the 5-HT_3 antagonist ondansetron (Zofran). Postgrad Med J 1996;72:688–689.

17 Yliorkala D, Kauppila A, Ollanketo ML: Intramuscular ACTH or placebo in the treatment of hyperemesis gravidarum. Acta Obstet Gynecol Scand 1979;58:453–455.

18 Safari HR, Fassett MJ, Souter IC, Alsulyman OM, Goodwin TM: The efficacy of methylprednisolone in the treatment of hyperemesis gravidarum: A randomized, double-blind, controlled study. Am J Obstet Gynecol 1998;179:921–924.

19 Taylor R: Successful management of hyperemesis gravidarum using steroid therapy. Q J Med 1996;89:103–107.

20 Moran P, Taylor R: Management of hyperemesis gravidarum: The importance of weight loss as a criterion for steroid therapy. Q J Med 2002;95:153–158.

21 Nelson-Piercy C, Fayers P, de Swiet M: Randomised, double-blind, placebo-controlled trial of corticosteroids for the treatment of hyperemesis gravidarum. BJOG 2001;108:9–15.

22 Fischer-Rasmussen W, Kjær SK, Dahl C, Asping U: Ginger treatment of hyperemesis gravidarum. Eur Obstet Gynecol Reprod Biol 1990;38:19–24.

23 Tesfaye S, Achari V, Yang YC, Harding S, Bowden A, Vora JP: Pregnant, vomiting and going blind. Lancet 1998;352:1594.

24 Hillborn M, Pyhtinen J, Pylvanen V, Sotaniemi K: Pregnant, vomiting and coma. Lancet 1999; 353:1584.

25 Sahakian V, Rouse D, Sipes S, Rose N, Niebyl J: Vitamin B_6 is effective therapy for nausea and vomiting of pregnancy: A randomized double-blind, placebo-controlled study. Obstet Gynecol 1991;78:33.
26 Vutyavanich T, Wongtrangan S, Ruangsri R: Pyridoxine for nausea and vomiting of pregnancy: A randomized double-blind, placebo-controlled trial. Am J Obstet Gynecol 1995;173:881.
27 Mazzotta P, Magee LA: A risk-benefit assessment of pharmacological and nonpharmacological treatments for nausea and vomiting of pregnancy. Drugs 2000;59:781–800.
28 Robinson JN, Banerjee R, Thiet MP: Coagulopathy secondary to vitamin K deficiency in hyperemesis gravidarum. Obstet Gynecol 1998;92:673–675.
29 Huxley RR: Nausea and vomiting of early pregnancy: Its role in placental development. Obstet Gynecol 2000;95:779–782.
30 Lumey LH: Compensatory placental growth after restricted maternal nutrition in early pregnancy. Placenta 1998;19:105–111.
31 Griggio MA, Luz J, Gorgulho AA, et al: The influence of food restriction during different periods of pregnancy. Int J Food Sci Nutr 1997;48:129–134.
32 Tsang IS, Katz VL, Wells SD: Maternal and fetal outcomes in hyperemesis gravidarum. Int J Gynaecol Obstet 1996;55:231–235.
33 Hallak M, Tsalamandris K, Dombrowski MP, Isaad NB, Pryda PG, Evans MI: Hyperemesis gravidarum. Effects on fetal outcome. J Reprod Med 1996;41:871–874.
34 Godsey RK, Newman RB: Hyperemesis gravidarum: A comparison of single and multiple admissions. J Reprod Med 1991;36:287–290.

N. Kemal Kuşcu, MD
Department of Obstetrics and Gynecology
Celal Bayar University, School of Medicine
TR–45020 Manisa (Turkey)
Tel. +90 236 2349070/297 or +90 532 3755566, Fax +90 236 2370213
E-Mail kemal.kuscu@bayar.edu.tr

Donnerer J (ed): Antiemetic Therapy.
Basel, Karger, 2003, pp 204–225

Hyperemesis gravidarum in the Clinical Setting

Rami Eliakim[a], *Ovadia Abulafia*[b], *David M. Sherer*[b]

[a] Division of Gastroenterology, Rambam Medical Center, Technion School of Medicine, Haifa, Israel, and
[b] Division of Maternal-Fetal Medicine, Department of Obstetrics and Gynecology, State University of New York, Downstate Medical Center, Brooklyn, N.Y., USA

Physiologic changes occurring during pregnancy commonly affect the gastrointestinal tract. Nausea and vomiting during pregnancy is common, affecting between 50 and 90% of gravidas [1]. Of women who experience nausea and vomiting during pregnancy, 70% sustain this symptomatology between the 4th and 7th week of pregnancy. Less than 10% of patients will note this occurrence before their missed period [2]. In approximately 90% of cases, vomiting ceases by the 16th week of gestation [2]. Nausea and vomiting in early pregnancy has a profound impact on women's general sense of well-being and day-to-day life activities [3]. The occurrence of nausea and vomiting during pregnancy is of such clinical significance that the National Institute of Child Health and Human Development (NICHD) and the Office of Rare Diseases Research at the National Institutes of Health (NIH), recently supported a conference pertaining solely to this topic. The meeting was the first of its kind and was designed to convene investigators representing medical disciplines including neuro-otology, gastroenterology, oncology, teratology, internal medicine, behavioral medicine, endocrinology, psychology, developmental biology, pediatrics, obstetrics and maternal-fetal medicine [4].

Hyperemesis gravidarum – pernicious vomiting of pregnancy – is a severe form of nausea and vomiting in pregnancy often associated with weight loss, ketonemia, ketonuria, electrolyte imbalance, dehydration and possible hepatic and renal damage which may persist throughout gestation [5, 6]. The true incidence of hyperemesis gravidarum has not been established, yet has been reported at between 0.3 and 2%, with most authors reporting an incidence of 0.5% [5, 7, 8].

The following chapter examines current data pertaining to epidemiology, etiology, clinical manifestations, differential diagnosis, complications, various treatment modalities, subsequent perinatal outcome, and recent developments.

Epidemiology

Hyperemesis gravidarum ranges in incidence between 0.3 and 2% of all deliveries. Annually in the USA more than 50,000 women are hospitalized with the diagnosis of hyperemesis gravidarum with an average hospital stay of 4 days per patient [9, 10].

Significant ethnic differences in the incidence of hyperemesis gravidarum have been noted among various populations. New Zealand Pacific Island women, United Kingdom Indian and Pakistani, and African American women have increased rates of occurrence in comparison with ethnic European women [11–13]. Increased incidences have been noted in association with nulliparity (odds ratio (OR) 1.6), adolescent patients, patients with increased body weight (Quetelet's index, $kg/m^2 \geq 24$, OR 1.5), multiple gestations (twins OR 1.5), gestational trophoblastic disease, fetal abnormalities including triploidy (partial mole), fetal central nervous system malformations (OR 4.0) and the occurrence of hyperemesis gravidarum in a previous pregnancy. Decreased incidences have been noted among patients with advanced maternal age (≥35 years of age, OR 0.5), maternal smokers (OR 0.6) and current fetal demise [11, 14].

Etiology

The precise underlying etiology of hyperemesis gravidarum remains elusive. Numerous etiologies have been considered and include: gestation-associated hormone levels, thyrotoxicosis, serotonin, upper gastrointestinal dysmotility, psychological factors, hepatic abnormalities, autonomic nervous dysfunction, nutritional deficiencies and *Helicobacter pylori* infection.

Hormonal Levels

Serum levels of β-human chorionic gonadotropin (β-hCG) peak early in gestation (10 weeks). Concurrent with the increase in serum β-hCG concentrations, levels of estradiol and progestins display a steep increase [15]. These facts and the increased incidence of hyperemesis gravidarum observed in association with both multiple gestations and gestational trophoblastic disease suggest that β-hCG, estradiol and 17-hydroxyprogesterone may play a pivotal role in the pathogenesis of this disease. In 1980, Soules et al. [16], in studying normal and molar gestations, were unable to demonstrate convincing relationships between these hormones and the incidence or severity of nausea and vomiting in pregnancy. Conversely, numerous authors have recently demonstrated an increase in serum levels of free β-hCG among patients with hyperemesis gravidarum versus control patients matched for age, weight and gestational age. Goodwin et al. [17] demonstrated an almost twofold increase of serum hCG, and threefold increase in free β-hCG serum levels, whereas α-hCG serum levels did not differ between the two groups studied. Furneaux et al. [18] recently reviewed the relationship between nauseas and vomiting of pregnancy and hCG.

hCG is also considered to cause direct elevation of thyroid hormone levels by hormone cross-talk to the thyrotropin (TSH) receptor [19]. Recently, Jordan et al. [20] noted a twofold increase in the mean serum total hCG levels among patients with hyperemesis gravidarum when compared with controls. The increase in hCG concentration was noted in the more acidic half of the chromatofocusing pH range correlating with significantly lower mean serum TSH levels in the study group and concluded that acidic isoforms of hCG may play a role in hyperemesis gravidarum and gestational thyrotoxicosis. Panesar et al. [21] compared sensitive thyroid-stimulating hormone, free thyroxine, free triiodothyronine and total β-hCG immunoassay levels of patients with hyperemesis gravidarum with those of healthy pregnant controls matched for gestational age. These authors concluded that hCG is not independently involved in the etiology of hyperemesis gravidarum but may be involved by its ability to stimulate the thyroid. It should be mentioned however that other authors have not been able to confirm the role of hCG as a thyroid stimulator in patients with hyperemesis gravidarum [22].

Similarly, Depue et al. [14] demonstrated that after adjusting for gestational age, mean levels of total estradiol and sex hormone binding globulin were 26 and 37% higher, respectively, among patients with hyperemesis gravidarum versus controls, suggesting that elevated estrogen levels are responsible for excessive vomiting in pregnancy.

Thyrotoxicosis

Diagnosis of thyroid disease and analysis of thyroid function tests in pregnant women is complex. Although autoimmune thyroid disease has traditionally been considered the most common etiology of thyrotoxicosis in pregnancy, recent studies indicate that increased production of β-hCG (as stated above) is the leading cause for thyroid function abnormalities during the first half of pregnancy [23]. Increased free thyroxin (T_4) index was observed in 24 (73%) of 33 women with hyperemesis gravidarum [24]. Other studies demonstrated an incidence ranging between 40 and 58% [25, 26]. Conversely, Wilson et al. [27]

in 1992 found no consistent pattern of thyroid function abnormality among patients with hyperemesis gravidarum compared with controls.

As women with hyperthyroidism rarely manifest vomiting, it appears unlikely that thyrotoxicosis (abnormal thyroid function) is the etiology of hyperemesis gravidarum. Recently, a link between hyperemesis gravidarum and thyroid stimulation during pregnancy has been related to β-hCG (lacking the carboxyl terminal of the intact hCG molecule) and has been termed transient/gestational hyperthyroidism as discussed previously [19, 20, 28, 29].

Serotonin

Central and peripheral serotonin receptors may play an important role in the vomiting reflex arc [30]. Serotonin exerts its physiologic effects on a variety of receptor subtypes in the central nervous system, gastrointestinal tract and other sites and is involved in many clinical conditions of emesis in humans [31]. Serotonin receptor compounds used for treatment of nausea and vomiting include 5-HT_3 receptor antagonists and 5-HT_4 receptor agonists [31]. Cases have been reported of successful application of ondansetron (Zofran) a 5-HT_3 receptor antagonist for intractable hyperemesis gravidarum [32, 33]. These cases led Borgeat et al. [34] to examine a possible relationship between hyperemesis gravidarum and liberation of serotonin. Urinary hydroxyindoleacetic acid (HIAA), a major urinary metabolite of serotonin, was measured in 13 patients with hyperemesis gravidarum, 10 normal controls and 10 nongravid women (matched for age, and not taking oral contraceptive medications). No differences in urinary excretion of HIAA were noted between the groups. The authors concluded that hyperemesis gravidarum was not associated with increased serotonin secretion. Subsequently, Sullivan et al. [30] conducted a double-blinded, randomized controlled study comparing intravenous ondansetron to promethazine among patients with hyperemesis gravidarum. No difference in response to the two medications was noted.

Upper Gastrointestinal Dysmotility

During pregnancy, esophageal gastric and small bowel motility are impaired as a result of smooth muscle relaxation due to increased levels of progesterone, factors which in concert may contribute to increased nausea and vomiting [1]. Hormonal changes alter low esophageal sphincter function manifested mainly by heartburn, but also by nausea and vomiting. Lower esophageal sphincter pressure gradually decreases during pregnancy. Van Thiel et al. [35] noted resting lower esophageal sphincter pressure to be low throughout all gestation with a nadir in the third trimester returning to normal postpartum.

Delayed gastric emptying during pregnancy contributes significantly to increased nausea and vomiting [1]. Koch et al. [36] measured gastric electric rhythm by recording electrogastrograms (EGG) in pregnant women with various degrees of nausea and vomiting of pregnancy and found gastric dysrhythmias in the vast majority of cases. Of 32 patients examined, 17 (53%) exhibited tachygastria and 9 (28%) exhibited bradygastria. The remaining patients had minimal nausea or vomiting and exhibited normal EGG studies as did 15/17 (94%) healthy nonpregnant patients. Six patients with nausea and abnormal EGG studies exhibited postpartum normalization of their EGG. Riezzo et al. [37] conducted EGG studies before and after consumption of a standardized meal in 9 women with first trimester nausea and vomiting and 2 months following elective termination of pregnancy and in 8 control pregnant women without nausea and vomiting. Among the patients with hyperemesis gravidarum, there was a higher incidence of unstable EGG activity and a reduced increase in postprandial power during pregnancy than after pregnancy termination. These authors concluded that gastric myoelectrical activity is normal although unstable, mainly after food ingestion in asymptomatic pregnant patients returning to normal after pregnancy termination. These characteristics are significantly more pronounced among symptomatic patients.

Maes et al. [38] investigated gastric emptying of solids in asymptomatic pregnant patients, patients recovering from hyperemesis gravidarum and healthy nonpregnant women, using ^{13}C-octnoic acid gastric emptying breath test. Gastric emptying of solids was not different among asymptomatic pregnant patients and nonpregnant controls. Gastric emptying of solids was significantly accelerated among patients recovering from hyperemesis gravidarum. These results led the authors to conclude that upper gastrointestinal disorders were not implicated in hyperemesis gravidarum. A detailed review of gastrointestinal factors in nausea and vomiting of pregnancy including a diagnostic approach and therapeutic options for treating nausea and vomiting of pregnancy based on understanding of gastric neuromuscular dysfunction has been outlined by Koch [39].

Helicobacter pylori *Infection*

H. pylori-associated gastritis may manifest clinically with nausea and vomiting. The incidence of *H. pylori* infection among women of childbearing age in the USA is low. An incidence of peptic ulcer disease of 6 per 23,000 deliveries was reported by Michaletz-Onody [40]. The incidence of seropositivity to *H. pylori* was 22% among 562 pregnant women studied [40].

Frigo et al. [41] demonstrated that 90.5% of women with hyperemesis gravidarum were seropositive to *H. pylori* (by enzyme-linked immunoassay using specific serum IgG antibodies) in comparison with 46.5% of pregnant controls, matched for gestational age. Recent case reports have suggested that eradication of *H. pylori* infection ameliorated clinical hyperemesis gravidarum

[42, 43]. Lanciers et al. [44] in 1999 assayed sera from 229 asymptomatic pregnant women for the presence of *H. pylori*-specific immunoglobulin G (IgG) and immunoglobulin M (IgM) antibodies by means of a commercially available serum ELISA test, and results compared with those previously obtained in symptomatic, healthy, nonpregnant individuals. 120/229 women (52.4%) and 55/118 nonpregnant subjects (46.6%) were seropositive for *H. pylori*-specific IgG antibodies ($p > 0.3$). Out of these 120 IgG antibody-positive women, 36 (30%) were positive for *H. pylori*-specific IgM antibodies, as were 25/109 (22.9%) in the IgG antibody-negative group ($p > 0.3$). Overall, 61/229 (26.6%) of the pregnant women had recently been infected with *H. pylori*, compared with 11% of the healthy, nonpregnant population ($p > 0.01$), confirming the possibility of an increased susceptibility of *H. pylori* infection in pregnancy [44].

Clearly at this stage, additional studies are required to further understand the immune response to *H. pylori* in pregnancy.

Hepatic Abnormalities

Throughout pregnancy, an increased load of steroid hormone production exists creating an increased physiologic burden on the liver which is the major site of steroid hormonal inactivation. Liver disease may manifest with nausea and vomiting. Liver test abnormalities are commonly noted in association with hyperemesis gravidarum. Morali and Braverman [45] in a retrospective analysis of 80 patients with hyperemesis gravidarum demonstrated abnormal liver enzymes (both GPT and GOT, approximately ≤4 times the normal) in 16% of cases. When patients with hyperemesis were analyzed according to the presence or absence of liver enzyme abnormality, the two groups differed significantly with regard to gestational age. The mean gestational age of the group with liver function abnormalities was 14 weeks ± 10 days versus 6.3 weeks ± 14.7 days in the group with normal liver function. Interestingly, in this study no correlation was noted between liver function abnormality and degree of ketonuria, thus suggesting factors other than starvation may produce the abnormal liver function in hyperemesis gravidarum [45]. An additional study by Wallstedt et al. [46] noted that 50% of patients hospitalized with hyperemesis gravidarum exhibited abnormal liver function. Larrey et al. [47] reported recurrent jaundice in a woman with hyperemesis gravidarum in three consecutive pregnancies. Rapid recovery after cessation of vomiting in this patient, suggested an association of hyperemesis gravidarum and jaundice [47]. A similar association between jaundice and hyperemesis was reported by Orazi et al. [48].

Taken together, the fact that liver abnormalities do not occur in all patients with hyperemesis gravidarum and are associated with a more severe disease course and resolve spontaneously concurrent with disease resolution, leads to the thought that liver dysfunction is a *secondary* event in hyperemesis gravidarum.

Lipid Metabolism

Modest differences in serum lipid and lipoproteins in association with hyperemesis gravidarum have been considered related to altered hepatic estrogen metabolism [15]. Signorello et al. [49] conducted a case-control study to investigate the effect of prepregnancy diet (and in particular dietary fat) on the risk of developing severe hyperemesis gravidarum. These authors noted that prepregnancy high daily intake of total fat increases the risk of hyperemesis gravidarum (OR 2.9 for each 25 g/day increase), which was driven primarily by saturated fat (OR 5.4 for each 15 g/day increase). No independent effect of total energy intake was noted.

Autonomic Nervous Dysfunction

Changes in autonomic functions that may be related to physiologic changes in pregnancy include changes in blood volume, temperature, heart rate and vascular resistance. When EGG abnormalities occur, these are associated with abnormalities of sympathetic adrenergic function [15]. Minagawa et al. [50] investigated the immunological status throughout gestation and found that activation of granulocytes, natural killer (NK) cells and extrathymic cells through sympathetic nerve activation are essential for the maintenance of pregnancy. Overactivation of the immunological state may be responsible for the onset of pregnancy-related disorders. Patients with pregnancy-related disorders including hyperemesis gravidarum exhibited higher blood and uterine levels of NK and/or extrathymic T cells [50].

Nutritional Deficiencies

Deficiencies of trace elements have been considered possible etiologies of hyperemesis gravidarum. A number of reports have demonstrated that patients with hyperemesis gravidarum are deficient in vitamin B_6 and propose that his deficiency is caused by increased need for the co-enzyme pyridoxale phosphate due to changes in protein metabolism during pregnancy [51]. Studies assessing serum zinc and copper levels of pregnant women have not noted differences between normal women and patients with hyperemesis gravidarum [52–54].

Psychological Factors

Psychological and psychiatric factors have been strongly implemented in association with hyperemesis gravidarum [5, 55, 56]. Frequent occurrence of hyperemesis gravidarum has been linked to both stress and emotional tension [55]. Hyperemesis gravidarum appears more common among immature, dependent, hysteric, depressed or anxious women [57]. Hyperemesis is considered a possible protest reaction against the pregnancy as a result of psychological conflicts especially from within the familial and home environment. The importance of psychological factors in the etiology of hyperemesis gravidarum is emphasized by the disappearance and recurrence of symptomatology in relation with separation or return to the family environment and by the fact that this disease is amenable to treatment with hypnosis and other forms of suggestion [57].

Eating disorders have been associated with hyperemesis gravidarum [58]. A series of 13 women in whom an eating disorder was precipitated during pregnancy, including 4 with hyperemesis gravidarum, were described indicating that the interaction between the two entities is variable and dependent upon the individual psychological characteristics of the patient [59].

Although few data support the hypothesis that nausea and vomiting in pregnancy is a true conversion disorder, evidence exists that supports psychological responses to the physiological conditions underlying this problem may become entrenched, or conditioned. An extensive review of psychological factors in the etiology and treatment of severe nausea and vomiting in pregnancy has been published by Buckwalter and Simpson [60].

Diagnosis

Clinical Manifestations

Hyperemesis gravidarum is a clinical diagnosis depending on typical presentation *and* exclusion of other causes. The disease typically occurs between the 4th and the 10th week of gestation, with resolution by the 20 weeks' gestation. While initially the nausea and vomiting are tolerable, gradual weight loss ($\geq$5% of body weight), dehydration accompanied by abnormal serum electrolyte levels, and ketosis may occur. Hypersalivation occurs frequently, yet rarely is a major complaint.

Physical Examination

Patients with hyperemesis gravidarum presenting to the emergency department are often significantly dehydrated. These patients may manifest orthostatic changes (both systolic blood pressure, mean change 8.3 $\pm$ 12.3 mm Hg, and heart rate changes, mean 26.8 $\pm$ 14.5 bpm) which improve upon rehydration [61]. However, the presenting orthostatic changes *lack* sufficient sensitivity to be effectively applied as a quantitative screening tool for the severity of dehydration [61]. In severe cases, a dry and furry tongue (resulting from severe hypovolemia) and ketotic breath may be noted [62]. Infrequently, patients may manifest jaundice [47, 48].

Laboratory Findings

Laboratory findings include evidence of dehydration: increased urine-specific gravity and ketonuria, increase serum blood urea nitrogen and hematocrit levels, electrolyte disturbances including hyponatremia, hypokalemia and hypochloremia, which may be found in 15–25% of patients [63]. Elevated serum amniotransferases and total bilirubin occur in between 15 and 50% of patients [45, 46]. Robertson and Miller [64] demonstrated that 24% of patients with hyperemesis gravidarum will exhibit elevated serum amylase levels with normal pancreatic amylase suggesting the source of the elevated amylase is salivary. Abnormalities in thyroid function, mainly elevated free T_4 index or suppressed TSH, are found in approximately 60% of patients [63]. A number of authors have noted decreased serum vitamin B_6 levels [51]. No alterations in serum zinc and copper metabolism were noted [53].

Differential Diagnosis

Numerous disease entities must be considered in the assessment of the pregnant patient presenting with nausea and vomiting (table 1). A thorough medical history should be obtained, meticulous physical examination and *targeted* laboratory examinations be performed. These include an electrocardiogram and pelvic ultrasound to document pregnancy viability, number of fetuses (gestational age and rule out gestational trophoblastic disease). At times, abdominal ultrasound and upper gastrointestinal endoscopy may be required. Unusual causes of nausea and vomiting such as intracranial tumor and central pontine myelinolysis should be considered [65, 66].

Maternal Complications

Prior to the 1940s (at which time fluid and electrolyte dynamics were not clear) maternal death complicating hyperemesis was not uncommon. In the distant past, due to the severity of potential complications of hyperemesis gravidarum, at times pregnancy termination was advocated [62]. Currently, hyperemesis gravidarum is rarely associated with death. Notwithstanding, serious *life-threatening* complications may occur. The most common serious reported complication involves the central nervous system. These include:

Wernicke's encephalopathy: This condition is manifested by confusion, gait ataxia, ophthalmoplegia or convulsions [67–73]. Wernicke's encephalopathy is due to a deficiency in of thiamine (vitamin B_1) an essential co-factor in carbohydrate metabolism. In the clinical setting of hyperemesis gravidarum this

Table 1. The differential diagnosis of hyperemesis gravidarum

Drug toxicity/side effects
Hepatic and gastrointestinal disorders
Viral hepatitis (A through E)
Fatty liver of pregnancy
Preeclampsia and HELLP syndrome peptic ulcer disease
Cholelithiasis
Gastroenteritis
Pancreatitis
Appendicitis
Genitourinary disorders
Gestational trophoblastic disease
Pyelonephritis
Nephrolithiasis
Uremia
Degeneration of uterine leiomyomas
Adnexal torsion
Neurological disorders
Pseudotumor cerebri
Vestibular disorders
Migraine
Central nervous system lesions
Conversion disorders
Metabolic disorders
Hyperthyroidism
Addison's disease
Diabetic ketoacidosis
Porphyria

deficiency is usually caused by replacement of fluid without thiamine supplementation. Most patients manifest only one or two of the above symptoms. Diagnosis of this uncommon complication may be assisted by cranial computed tomography or magnetic resonance imaging which may reveal symmetrical periventricular lesions in the mediodorsal nuclei of the thalami, hypothalamus and periaqueductal gray matter [67, 69, 74].

Central pontine myelinolysis (osmotic demyelination syndrome): This uncommon disorder is associated with rapid correction of severe hyponatremia ($<$120 mEq/l) and has been reported in association with hyperemesis gravidarum with or without Wernicke's encephalopathy [75–78]. Central pontine myelinolysis may be associated with permanent brain damage or death [79].

Vasospasm of cerebral arteries: Two patients with severe hyperemesis gravidarum refractory to intravenous fluid and multivitamin replacement were noted to have vasospasm of the middle cerebral arteries by magnetic resonance imaging. In both cases, vasospasm diminished following improvement of the hyperemesis. The authors speculated that increased sympathetic nervous system activity led to the vasospasm [80].

Pneumomediastinum/esophageal rupture: Rare reports of spontaneous pneumomediastinum complicating hyperemesis gravidarum have been reported [81–83]. Most likely considered causes of this complication were esophageal or alveolar rupture. Spontaneous esophageal rupture (common in alcoholics) has been reported complicating hyperemesis gravidarum [84].

Others: Unusual complications of hyperemesis gravidarum include rhabdomyolysis, coagulopathy secondary to vitamin K deficiency and peripheral neuropathy caused by either vitamin B_6 or B_{12} deficiency [63, 85, 86].

Treatment

Fluid Electrolyte and Vitamin Resuscitation

Current conventional treatment is summarized in table 2. Caution must be taken during fluid and electrolyte restitution in that rapid correction of hyponatremia has led to development of central pontine myelinolysis. Lack of attention to vitamin deficiencies or inadequate supplementation may lead to Wernicke's encephalopathy, peripheral neuropathy or coagulopathy [71]. Thiamine replacement should be administered [63]. Vitamin B_6 (pyridoxine) is the most commonly studied drug in hyperemesis gravidarum. It is usually administered in conjunction with antihistamines, but it is likely that it is effective by itself. Meticulous measurements of input, output, and daily weight are keystone elements in management. During the initial therapeutic period, food intake should be restricted and gradually restituted initially with oral fluid intake, followed by small carbohydrate meals and total avoidance of fatty foods. Many patients may benefit from psychological, emotional support and reassurance.

Antiemetics

For patients experiencing continued nausea and vomiting despite institution of the above conservative treatment, pharmacological measures may be indicated, including medications with antihistaminic, antiserotonin or sedative/hypnotic properties or both.

Randomized controlled studies of antiemetic medications showing beneficial results of drugs administered for hyperemesis gravidarum include: Bendectin = Debendox (contained doxylamine, ±dicyclomine, pyridoxine), meclizine, metoclopramide, promethazine, hydroxyzine, trimethobenzamine,

Table 2. Treatment of hyperemesis gravidarum

Nonspecific measures	
	Intravenous fluid replacement
	Correction of electrolyte imbalance (avoid rapid correction of hyponatremia)
	Vitamin supplementation
	Thiamine replacement (100 mg IV or IM)
	Vitamin B_6 (pyridoxine) (10–50 mg q 8 h)
	Acupuncture
Antiemetics	
	Bendectin = Debendox (contained doxylamine, ±dicyclomine, pyridoxine)
	Meclizine
	Metoclopramide (10 mg q 6–8 h PO/IM/IV, SC)
	Promethazine (25 mg q 4 h PO/PR)
	Hydroxyzine
	Trimethobenzamine (200 mg q 6 h PR)
	Thielpyrazine
	Mepyramine
	Dimenydrinate
	Droperidol (50 mg per admission, continuous IV)
	Diphenylhydramine
	Ondansetron (10 mg q 8 h IV)
Steroids	
	Methylprednisolone (16 mg q 8 h, PO)
Alternative treatment	
	Ginger (1 g/day for 4 days)
Enteral nutrition	
	Nasogastric tube
	Jejunostomy or
	Percutaneous endoscopic gastrostomy
Parenteral nutrition	

thielpyrazine, mepryramine, dimenhydrinate, droperidol and diphenylhydramine (table 2) [1, 87–92].

Bendectin, the only FDA-approved drug for nausea and vomiting in pregnancy yet, was removed by the manufacturer due to concerns regarding congenital malformations, though both retrospective and prospective studies failed to *prove* teratogenicity [1]. However, various components of Bendectin such as pyridoxine and doxylamine have been continuously available over the counter [1]. Droperidol is a dopamine antagonist more potent than the phenothiazines with fewer side effects. Diphenylhydramine exhibits antihistamine, anticholinergic and sedative effects. Benefits of the two latter drugs administered together include synergistic antiemetic properties with fewer side effects. Droperidol (50 mg per admission) in continuous intravenous infusion for a mean duration of 50 h in conjunction with bolus intravenous Diphenylhydramine administration shortened hospitalization duration by approximately 1 day, as well as fewer days per pregnancy hospitalized and decreased re-admissions [90].

Metoclopramide (a dopamine antagonist) was shown to be associated with improved symptomatology in 79% of patients in a controlled study [92].

Recently, Buttino et al. [93] retrospectively analyzed utilization of subcutaneous (s.c.) metoclopramide in the outpatient treatment of 646 women with hyperemesis gravidarum, identifying included patients from a national database. A total of 413 patients (63.9%) exhibited complete resolution of symptoms. Seventy-five percent of patients had received one or more antiemetic medication before initiation of s.c. metoclopramide. A total of 192 patients (30.5%) reported at least one side effect related to treatment. The majority of reported side effects were considered mild and did not require discontinuation of treatment [93]. All the above-mentioned medications are FDA class B or C drugs.

Ondansetron (intravenous 10 mg q 8 h), a 5-hydroxytryptamine receptor antagonist, is effective in treating severe nausea and vomiting. Sullivan et al. [30] compared the effectiveness to promethazine in 30 women and failed to demonstrate and increased benefit among patients with hyperemesis gravidarum.

Finally, the reader is referred to two recent review articles: the first pertaining to the safety and effectiveness of available antiemetics for treatment of nausea and vomiting of pregnancy by Magee et al. [94], and the second, a comprehensive review regarding the perceived versus true risk of the teratogenicity of drugs for nausea and vomiting of pregnancy, by Koren and Levichek [95].

Steroids

A number of *recent* randomized clinical trials support the administration of steroids in the treatment of hyperemesis gravidarum. Corticosteroids are thought to exert an antiemetic effect via a chemoreceptor trigger zone located in the brainstem and have demonstrated beneficial effects in chemotherapy-induced emesis. An alternative explanation for the positive effect of corticosteroids in hyperemesis gravidarum is a 'relative adrenal insufficiency' which develops as a result of the inability of the hypothalamic-pituitary-adrenal axis to respond the increased demands for adrenal output during early pregnancy [80].

Safari et al. [96] administered oral doses of methylprednisolone (48 mg/day) to women with intractable hyperemesis gravidarum, for 3 consecutive days, followed by a tapering dose over 2 weeks, and no longer than 1 month. These authors demonstrated a 94% relief of symptomatology within 3 days and concluded that a short course of oral methylprednisolone appeared a reasonable therapeutic alternative for intractable hyperemesis gravidarum [96].

Subsequently, this group conducted the largest double-blind, randomized controlled study evaluating medical treatment for hyperemesis gravidarum comparing oral methylprednisolone (16 mg q 8 h) to oral promethazine (25 mg q 8 h) in the treatment of hyperemesis gravidarum. After 3 days, methylprednisolone was tapered during the course of 2 weeks whereas the dose of promethazine was not altered. This study demonstrated that the short course of oral methylprednisolone is more effective than promethazine for the treatment of hyperemesis [97]. These authors currently recommend that methylprednisolone be utilized in patients whose symptomatology does not respond favorably to conventional intravenous hydration and promethazine. A short course of oral methylprednisolone appears to be a simple and effective alternative to inpatient therapy [97].

Nelson-Piercy et al. [98] performed a multicenter, double-blind, randomized, placebo-controlled trial designed to assess the efficacy of corticosteroids in the treatment of severe hyperemesis gravidarum refractory to conventional management. Twenty-five women were randomized to receive either 40 mg prednisolone daily in two divided doses, or equivalent placebo tablets. If after 3 days the patient was still vomiting, medication was changed to the equivalent intravenous alternative (hydrocortisone 100 mg twice daily or normal saline injections). Frequency of vomiting and the dependence on intravenous fluid replacement therapy after 1 week of treatment was the main outcome measure. A nonsignificant trend towards improved nausea and vomiting and reduced dependence on intravenous fluids was observed. However, steroid therapy led to an improved sense of well-being ($p = 0.021$), improved appetite ($p = 0.039$) and increased weight gain ($p = 0.025$), compared with placebo. There was no difference in pregnancy outcome between the treatment and placebo groups. Although overall the study supported a beneficial role for the administration steroids in severe hyperemesis gravidarum, the authors were unable to validate their hypothesis that steroids will lead to rapid and complete remission of symptoms and the study did not demonstrate a significant improvement in primary outcome measures assessed [98].

Alternative Treatment

Ginger

Gastrointestinal symptoms in motion sickness resemble those of hyperemesis gravidarum. Report of the beneficial effect of ginger as the rhizome of *Zingiber officinale* on motion sickness inspired a double-blind, randomized, cross-over study in which ginger 1 g/day for 4 days was noted to be superior to placebo in eliminating symptoms of hyperemesis gravidarum [99].

Enteral Nutrition

Patients with intractable hyperemesis gravidarum, nonresponsive to all the above therapeutic measures, are candidates for enteral or parentral nutrition.

Hsu et al. [100] reported their experience in treating hyperemesis gravidarum with nasogastric enteral feeding in 7 women (using an 8-Fr nasogastric feeding tube) as a continuous infusion beginning with a rate of 25 ml/h, and increased in a daily fashion until nutritional requirements were met. Nausea and vomiting improved within 24 h of nasogastric tube placement and patients were discharged within 8 days and continued enteral feeding in an outpatient setting for a mean of 43 days after which oral feeding was resumed.

An extreme alternative to nasogastric tube nutrition is treatment via a jejunostomy or percutaneous endoscopic gastrostomy (PEG) [101, 102].

Parenteral Nutrition

Van Stuijvenberg et al. [87] assessed the nutritional status of 20 patients with hyperemesis gravidarum with gestational age matched controls and noted that more than 60% of patients had suboptimal biochemical status of thiamine, riboflavin, vitamin B_6, vitamin A, and retinol-binding protein. Treatment consisting of intravenous normal saline solution together with an ampule of intravenous multivitamin preparation administered over 8 h was continued for 10 days, with oral fluid and food restriction. After 10 days, patients were discharged and supplied with oral vitamin and mineral supplement to be taken daily for another 10 days. Treatment was associated with cessation of nausea and vomiting and improvement of nutritional status. Zibel-Frisk et al. [103] administered parenteral nutrition support (including daily lipids) to 23 patients with severe hyperemesis gravidarum. The regimen was based on individual calculated requirements in addition to 300 kcal for pregnancy (50% of the non-protein calories were provided by lipids). Mean duration of therapy was 2.7 weeks, mean weight gain was 2.4 lb, 84% of patients were able to gain appropriate weight to maintain pregnancy. These authors concluded that parenteral nutrition provides a safe means of maintaining adequate maternal nutrition and continued fetal growth. Naef et al. [104] retrospectively compared intravenous nutritional support at home as an alternative to hospitalization in 50 patients versus 47 hospitalized patients (matched for gravidity, gestational age and weight loss from prepregnancy weight). Patients had similar days of intravenous therapy and similar mean weight change following therapy, with 90% efficacy of treatment of both groups. Cost of therapy was fourfold less in home treated patients [104].

Acupuncture

Acupuncture on the point PC6 above the wrist on the palmar side has been found previously to prevent some types of nausea and vomiting. Carlsson et al.

[105] in 2000 studied 33 women with hyperemesis gravidarum in a randomized, single-blind, crossover comparison of two methods of acupuncture, active (deep) PC6 acupuncture or placebo (superficial) acupuncture. The women estimated their degree of nausea on a visual analogue scale (VAS). The daily number of emesis episodes were documented. Crossover analyses showed that there was a significantly faster reduction of nausea (VAS) and more women who stopped vomiting after active acupuncture than after placebo acupuncture [105].

Similarly, Slotnick [106] studied the effectiveness of P-6 acustimulation for the relief of nausea and vomiting associated with early pregnancy and concluded that P-6 acustimulation may prove to be of a significant therapeutic alternative in this clinical setting.

Conversely, Knight et al. [107] in 2001 in a subject- and observer-masked, randomized, controlled trial, treated 55 women with nausea of pregnancy between 6 and 10 weeks' gestation traditional-style acupuncture or sham treatment with a cocktail stick on three or four occasions over 3 weeks. The main outcome measure was nausea score, as determined by subject report on a VAS in a daily diary. The study design had a 95% power to detect significant results in nausea scores. Anxiety and depression were also assessed. The study demonstrated that nausea scores decreased from a median of 85.5 (interquartile range 71.25–89.75) to 47.5 (interquartile range 29.25–69.5) in the acupunture group and from 87.0 (interquartile range 73.0–90.0) to 48 (interquartile range 14.0–8.0) in the sham treatment group. There was strong evidence of a time effect ($p < 0.001$) but no evidence of a group effect ($p = 0.9$), or a group interaction ($p = 0.8$). Similarly, there was evidence of time effects in scores for anxiety and depression but no group differences. The authors concluded that acupuncture was as effective in treating nausea of pregnancy as a sham procedure.

Others

Recently an association of increased seropositivity to *H. pylori* among patients with hyperemesis gravidarum versus asymptomatic healthy pregnant controls was reported [41]. Several case reports have suggested a beneficial effect of *H. pylori* eradication [43].

Gastric dysmotility has also been demonstrated among patients with hyperemesis gravidarum [36]. Several serendipitous cases in which erythromycin administered for other indications were associated with complete resolution of otherwise intractable hyperemesis gravidarum [42]. It is possible the benefit resulted from the motilin-like actions of erythromycin.

Systemic Review

Jewell and Young [108] performed a review of randomized trials of any treatment for nausea and vomiting in early pregnancy inclusive through

October 2001. Twenty-three trials of variable quality were included. Nausea treatments were different antihistamine medications, vitamin B_6 (pyridoxine), the combination tablet Debendox (Bendectin) and P-6 acupressure. For hyperemesis gravidarum, five trials were identified with oral ginger root extract, oral corticosteroids, or injected adenocorticotropic hormone (ACTH) and intravenous diazepam. Based on 13 trials there was an overall reduction in nausea from antiemetic medication (OR 0.17, 95% confidence interval 0.13–0.21). Of the newer treatments, pyridoxine (vitamin B_6) appears to be more effective in reducing nausea. These authors found that no trials of treatments of hyperemesis gravidarum show evidence of benefit! [108]

Perinatal Outcome

Fetal outcome among patients experiencing hyperemesis gravidarum has been debated in a number of studies. Gross et al. [109] followed perinatal outcome of 64 patients with hyperemesis gravidarum classifying patients into two groups. Patients with weight loss >5% of prepregnancy weight at the time of admission for hyperemesis gravidarum (severe) were compared with the others. Infants of women with severe hyperemesis gravidarum were significantly smaller at birth, had a higher incidence of fetal growth restriction (<10th centile at birth), and significantly lesser incidence of macrosomia. These authors suggested the group with severe disease may constitute a distinct entity at increased risk for adverse perinatal outcome [109]. Godsey and Newman [110] compared 140 patients with single versus multiple admissions for hyperemesis gravidarum. Of these, 39 patients had multiple admissions. Interestingly, women admitted repeatedly had more severe nutritional disturbances, reduced maternal weight gain and neonatal birth weight (2,806 ± 76 vs. 3,071 ± 477 g), arguing for increased fetal surveillance in cases of severe hyperemesis gravidarum requiring multiple admissions [110].

In contrast, other authors have not been able to confirm these observation. Hallak et al. [111] studied 138 patients with hyperemesis gravidarum, stratified according to severity of disease. Forty patients with mild hyperemesis gravidarum were compared to 98 patients with severe disease and 12,335 controls. No differences were noted in birth weight, incidence of congenital malformations, prematurity or other perinatal outcomes including frequency of 5 min Apgar score <7, or neonatal intensive care unit admissions. Similar nonsignificant differences were demonstrated by Tsang et al. [112] among 193 patients with hyperemesis gravidarum versus 12,860 controls. Depue et al. [14] compared 419 patients with hyperemesis gravidarum to 836 matched controls. Patients with hyperemesis gravidarum had significantly reduced risk of fetal loss, however their infants had a significantly higher risk of central nervous system malformations. Bashiri et al. [8] compared perinatal outcomes of 164 patients with hyperemesis gravidarum to 209 control patients. These authors noted a lower incidence (3.1%) of spontaneous early pregnancy loss among women with hyperemesis gravidarum in comparison to 15% among the general population. Perinatal outcome or the incidence of pregnancy complications did not differ between the two groups however [8].

References

1 Broussard CN, Richter JE: Nausea and vomiting of pregnancy. Gastroenterol Clin North Am 1998;27:123–151.
2 Gadsby R, Barnie-Adshead AM, Jagger C: A prospective study of nausea and vomiting during pregnancy. Br J Gen Pract 1993;43:245–248.
3 Smith C, Crowther C, Beilby J, Dandeaux J: The impact of nausea and vomiting on women: A burden of early pregnancy. Aust NZ J Obstet Gynaecol 2000;40:397–401.
4 Goodwin TM, Romero R: Understanding and treating nausea and vomiting in pregnancy. Am J Obstet Gynecol 2002;186:S181–S266.
5 Fairweather DV: Nausea and vomiting in pregnancy. Am J Obstet Gynecol 1968;102:135–175.
6 Cruikshank DP, Wigton TR, Hays PM: Maternal physiology in pregnancy; in Gabbe SG, Niebyl JR, Simpson JL (eds): Obstetrics Normal and Problem Pregnancies, ed 3. New York, Churchill Livingstone, 1996, pp 91–109.
7 Kallen B: Hyperemesis during pregnancy and delivery outcome: A registry study. Eur J Obstet Gynecol Reprod Biol 1987;26:292–302.
8 Bashiri A, Newmann L, Maymon E, Katz M: Hyperemesis gravidarum: Epidemiologic features, complications and outcome. Eur J Obstet Gynecol Reprod Biol 1995;63:135–138.
9 Pokras R: Vital and Health Statistics: Detailed Diagnoses and Procedures, National Hospital Discharge Survey. DHHS Publ No (PHS) 87-1751, Series 13, No 90. Rockville, US Department of Health and Human Services, 1985.
10 Commission on Professional and Hospital Activities: Length of Stay by Diagnosis, Northeastern Region. Ann Arbour, CPH Publications, 1986, p 150.
11 Klebanoff MA, Koslowe PA, Kaslow R, Rhodes GG: Epidemiology of vomiting in early pregnancy. Obstet Gynecol 1985;66:612–616.
12 Price A, Davies R, Heller SR, Milford-Ward A, Weetman AP: Asian women are at risk of gestational thyrotoxicosis. J Clin Endocrinol Metab 1996;81:1160–1163.
13 Jordan V, MacDonald J, Crichton S, Stone P, Ford H: The incidence of hyperemesis gravidarum is increased among Pacific Islanders living in Wellington. NZ Med J 1995;108:342–344.
14 Depue RH, Bernstein L, Ross RK, Judd HL, Henderson BE: Hyperemesis gravidarum in relation to estradiol levels, pregnancy outcome, and other maternal factors: A seroepidemiology study. Am J Obstet Gynecol 1987;156:1137–1141.
15 Abell TL, Riel CA: Hyperemesis gravidarum. Gastroenterol Clin North Am 1992;21:835–849.
16 Soules MR, Hughes CL, Garcia JA, et al: Nausea and vomiting in pregnancy: Role of human chorionic gonadotropin and 17-hydroxyprogesterone. Obstet Gynecol 1980;55:696–700.
17 Goodwin TM, Hershman JM, Cole L: Increased concentration of the free β-subunit of human chorionic gonadotropin in hyperemesis gravidarum Acta Obstet Gynecol Scand 1994;73:770–772.
18 Furneaux EC, Langley-Evans AJ, Langley-Evans SC: Nausea and vomiting of pregnancy: Endocrine basis and contribution to pregnancy outcome. Obstet Gynecol Surv 2001;56:775–782.
19 Kimura M, Amino N, Tamaki H, Ito E, Mitsuda N, Miyai K, Tanizawa O: Gestational thyrotoxicosis and hyperemesis gravidarum: Role of hCG with higher stimulating activity. Clin Endocrinol 1993;38:345–350.

20 Jordan V, Grebe SKG, Cooke RR, Ford HC, Larsen PD, Stone PR, Salmond CE: Acidic forms of chorionic gonadotropin in European and Samoan women are associated with hyperemesis gravidarum and may be thyrotropic. Clin Endocrinol 1999;50:619–627.
21 Panesar NS, Li Cy, Rogers MS: Are thyroid hormones or hCG responsible for hyperemesis gravidarum? A matched paired study in Chinese women. Acta Obstet Gynecol Scand 2001;80:519–524.
22 Kennedy RL, Darne J, Davies R, Price A: Thyrotoxicosis and hyperemesis gravidarum associated with a serum activity which stimulates human thyroid cells in vitro. Clin Endocrinol 1992;36:83–89.
23 Mestman JH: Hyperthyroidism in pregnancy. Endocrinol Metab Clin North Am 1998;27:127–149.
24 Boullion R, Naesens M, van Assche FA, De Keyser L, De Moor P, Renaer M, de Vos P, De Roo M. Thyroid function in patients with hyperemesis gravidarum Am J Obstet Gynecol 1982;143:922–926.
25 Bober SA, McGill AC, Tunbridge WMG: The thyroid function in hyperemesis gravidarum. Acta Endocrinol 1986;111:404–410.
26 Valbo A, Jerve F: A study of thyroid hormones in women suffering from vomiting in pregnancy. Acta Eur Fertil 1987;18:381–383.
27 Wilson R, McKillop JH, MacLean M, Walker JJ, Fraser WD, Gray C, Dryburgh F, Thomson JA: Thyroid function test are rarely abnormal in patients with severe hyperemesis gravidarum. Clin Endocrinol 1992;37:331–334.
28 Goodwin TM, Montoro M, Mestman JH: Transient hyperthyroidism and hyperemesis gravidarum: Clinical aspects. Am J Obstet Gynecol 1992;167:649–652.
29 Goodwin TM, Montoro M, Mestman JH, Pekary AE, Hershman JM: The role of chorionic gonadotropin in transient hyperthyroidism of hyperemesis gravidarum. J Clin Endocrinol Metab 1992;75:1333–1337.
30 Sullivan CA, Johnson CA, Roach H, Martin RW, Stewart DK, Morrison JC: A pilot study of intravenous ondansetron for hyperemesis gravidarum. Am J Obstet Gynecol 1996;174:1565–1568.
31 Hasler WL: Serotonin receptor physiology: Relation to emesis. Dig Dis Sci 1999;44:108S–118S.
32 Guikontes E, Spantideas A, Diakadis J: Ondansetron and hyperemesis gravidarum. Lancet 1992; 340:1223.
33 World MJ: Ondansetron and hyperemesis gravidarum. Lancet 1993;341:185.
34 Borgeat A, Fathi M, Valiton A: Hyperemesis gravidarum: Is serotonin implicated. Am J Obstet Gynecol 1997;176:476–477.
35 Van Thiel DH, Gravaler JS, Joshi SN, Sarah RK, Stremple J: Heartburn in pregnancy. Gastroenterology 1977;72:666–668.
36 Koch KL, Stern RM, Vasey M, Otti JJ, Creasy GW, Dwyer A: Gastric dysrhythmias and nausea of pregnancy. Dig Dis Sci 1990;35:961–968.
37 Riezzo G, Pezzolla F, Darconza G, Giorgio I: Gastric myoelectrical activity in the first trimester of pregnancy: A cutaneous electrogastrographic study. Am J Gastroenterol 1992;87:702–707.
38 Maes BD, Spitz B, Ghoos YF, Hiele MI, Evenepoel P, Rutgeerts PJ: Gastric emptying in hyperemesis gravidarum and non-dyspeptic pregnancy. Aliment Pharmacol Ther 1999;13:237–243.
39 Koch KL: Gastrointestinal factors in nausea and vomiting of pregnancy. Am J Obstet Gynecol 2002;186:S198–S203.
40 Michaletz-Onody PA: Peptic ulcer disease in pregnancy. Gastroenterol Clin North Am 1992;21: 817–826.
41 Frigo P, Lang C, Reisenberger K, Kolbl H, Hirschl AM: Hyperemesis gravidarum associated with *Helicobacter pylori* seropositivity. Obstet Gynecol 1998;91:615–617.
42 El Younis CM, Abulafia O, Sherer DM: Rapid response of severe hyperemesis gravidarum to oral erythromycin. Am J Perinatol 1998;15:533–534.
43 Jacoby EB, Porter KB: *Helicobacter pylori* infection and persistent hyperemesis gravidarum. Am J Perinatol 1999;16:85–88.
44 Lanciers S, Despinasse B, Mehta DI, Blecker U: Increased susceptibility to *Helicobacter pylori* infection in pregnancy. Infect Dis Obstet Gynecol 1999;7:195–198.
45 Morali JA, Braverman DZ: Abnormal liver enzymes and ketonuria in hyperemesis gravidarum: A retrospective review of eighty patients. J Clin Gastroenterol 1990;12:303–305.
46 Wallstedt A, Riely CA, Shaver D, et al: Prevalence and characteristics of liver dysfunction in hyperemesis gravidarum. Clin Res 1990;38:970–972.

47 Larrey D, Rueff B, Feldman G, Degott C, Danan G, Benhamou JP: Recurrent jaundice caused by recurrent hyperemesis gravidarum. Gut 1984;25:1414–1415.
48 Orazi G, Dufour PH, Puech F: Jaundice induced by hyperemesis gravidarum. Int J Gynecol Obstet 1998;61:181–183.
49 Signorello LB, Harlow BL, Wang S, Erick MA: Saturated fat intake and the risk of severe hyperemesis gravidarum. Epidemiology 1998;9:636–640.
50 Miagawa M, Narita J, Tada T, Maruyama S, Shimuzu T, Bannai M, Oya H, Hatakeyama K, Abo T: Mechanisms underlying immunologic states during pregnancy: Possible association of the sympathetic nervous system. Cell Immunol 1999;196:1–13.
51 Reinken L, Gant H: Vitamin B_6 nutrition in women with hyperemesis gravidarum during the first trimester of pregnancy. Clin Chem Acta 1974;55:101–102.
52 Tabbakh GE, Darwish E, Sebaie FE, et al: Study of serum copper and zinc in serum of patients with hyperemesis gravidarum. Int J Gynecol Obstet 1989;29:202–207.
53 Lao TT, Chin RKH, Mak YT, Panesar NS: Plasma zinc concentration and thyroid function in hyperemetic pregnancies. Acta Obstet Gynecol Scand 1988;67:599–604.
54 Chin RKH, Lao TT, Swaminathan R, Mak YT: A longitudinal study of changes in erythrocyte zinc concentration in hyperemesis gravidarum. Gynecol Obstet Invest 1990;29:22–25.
55 Guze B, DeLong WB, Majerus PW, et al: Association of clinical psychiatric disease with hyperemesis gravidarum. N Engl J Med 1957;261:136–138.
56 Katon WJ, Ries RK, Bokan LA, et al: Hyperemesis gravidarum: A biopsychological perspective. Int J Psychiatry Med 1980;10:151–162.
57 Iancu I, Kotler M, Spivak B, Radvan M, Weizman A: Psychiatric aspects of hyperemesis gravidarum. Psychother Psychosom 1994;61:143–149.
58 Stewart DE: Reproductive functions in eating disorders. Ann Med 1992;24:287–291.
59 Lingham R, McCluskey S: Eating disorders associated with hyperemesis gravidarum. J Psychosom Res 1996;40:231–234.
60 Buckwalter JG, Simpson SW: Psychological factors in the etiology and treatment of severe nausea and vomiting in pregnancy. Am J Obstet Gynecol 2002;186:S210–S214.
61 Johnson DR, Douglas D, Hauswald M, Tandberg D: Dehydration and orthostatic vital signs in women with hyperemesis gravidarum. Acad Emerg Med 1995;2:692–697.
62 Hod M, Orvieto R, Kaplan B, Friedman S, Ovadia J: Hyperemesis gravidarum: A review. J Reprod Med 1994;39:605–612.
63 Goodwin TM: Hyperemesis gravidarum. Clin Obstet Gynecol 1998;41:597–605.
64 Robertson C, Miller H: Hyperamylasemia in bulimia nervosa and hyperemesis gravidarum. Int J Eat Disord 1999;26:223–227.
65 Van Calenbergh SG, Poppe WA, Van Calenbergh F: An intracranial tumor – An uncommon cause of hyperemesis gravidarum. Eur J Obstet Gynaecol Reprod Biol 2001;95:182–183.
66 Valiulis B, Kelley RE, Hardjasudarma M, London S: Magnetic resonance imaging detection of a lesion compatible with central pontine myelinolysis in a pregnant patient with recurrent vomiting and confusion. J Neuroimaging 2001;11:441–443.
67 Omer SM, al Kawi MZ, al Watban J, Bohelga S, McLean DR, Miller G: Acute Wernicke's encephalopathy associated with hyperemesis gravidarum: Magnetic resonance imaging findings. J Neuroimaging 1995;5:251–253.
68 Rotman P, Hassin D, Mouallem M, Barkai G, Farfel Z: Wernicke's encephalopathy in hyperemesis gravidarum: Association with abnormal liver function. Israel J Med Sci 1994;30: 225–228.
69 Gardian G, Voros E, Jardanhazy T, Ungurean A, Vecsei L: Wernicke's encephalopathy induced by hyperemesis gravidarum. Acta Neurol Scand 1999;99:196–198.
70 Rees JH, Ginsberg L, Schapira HV: Two pregnant women with vomiting and fits. Am J Obstet Gynecol 1997;177:1539–1540.
71 Spruill SC, Kuller JA: Hyperemesis gravidarum complicated by Wernicke's encephalopathy. Obstet Gynecol 2002;99:875–877.
72 Togay-Isikay C, Yigit A, Mutluer N: Wernicke's encephalopathy due to hyperemesis gravidarum: An under-recognized condition. Aust NZ J Obstet Gynaecol 2001;41:453–456.

73 Accetta SG, Abeche AM, Buchabqui JA, Hammes L, Pratti R, Afler T, Capp E: Memory loss and ataxia after hyperemesis gravidarum: A case of Wernicke-Korsakoff syndrome. Eur J Obstet Gynecol Reprod 2002;102:100–101.
74 Ohkoshi N, Ishii A, Shoji S: Wernicke's encephalopathy induced by hyperemesis gravidarum, associated with bilateral caudate lesions on computed tomography and magnetic resonance imaging. Eur Neurol 1994;34:177–180.
75 Peeters A, van de Wyngaert F, Van Lierde M, Sindic CJ, Laterre EC: Wernicke's encephalopathy and central pontine myelinolysis induced by hyperemesis gravidarum. Acta Neurol Belg 1993;93: 276–282.
76 Bergin PS, Harvey P: Wernicke's encephalopathy and central pontine myelinolysis associated with hyperemesis gravidarum. Br Med J 1992;305:517–518.
77 Castillo RA, Ray RA, Yaghmai F: Central pontine myelinolysis and pregnancy. Obstet Gynecol 1989;73:459–461.
78 Fraser D: Central pontine myelinolysis as a result of treatment of hyperemesis gravidarum. Case report. Br J Obstet Gynaecol 1988;95:621–623.
79 Arieff AI: Hyponatremia, convulsions, respiratory arrest and permanent brain damage after elective surgery in healthy women. N Engl J Med 1986;314:1529–1534.
80 Kanayama N, Khatun S, Belayet HM, Yamashita M, Yonezawa M, Kobayashi T, Terao T: Vasospasms of cerebral arteries in hyperemesis gravidarum. Gynecol Obstet Invest 1998;46: 139–141.
81 Schwartz M, Rossoff L: Pneumomediastinum and bilateral pneumothoraces in a patient with hyperemesis gravidarum. Chest 1994;106:1904–1906.
82 Gorbach JS, Counselmann FL, Mendelson MH: Spontaneous pneumomediastinum secondary to hyperemesis gravidarum. J Emerg Med 1997;15:639–643.
83 Liang SG, Ooka F, Santo A, Kaibara M: Pneumomediastinum following esophageal rupture associated with hyperemesis gravidarum. J Obstet Gynaecol Res 2002;28:172–175.
84 Chirino O, Kovac R, Bale D, Blythe JG: Barogenic rupture of the esophagus associated with hyperemesis gravidarum. Obstet Gynecol 1978;52:51S–53S.
85 Fukada Y, Ohta S, Mizuno K, Hoshi K: Rhabdomyolysis secondary to hyperemesis gravidarum. Acta Obstet Gynecol Scand 1999;78:71–73.
86 Robinson JN, Banerjee R, Thiet MP: Coagulopathy secondary to vitamin K deficiency in hyperemesis gravidarum. Obstet Gynecol 1998;92:673–675.
87 Van Stuijvenberg ME, Schabort I, Labadarios D, Nel JT: The nutritional status and treatment of patients with hyperemesis gravidarum. Am J Obstet Gynecol 1995;172:1585–1591.
88 Greenspoon JS, Rosen DJ, Ault M: Use of the peripherally inserted central catheter for parenteral nutrition during pregnancy. Obstet Gynecol 1993;81:831–834.
89 Sahakian V, Rouse D, Sipes S, et al: Vitamin B_6 is effective therapy for nausea and vomiting of pregnancy: A randomized, double-blind, placebo-controlled study. Obstet Gynecol 1991;78: 33–36.
90 Nageotte MP, Briggs GG, Towers CV, Asrat T: Droperidol and diphenhydramine in the management of hyperemesis gravidarum. Am J Obstet Gynecol 1996;174:1801–1805.
91 Leathem A: Safety and efficacy of antiemetics used to treat nausea and vomiting of pregnancy. Clin Pharm 1986;5:660–668.
92 Desmond PV, Watson KJR: Metoclopramide – A review. Med J Aust 1986;144:366–369.
93 Buttino L, Coleman SK, Bergauer NK, Gambon C, Stanziano GJ: Home subcutaneous metoclopramide therapy for hyperemesis gravidarum. J Perinatol 2000;20:359–362.
94 Magee LA, Mazzotta P, Koren G: Evidence-based view of safety and effectiveness of pharmacologic therapy for nausea and vomiting of pregnancy. Am J Obstet Gynecol 2002;186: S256–S261.
95 Koren G, Levichek Z: The teratogenicity of drugs for nausea and vomiting of pregnancy: Perceived versus true risk. Am J Obstet Gynecol 2002;186:S248–S252.
96 Safari HR, Alsulyman OM, Gherman RB, Goodwin TM: Experience with oral methylprednisolone in the treatment of refractory hyperemesis gravidarum. Am J Obstet Gynecol 1998;178: 1054–1058.

97 Safari HR, Fassett MJ, Souter IC, Alsulyman OM, Goodwin TM: The efficacy of methylprednisolone in the treatment of hyperemesis gravidarum: A randomized, double blind, controlled study. Am J Obstet Gynecol 1998;179:921–924.
98 Nelson-Piercy C, Fayers P, de Swiet M: Randomised, double-blind, placebo-controlled trial of corticosteroids for the treatment of hyperemesis gravidarum. Br J Obstet Gynaecol 2001;108:9–15.
99 Fisher-Rasmussen W, Kjær S, Dahl C, Asping U: Ginger treatment of hyperemesis gravidarum. Eur J Obstet Gynecol Reprod Biol 1990;38:19–24.
100 Hsu JJ, Clark-Glena R, Nelson DK, Kim CH: Nasogastric enteral feeding in the management of hyperemesis gravidarum. Obstet Gynecol 1996;88:343–346.
101 Erick M: Nutrition via jejunostomy in refractory hyperemesis gravidarum: A case report. J Am Diet Assoc 1997;97:1154–1156.
102 Godil A, Chen YK: Percutaneous endoscopic gastrostomy for nutrition support in pregnancy associated with hyperemesis gravidarum and anorexia nervosa. J Parenter Enteral Nutr 1998;22: 238–241.
103 Zibell-Frisk D, Jen KLC, Rick J: Use of parenteral nutrition to maintain adequate nutritional status in hyperemesis gravidarum. J Perinatol 1990;10:390–395.
104 Naef RW, Chauhan SP, Roach H, Roberts WE, Travis KH, Morrison JC: Treatment for hyperemesis gravidarum in the home: An alternative to hospitalization. J Perinatol 1995;15:289–292.
105 Carlsson CP, Axemo P, Bodin A, Carstensen H, Ehrenroth B, Madegard-Lind I, Lavander C: Manual acupuncture reduces hyperemesis gravidarum: A placebo-controlled, randomized, single-blind, cross-over study. J Pain Symptom Manage 2000;20:273–279.
106 Slotnik RN: Safe, successful nausea suppression in early pregnancy with P-6 acustimulation. J Reprod Med 2001;46:811–814.
107 Knight B, Mudge C, Openshaw S, White A, Hart A: Effect of acupuncture on nausea of pregnancy: A randomized, controlled trial. Obstet Gynecol 2001;97:184–188.
108 Jewell D, Young G: Interventions for nausea and vomiting in early pregnancy. Cochrane Database Syst Rev 2002;1:CD000145.
109 Gross S, Librach C, Cecutti A: Maternal weight loss associated with hyperemesis gravidarum: A predictor of fetal outcome. Am J Obstet Gynecol 1989;160:906–909.
110 Godsey RK, Newman RB: Hyperemesis gravidarum: A comparison of single and multiple admissions. J Reprod Med 1991;36:287–290.
111 Hallak M, Tsalamandris K, Drombrowski MP, Isada NB, Pryde PG, Evans MI: Hyperemesis gravidarum: Effects on fetal outcome. J Reprod Med 1996;41:871–874.
112 Tsang IS, Katz VL, Wells SD: Maternal and fetal outcomes in hyperemesis gravidarum. Int J Gynecol Obstet 1996;55:231–235.

David M. Sherer, MD
Division of Maternal-Fetal Medicine, Department of Obstetrics and Gynecology
State University of New York (SUNY), Downstate Medical Center
455 Lenox Road, Box 24, Brooklyn, NY 11203 (USA)
Tel. +1 718 2702081, Fax +1 718 2704122, E-Mail dmsherer@aol.com

Author Index

Subject Index